HIGH-YIELD
ORTHOPAEDICS

HIGH-YIELD
ORTHOPAEDICS

Javad Parvizi, MD, FRCS

Professor of Orthopaedic Surgery
Rothman Institute of Orthopaedics
Thomas Jefferson University Hospital
Philadelphia, Pennsylvania

Gregory K. Kim, MD, Associate Editor

Research Fellow
Rothman Institute of Orthopaedics
Thomas Jefferson University Hospital
Philadelphia, Pennsylvania

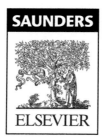

SAUNDERS

ELSEVIER

SAUNDERS
ELSEVIER

1600 John F. Kennedy Blvd.
Ste 1800
Philadelphia, PA 19103-2899

HIGH-YIELD ORTHOPAEDICS   ISBN:978-1-4160-0236-9
Copyright © 2010 by Saunders, an imprint of Elsevier Inc.

Notice

Knowledge and best practice in this field are constantly changing. As new research and experience broaden our knowledge, changes in practice, treatment and drug therapy may become necessary or appropriate. Readers are advised to check the most current information provided (i) on procedures featured or (ii) by the manufacturer of each product to be administered, to verify the recommended dose or formula, the method and duration of administration, and contraindications. It is the responsibility of the practitioner, relying on his or her own experience and knowledge of the patient, to make diagnoses, to determine dosages and the best treatment for each individual patient, and to take all appropriate safety precautions. To the fullest extent of the law, neither the publisher nor the authors assume any liability for any injury and/or damage to persons or property arising out of or related to any use of the material contained in this book.

The Publisher

Library of Congress Cataloging-in-Publication Data

Parvizi, Javad
  High-yield orthopaedics / Javad Parvizi.—1st ed.
    p. ; cm.
  ISBN 978-1-4160-0236-9
  1. Orthopedics—Encyclopedias. I. Title.
  [DNLM: 1. Musculoskeletal Diseases. 2. Musculoskeletal System. 3. Orthopedics.
  WE 100 P276h 2010]
  RD723.P37 2010
  616.7003—dc22

                                                    2008006781

Acquisitions Editors: Daniel Pepper, Pamela Hetherington
Publishing Services Manager: Tina Rebane
Senior Project Manager: Linda Lewis Grigg
Design Direction: Louis Forgione

Working together to grow
libraries in developing countries
www.elsevier.com | www.bookaid.org | www.sabre.org

Printed in the United States of America

ELSEVIER   BOOK AID International   Sabre Foundation

Last digit is the print number: 9 8 7 6 5 4 3 2 1

*To my wife, Fariba, who sees only the good
and never the bad side of human nature.*

*To my energetic children, Niosha and Cyrus,
who, despite their youth, understand me
and give me latitude to do what I do in my work
by allowing me to steal time from them.*

Preface

Orthopaedic surgery is one of the most exciting surgical fields. The immense popularity of this surgical discipline among medical students and the fierce competition to get into orthopaedic residency attest to this fact. There is a multitude of reasons for the popularity of orthopaedic surgery. I will highlight one.

Orthopaedic surgery is a surgical discipline in growth, which is much different from other surgical specialties. The growth of orthopaedic surgery in turn is due to the effectiveness of the surgical and nonsurgical care for various conditions afflicting the population and also the "development" of many innovative and novel strategies to improve the well-being of humankind who suffer from orthopaedic conditions. Examples abound. Joint replacement of major and nonmajor joints, ligament reconstruction, effective trauma care, correction of deformities in children, and successful surgical treatment of musculoskeletal oncologic conditions are just a few examples of how orthopaedics has become so exciting to practice on a daily basis.

The growth of this surgical discipline, or any discipline for that matter, cannot be achieved without an investment in time and energy to scientifically explore the basis of diseases. Musculoskeletal scientists and clinicians have been actively engaged in understanding the pathomechanism, mostly at the molecular level, for so many of these conditions. In other words, the frontier of science has moved far in the field of orthopaedic surgery and continues to advance further.

The impetus behind this book was mainly twofold. First, we attempted to capture the most recent and important information for each topic. The material in each chapter is a result of extensive research to identify all the latest science and discoveries for each topic. The second and just as important intention was to provide all the information for each topic in a concise and easy-to-read manner. The information was further highlighted by inclusion of relevant diagrams, figures, radiographs, and histologic slides. During my residency and preparation for examinations, I always yearned for a book that had all the relevant information on topics that were "popular" in the examination. Thus, the "High-Yield" part of this book is a result of looking through 15 years' worth of examination material to identify the subjects that were important both for examination purposes and for clinical practice. I recall a mentor of mine saying: "If Watson and Crick could describe the double stranded structure of DNA in two pages, one could talk about Paget's disease in one page." That is exactly what we have tried to do. I hope you will agree.

This first edition of the book is likely to suffer from many shortfalls. I hope you will forgive us for the shortcomings. I very much hope you will communicate your input with the publisher or myself. I will be most grateful to you for doing so.

I want to thank you for choosing this book and wish you success in your endeavors in practicing this most exciting surgical discipline.

JAVAD PARVIZI, MD
Philadelphia, Pennsylvania

Acknowledgments

The compilation of this book would not have been possible without the help of numerous medical students who worked tirelessly to gather data for each topic. Most if not all of the chapters were initially written by medical students, mostly at Thomas Jefferson University. I am most grateful to every one of them.

I am, in particular, most grateful to my Associate Editor, Gregory K. Kim, who spent an entire year collecting images, editing chapters, and updating the material for each chapter. Besides his incredible intellect, Greg contributed immensely to each chapter by providing his clinical insight. He invested immense energy to ensure that every chapter contained the most useful and updated material. He performed an outstanding job and was elemental for completion of this book.

Contents

Definition: The abductor mechanism consists of the gluteus medius, gluteus maximus, and tensor fascia lata (TFL). The superior gluteal nerve (L4, L5, and S1 roots) supplies the TFL and gluteus medius, whereas the inferior gluteal nerve (L5, S1, and S2) supplies the gluteus maximus. The superior gluteal artery supplies the TFL and gluteus medius, whereas the inferior and superior gluteal arteries and the first perforating branch of the profunda femoris artery supply the gluteus maximus. The abductor mechanism stabilizes the pelvis during the single leg phase of gait and enables foot clearance in the swing phase loading the hip joint with several times the body weight. An individual might take an average of one million gait cycles per year.

Trendelenburg Gait/Duchenne Limp: Failure of the abductor mechanism may occur through neurologic injury, pain inhibition, cuff tear of the hip, or mechanical factors such as a decreased hip offset as seen in coxa valga. The characteristic gait compensates for the abductor weakness by shifting the center of gravity over the standing leg. This decreases the moment arm of the gravitational force and hence decreases the force required from the abductors. This diminished force in the abductors also decreases the joint reaction force in the hip.

Trendelenburg Sign: As the patient stands facing the surgeon, palpate the iliac crests and allow the patient to steady himself on the surgeon. Then ask the patient to bend one knee, taking all his weight through the side being tested. Sign is positive when the pelvis drops on the opposite side.

Surgical Anatomy: The superior gluteal nerve arises from nerve roots L4, L5, and S1. It leaves the pelvis through the greater sciatic foramen and then travels *superior* to the piriformis, accompanied by the superior gluteal vessels (inferior gluteal—L5, S1, and S2—to the piriformis and gluteus maximus). It then divides into superior and inferior branches. The superior branch travels to the deep division of the superior gluteal artery supplying the gluteus minimus. The inferior branch runs with the lower branch of the deep division of the superior gluteal artery and supplies the gluteus medius and minimus, as well as the TFL. The relevance of this anatomy is seen when a split of the gluteus medius is performed during an anterolateral approach. If it is extended more than 4 to 5 cm proximally (varies with height), the gluteus medius may be denervated.

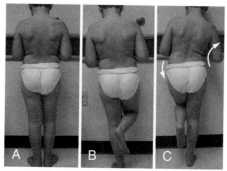

Fig. 1-1 Trendelenburg sign: In a patient with a hip disorder, the abductor muscle mechanism of the affected hip is not able to keep the pelvis stable when the patient stands only on the affected limb. **A,** When the patients stands on both feet, the shoulders and pelvis are level. **B,** When the patient stands on the unaffected left limb, the level positions of the shoulders and pelvis are maintained. **C,** However, when the patient stands on the affected right limb, the pelvis tilts down to the left *(arrow)* and there is compensatory leaning *(to the right)* of the trunk *(arrow)* over the affected hip to maintain balance. *(From Dormans JP: Pediatric Orthopaedics and Sports Medicine: The Requisites, 1st ed. St. Louis, Mosby, 2004.)*

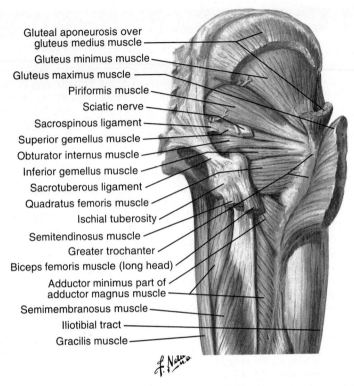

Gluteal aponeurosis over gluteus medius muscle

Gluteus minimus muscle

Gluteus maximus muscle

Piriformis muscle

Sciatic nerve

Sacrospinous ligament

Superior gemellus muscle

Obturator internus muscle

Inferior gemellus muscle

Sacrotuberous ligament

Quadratus femoris muscle

Ischial tuberosity

Semitendinosus muscle

Greater trochanter

Biceps femoris muscle (long head)

Adductor minimus part of adductor magnus muscle

Semimembranosus muscle

Iliotibial tract

Gracilis muscle

Fig. 1-2   Deeper dissection of the hip. *(From Netter F: Atlas of Human Anatomy, 3rd ed. Philadelphia, Saunders, 2003.)*

Definition: Fracture of the acetabulum resulting from a variable amount of energy transfer to the acetabular region.

Incidence: True incidence is unknown.

Age: Older patients and those with osteoporosis may occasionally have acetabular fractures as a result of low-energy trauma (e.g., falls from a standing height). In the young patient population, acetabular fractures typically result from high-energy trauma such as a motor vehicle accident and can be associated with hip dislocation.

Gender: No predilection.

Anatomy: Acetabulum formed by ilium, ischium, and pubis. Letournel: acetabulum = inverted Y with a posterior and anterior column. Anterior column (AC) = pelvic rim, anterior wall (AW), superior pubic ramus, anterior border of iliac wing. Posterior column (PC) = greater and lesser sciatic notch, posterior wall (PW), ischial tuberosity, majority of quadrilateral surface.

Radiographic Evaluation: Anteroposterior (AP), obturator oblique (OO), iliac oblique (IO). Computed tomography (CT) scan: OO—fractured side rotated 45 degrees toward x-ray beam, profile of AC medially and PW laterally. IO—fractured side rotated 45 degrees away from x-ray beam, profile of PC medially and AW laterally.

Measurements: Examine all plain views for subtle subluxations and incongruity of the femoral head. Step-off of 1 mm can lead to post-traumatic arthritis. Roof-arc angle = angle between a plumb line drawn through the center of the acetabulum parallel to the patient and a line through the fracture site and the center of the acetabulum. The angle is drawn on each view of the plain films (AP, OO, IO).

Signs: *Gull*—on AP view, the PW fragment hinges laterally in PW fracture. *Spur*—on OO x-ray studies, spur = the intact iliac wing in the anatomic position when the dome of the acetabulum and femoral head have translated medially.

Fracture Classification: Letournel

Simple: 1—PW; 2—AW; 3—PC; 4—associated PC and PW; 5—transverse.

Complex: 1—Associated PC and PW; 2—associated PW and transverse; 3—T-shaped; 4—associated AW or AC and posterior hemitransverse; 5—both columns.

Treatment:

Operative Indications: 2-mm or greater step-off, roof-arc angle less than 45 degrees, involvement of superior 10 mm of dome on CT scan, instability due to posterior wall fractures, loss of congruency between acetabulum and femoral head.

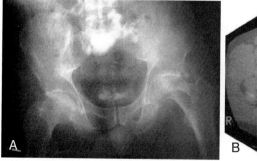 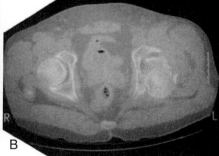

Fig. 2-1 Anteroposterior pelvic radiograph (**A**) and CT scan (**B**) of irreducible hip dislocation with posterior wall acetabular fracture. Posterior wall fragment is incarcerated, blocking reduction. *(From Canale ST, Beaty JH: Campbell's Operative Orthopaedics, 11th ed. Philadelphia, Mosby, 2007.)*

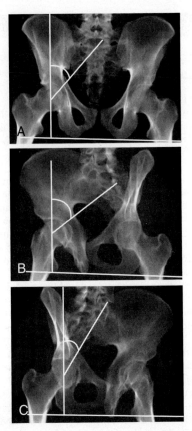

Fig. 2-2 A-C The measurements of acetabular fracture roof arc angles are shown on these three pelvic films. **A,** On the anteroposterior (AP) pelvic film, the right ischial tuberosity is involved by the fracture, so the horizontal standard line must be estimated. The femoral head is slightly subluxated on the AP view, so the center hip joint determination accounts for this. A vertical perpendicular line is drawn from the horizontal standard line through the hip joint center. Next and from the hip center, a line is drawn to the acetabular fracture edge. The angle between the perpendicular vertical and fracture edge lines is the roof arc angle. **B, C,** The process is repeated for the obturator and iliac oblique images. *(From Browner, BD et al: Trauma, 4th ed. Philadelphia, Saunders, 2008.)*

Nonoperative Indications: Secondary congruence on column fracture, infection, severe osteoporosis, nondisplaced fractures, and roof-arc angle greater than 45 degrees.
Operative Approaches:
• Kocher-Langenbeck—access to PC.
• Ilioinguinal—full access to AC and limited access to PC. Required for AW, AC, and most associated AW/AC, posterior hemitransverse, or both columns.
• Extended iliofemoral—access to PC and AC. Required for associated transverse and PW and some transtectal fractures, some associated AW or AC, and posterior hemitransverse and some T fractures.
Complications: Wound complications, nerve palsy, deep vein thrombosis, heterotopic ossification.

Definition: Complete or partial split of the Achilles tendon, most commonly at the musculus-tendinous junction. This rupture occurs less commonly as an avulsion from the posterior calcaneal tuberosity.

Etiology: Usually involves eccentric loading on a dorsiflexed ankle with the knee extended. Ruptures are commonly seen in relation to an atrophied soleus muscle in recreationally active athletes ("weekend warriors"). Consider gout or hyperparathyroid in pure avulsions. Steroid injections and fluoroquinolones can also be etiologic factors.

Incidence: Unknown.

Age: 3rd to 5th decade of life.

Gender: Male preponderance.

Symptoms: Patients experience acute episode of sharp pain behind the heel (described as being kicked or shot in the back of the leg) followed by an area of tender swelling. An area of nodularity may develop in a partial rupture.

Clinical Findings: The Thompson test is positive (squeezing the calf does not cause plantar flexion). A palpable depression is consistent with a complete rupture.

Diagnostic Studies: Ultrasonography is a fast, inexpensive way to determine the defect gap and tendon thickness. It can also be used for dynamic testing. Magnetic resonance imaging is better for detection of incomplete tears and chronic degenerative changes in the tendon, or to monitor healing.

Treatment: Goals of treatment are to restore length and tension of the tendon and ultimately optimize functional strength. This can be achieved both by nonoperative and operative means.

Nonoperative: Ultrasound can be used to observe appropriate tendon apposition with less than 20 degrees of plantar flexion. Next, splint immobilization is used for 2 weeks, followed by a short leg cast or boot for 6 to 8 weeks. The patient is weaned from the boot with passive range-of-motion (ROM) exercises progressing to calf resistance exercises at 8 to 10 weeks. Return to running is accomplished at 4 to 6 months. Full plantar flexion power can take 12 months to achieve, but and residual weakness is common.

Operative: Preferred treatment in younger, athletic patients or in those in whom adequate apposition cannot be achieved by closed means. Technique involves exposing tendon stumps and approximating with 2-4 nonabsorbable sutures using the Krachow, Bunnell, or other technique. Postoperatively, passive ROM exercise can begin as early as 3 to 7 days. Again, a short leg cast

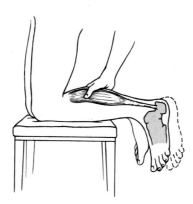

Fig. 3-1 Thompson's test. Compression of the calf muscles normally produces plantar flexion of the ankle. If the Achilles tendon is ruptured, this response is greatly diminished or absent. *(From Browner BD, et al: Skeletal Trauma: Basic Science, Management, and Reconstruction, 3rd ed. Philadelphia, Saunders, 2003.)*

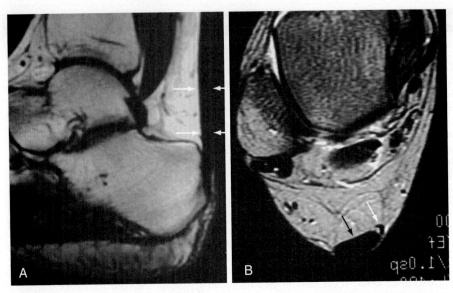

Fig. 3-2 **A,** Sagittal T$_1$-weighted magnetic resonance image of a normal Achilles tendon shows homo-geneously black tendon *(white arrows).* **B,** Axial T$_2$-weighted magnetic resonance image shows normal oval shape and homogeneous black signal of a normal Achilles tendon *(black arrow)* and adjacent plantaris tendon *(white arrow). (From DeLee D, Drez D (eds): DeLee and Drez's Orthopaedic Sports Medicine, 2nd ed. Philadelphia, Saunders, 2003.)*

or boot should be used for 6 to 8 weeks, followed by progressive resistance exercises at 8 to 10 weeks with progression to running at 4 to 6 months. A slight advantage in plantar flexion strength has been observed when compared with nonoperative treatment.

Complications: Re-rupture occurs in 0% to 2% of operative treated patients and 8% to 39% of nonoperative treated patients. Wound infection, skin necrosis, and nerve injury are additional complications reported with operative treatment.

Anatomy of the Achilles Tendon

The Achilles tendon is the strongest tendon in the body. It is made up of the distal aponeurosis of the gastrocnemius-soleus musculotendinous unit. The tendon inserts onto the middle part of the posterior surface of the calcaneus. The nearby retrocalcaneal bursa helps prevent excessive friction in this area. The Achilles tendon is surrounded throughout its length by the paratendon, which consists of several thin gliding membranes, and functions as a sheath that permits free movement of the tendon within the surrounding tissues. Under the paratendon, the entire tendon is surrounded by a smooth connective tissue sheath called the *epitenon.* Deep to the epitenon are the collagen fibers of the tendon itself, an integral network of vascular and lymphatic channels and requisite neural elements. The Achilles tendon receives blood supply (1) proximally, from the musculotendon junction, (2) through the surrounding paratenon vessel (most important blood supply to the tendon), and (3) distally, from vessels supplying the calcaneotendinous insertion.

The few intratendinous vessels are found within the tendon substance itself, running longitudinally between the collagen bundles. It has been demonstrated by angiography that a zone of relative avascularity exists in the middle one third of the tendon, approximately 2 to 6 cm proximal to the tendon insertion. The Achilles tendon is innervated by nerves supplying the gastrocnemius-soleus and by branches from nearby cutaneous nerves. Despite this paucity of intratendinous nerves, pain receptors are abundant in the paratenon.

Pathologic Changes in the Tendon

Paratendonitis and Peritendonitis: True inflammation in the paratenon or surrounding peritendinous tissue. Tendon itself is normal. Inflammatory cells and fibrinous exudates may exist, often causing thickening and adhesions between the tendon and the paratenon.

Tendinitis: Symptomatic degeneration of the tendon, characterized histologically by vascular disruption and an inflammatory repair response. Example: Insertional tendinitis—a clinical diagnosis not yet described histologically. Begins insidiously, with onset of pain at the insertion that worsens. May find spurring or erosion at the insertion on radiographic study although not diagnostic. Must be distinguished from retrocalcaneal bursitis.

Tendinosis: Chronic intratendinous degeneration and alteration of tendon architecture, with histologic findings of noninflammatory collagen degeneration, fiber disorientation, hypocellularity, scattered vascular ingrowth, and occasionally local necrosis or calcification. Tendinosis may be asymptomatic or may become painful with acute insult or chronic overuse. With aging, such degeneration will eventually occur to some degree in almost everyone.

Fig. 4-1 Lateral view. *(From Netter F: Atlas of Human Anatomy, 3rd ed. Philadelphia, Saunders, 2003.)*

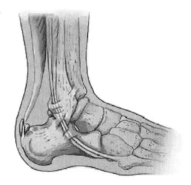

Proposed Etiologic Factors

Achilles peritendinitis and tendinosis are overuse phenomena and are the result of accumulative impact loading and repetitive microtrauma to the tendon. There are, however, both intrinsic and extrinsic factors that predispose an athlete to these injuries. Intrinsic factors include areas of decreased vascularity, aging and degeneration of the tendon, and anatomic deviations such as heel-leg or heel-forefoot malalignment, and poor gastrocnemius-soleus flexibility. Extrinsic factors that predispose an athlete to tendinitis include a sudden increase in training intensity, interval training, change of surface (soft to hard), and inappropriate or worn-out footwear. Systemic inflammatory diseases such as rheumatoid arthritis, ankylosing spondylitis, and Reiter's syndrome must be suspected especially in bilateral cases.

Clinical and Radiographic Diagnosis

Clinically, Achilles tendonopathy commonly manifests with gradual onset of pain during tendon loading and with morning stiffness in the tendon. Complaints of weakness and intermittent swelling are common. Clinical examination often reveals localized pain and swelling in the tendon, often in the middle third where blood supply is tenuous. Thickening and nodularity on palpation may be signs of chronic tendonosis or partial rupture. Hypoechoic areas on ultrasound and areas with increased signal intensity on MRI have been shown to correlate with altered collagen fiber structure and increased interfibrillar ground substance (hydrophilic glycosaminoglycans).

Treatment Options

Nonoperative: Therapy aims at identification and correction of possible etiologic factors. Stretching regimens and activity as symptoms allow are conservative options. Cold therapy, heat, massage, electrical stimulation, and laser therapy have all been used with little scientific evidence in support. Nonsteroidal anti-inflammatory drugs (NSAIDs) are often used despite any evidence of ongoing chemical inflammation. Corticosteroids are controversial, and some studies suggest a correlation with steroid injections and increased incidence of tear and the need for surgical repair.

Ultrasound Treatment: Recent studies have shown that ultrasound may increase collagen synthesis and tendon strength.

Eccentric Calf Muscle Training: Recent studies have shown that regular training with eccentric contractions may decrease pain and the need for surgery, with improved clinical result.

Operative: Various surgical techniques in cases of advanced disease and rupture. Most procedures involve straight longitudinal incision with identification and excision of the hypertrophic paretenon, as well as macroscopic identification and tenotomy of the portion of the tendon with tendonosis.

Recent Research

CDNA arrays have found down-regulation of MMP-3 (matrix-metallo-proteinase-3) genes and up-regulation of types I and III collagen in tendons with chronic tendonopathy. Also, up-regulation of MMP-2 (destructive enzyme) FNRB (fibronectin receptor involved in healing response), and VEGF (vascular endothelial growth factor) in painful tendinosis tissue.

Recent studies have placed a percutaneous microdialysis catheter to evaluate certain metabolites in the Achilles tendon:
- Concentrations of inflammatory prostaglandins were not found in higher concentrations in tendons with tendonosis versus healthy tendons. Study casts doubt over use of NSAIDs in treatment.

- Significantly elevated levels of lactate suggest anaerobic conditions and associated ischemia.
- Increased concentrations of glutamate were found in injured tendons.

Ultrasonography and Doppler studies have demonstrated increased neovascularization in injured tendonosed Achilles tendons. Neurotransmitter glutamate may be involved with proliferation of new neurovascular bundles found to innervate tendon in tendonosis. New innervation may cause increased pain and discomfort.

Definition: Anterior cruciate ligament (ACL) tears are most often a result of low-velocity, noncontact, deceleration injuries or contact injuries with a rotational component.

Frequency: An estimated 200,000 ACL injuries occur annually in the United States. Approximately 60,000 to 75,000 ACL reconstructions are performed annually.

Methods: ACL reconstruction is being performed with an autograft, allograft (cadaveric tissue), or a synthetic graft and is typically performed by knee arthroscopy.

Autograft: It is the most common graft chosen for reconstruction. Commonly used autografts are the mid-third of the patellar tendon with bone attached at both ends, one or two medial hamstrings, or the quadriceps tendon with bone at one end.

Allograft: Less operative time and not dealing with harvest site pain and morbidity are the advantages of using allograft tendons. The typical candidate for allograft ACL reconstruction is an active person who wishes to avoid graft harvest site pain. Infections with hepatitis B and C and with human immunodeficiency virus have been reported after ACL reconstruction using allografts; however, the risks of disease transmission seem to have become infinitely small.

Synthetic Grafts: The advantages of synthetic grafts are the lack of harvest site pain and and no disease transmission. However, the failure rates of synthetic grafts tested in the United States to date have been unacceptable. Synthetic graft engineering continues to occur with improvements to less successful modalities at the focus of the design.

Complications: The current failure rate is 8%. The major complications in ACL reconstructions are:

- Surgical wound infection
- Arthrofibrosis (due to inflammation of the synovium and fat pad)
- Lack of full range of motion after surgery
- Recurrent instability, secondary to significant laxity in the reconstructed ligament
- Risk of developing osteoarthritis
- Lack of graft incorporation, secondary to rejection or stress shielding
- Graft failure from re-injury or aggressive rehabilitation (graft rupture incidence = 2.5%)
- Patella fractures and patellar tendon ruptures

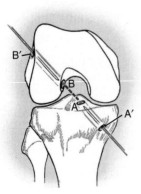

Fig. 5-1 Anterior cruciate ligament reconstruction with hamstrings. Lines A-A' and B-B' coincide with anatomic center of normal ACL. *(From Hendler RC: Intraarticular semitendinosus cruciate ligament reconstruction. In Scott WN (ed): The Knee. St. Louis, Mosby, 1994.)*

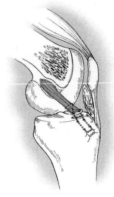

Fig. 5-2 Repair of avulsion of tibial attachment of anterior cruciate ligament with fragment of bone. Crater in tibia should be deepened, and bone fragment on end of ligament is pulled into crater depth to restore tension in avulsed ligament. *(From Canale ST and Beaty JH: Campbell's Operative Orthopaedics, 11th ed. St. Louis, Mosby 2007.)*

- Postoperative deep vein thrombosis
- Postoperative pain at donor site (autograft)

Prognosis: Patients treated with surgical reconstruction of the ACL have long-term success rates of 82% to 95%. Activities such as return to work are restored between a few days and a few months depending on the patient's occupation. A full return to activities and sports generally takes from 4 to 6 months.

Background:
- Acromioclavicular (AC) joint pathology was first delineated from glenohumeral joint pathology by Hippocrates.
- Injuries most commonly occur in athletic/active young adults.

Anatomy:
- AC joint is composed of the articular surfaces of the clavicle and the acromion, a surrounding capsule, and the AC and coracoclavicular (CC) ligaments.
- AC ligament is the principal restraint to anteroposterior translation.
- CC ligament is composed of the conoid and trapezoid ligaments, which together form a strong band that provides vertical stability.

Mechanism of Injury: Result from a force applied downward on the acromion, most commonly a fall directly onto the dome of the shoulder

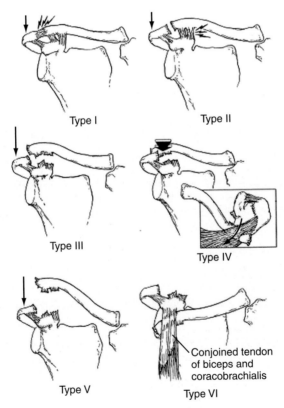

Fig. 6-1 Classification of acromioclavicular injuries. Type I, neither acromioclavicular nor coracoclavicular ligaments are disrupted. Type II, acromioclavicular ligament is disrupted, and coracoclavicular ligament is intact. Type III, both ligaments are disrupted. Type IV, ligaments are disrupted, and distal end of clavicle is displaced posteriorly into or through trapezius muscle. Type V, ligaments and muscle attachments are disrupted, and clavicle and acromion are widely separated. Type VI, ligaments are disrupted, and distal clavicle is dislocated inferior to coracoid process and posterior to biceps and coracobrachialis tendons. *(Redrawn from Rockwood CA Jr: Subluxations and dislocations about the shoulder. In Rockwood CA Jr, Green DP [eds]: Fractures in Adults, 2nd ed. Philadelphia, JB Lippincott,1984; from Canale ST and Beaty JH Campbell's Operative Orthopaedics, 11th ed. St. Louis, Mosby, 2007.)*

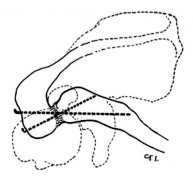

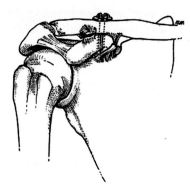

Fig. 6-2 Acromioclavicular ligament repair. The acromioclavicular joint is fixed internally with two unthreaded Kirschner wires. The wires are generally removed approximately 8 weeks after surgery. *(From Justis EJ Jr: Traumatic disorders. In Canale ST (ed): Campbell's Operative Orthopedics, 7th ed, vol 3. St. Louis, Mosby, 1987.)*

Fig. 6-3 Modified Bosworth technique for reduction and fixation of acromioclavicular dislocation. *(From Canale ST and Beaty JH: Campbell's Operative Orthopaedics, 11th ed. St. Louis, Mosby, 2007.)*

Physical Examination Findings: Pain, swelling, unstable AC joint with a mobile distal clavicle

Rockwood Classification:
- *Type I:* Minor sprain of AC ligament, intact joint capsule, intact CC ligament, intact deltoid and trapezius
- *Type II:* Rupture of AC ligament and joint capsule, sprain of CC ligament but CC interspace intact, minimal detachment of deltoid and trapezius
- *Type III:* Rupture of AC ligament, joint capsule, and CC ligament; clavicle elevated (as much as 100% displacement); detachment of deltoid and trapezius
- *Type IV:* Rupture of AC ligament, joint capsule, and CC ligament; clavicle displaced posteriorly into the trapezius; detachment of deltoid and trapezius
- *Type V:* Rupture of AC ligament, joint capsule, and CC ligament; clavicle elevated (more than 100% displacement); detachment of deltoid and trapezius
- *Type VI (Rare):* Rupture of AC ligament, joint capsule, and CC ligament; clavicle displaced behind the tendons of the biceps and coracobrachialis

Treatment:
- *Type I (Nonsurgical):* Rest, Ice, Compression, Elevate, early ROM, activity as tolerated
- *Type II:* Similar to type I; average 6 weeks of rest before return to contact sports
- *Type III:* Controversial, (nonsurgical) full recovery of strength/ROM for ADLs, elite athletes report pain with throwing and contact sports (surgery may be needed)
- *Types IV, V, VI (Surgical):* Any procedure should fulfill three requirements: (1) the AC joint must be exposed/débrided, (2) the CC and AC ligaments must be repaired, and (3) stable reduction of the AC joint must be obtained. Procedures that accomplish these three goals, no matter how the joint is fixed, should produce acceptable results.

Definition: An adamantinoma is a slow-growing (low-grade), malignant bone tumor that is most often found in the diaphyseal region of the tibia or the mandible.

Etiology: Unknown.

Associations: A history of trauma is frequent, and many affected patients describe local swelling with or without pain.

Incidence: It is a rare tumor (200 cases in the United States). It is most common in long bones (97%), especially the tibia (80% to 85%). Other bones involved in decreasing frequency: the humerus (6%), ulna (4%), femur (3%), fibula (3%), and radius (1%); rarely in the innominate bone, ribs, spine, hands, or feet. Within the long bone, it is most common in the diaphyseal region.

Age and Gender: Adamantinomas are slightly more common in men than in women (5:4) with age ranging from the second to the sixth decade. Classic variety occurs in persons older than 20 years; differentiated variety occurs in persons younger than 20 years.

Clinical Findings: Insidious onset of pain. Slow-growing tumor of the jaw or tibia.

Symptoms: Localized, insidious, aching pain and/or gradual swelling and deformity of the affected limb. Limping. Increased pain with activity or weight bearing.

Signs: Advanced or recurrent lesions may be associated with a soft tissue mass (15%).

Diagnostic Studies: Radiographs are best. Isotope scan, computed tomography, and magnetic resonance imaging are used to assess the extent of the lesion.

Pathology: Adamantinoma is a locally aggressive osteolytic tumor that is found 90% of the time in the diaphysis of the tibia with the remaining lesions found in the fibula and long tubular bones. Microscopically there are epithelial-like and fibrous components. There are variety of epithelial-like cells intermixed within a fibrous stroma. Four basic forms are found in varying combinations: basaloid, squamous, spindle, and tubular.

Treatment: Wide surgical resection is the mainstay of treatment. Radiation therapy or chemotherapy is not very effective. Because of the extensive involvement, some patients are treated by amputation. Limb salvage is an option, if the surgeon can completely remove the tumor. Local recurrence is common if the tumor is not completely removed. Metastases may occur to lymph nodes and the lungs.

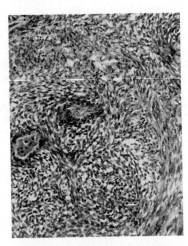

Fig. 7-1   Adamantinoma. Low-power photomicrograph (×250) shows biphasic differentiation, with spindle cells and epithelioid cells. *(From Miller M: Review of Orthopaedics, 5th ed. Philadelphia, Saunders, 2008.)*

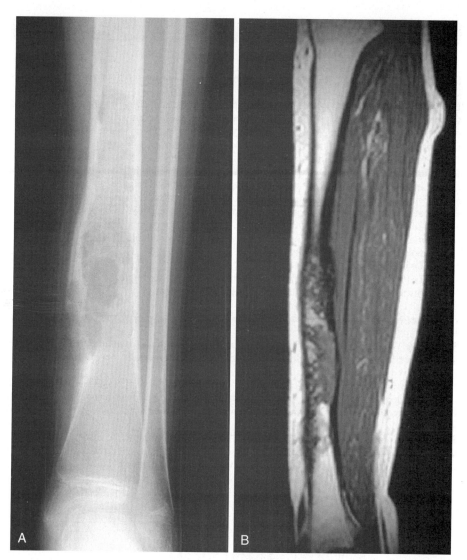

Fig. 7-2 Adamantinoma. **A,** AP radiograph of the tibia showing a multiloculated, lytic lesion expanding the cortex. **B,** Sagittal T1-weighted MRI showing a lobulated diaphyseal lesion with extension into the medullary cavity. *(From Adam A, et al: Grainger & Allison's Diagnostic Radiology, 5th ed. Philadelphia, Churchill Livingstone, 2008.)*

Definition: Deformity caused by plantar flexion of the medial foot, hindfoot varus, and forefoot valgus.

Etiology: The three major etiologies accounting for 80% of the adult cavovarus foot are neurologic, traumatic, and the result of malunion of calcaneal or talar fractures. Additionally, idiopathic etiologies comprise the remaining 20% of this deformity. The most common neuromuscular condition manifesting with a varus deformity is Charcot-Marie-Tooth disease.

Signs and Symptoms: Painful plantar callosities and ulceration under the metatarsal heads, lateral ankle instability, metatarsal stress fractures, peroneal tendonitis, and degenerative joint disease in overloaded joints are some of the symptoms and signs. The Coleman block test is used to determine the hindfoot flexibility. Clawing of the toes can also be found on examination.

Diagnostic Studies: Weight-bearing anteroposterior and lateral views of the foot and ankle along with a calcaneal axial view are required. Patients often have a degenerative spur in the posterior aspect of the subtalar joint. In the weight-bearing radiograph:

- Metatarsals are excessively plantar flexed.
- Midfoot is elevated.
- Hindfoot is in varus position with reduced plantar flexion of the talus.
- Dorsiflexion of the metatarsophalangeal joints is also apparent.

CT scan of the foot is more accurate in the assessment of the degenerative changes of the overloaded joints.

Pathology: The strong peroneus longus and tibialis posterior muscles put the hindfoot in varus and forefoot in valgus position. In children, the deformity is usually flexible but the patient develops fixed deformity with time.

Treatment: Surgical treatment is based on rigidity of the foot. Some of the techniques advocated include tendon lengthening and transfer, plantar fascia release, first metatarsal osteotomy, calcaneal osteotomy, and triple arthrodesis. Nonsurgical treatments include orthotic devices and shoe wear.

Sequelae: Compartment syndrome, residual clubfoot, and neuromuscular disease.

Complications: Nonunion, malunion, infection, undercorrection, overcorrection, recurrence of the deformity, progression of the deformity, nerve injury, and continued pain.

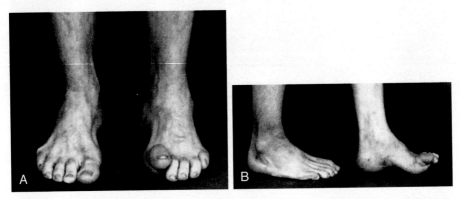

Fig. 8-1 Cavovarus foot deformity in Charcot-Marie-Tooth disease. **A,** Clawing of left great toe. **B,** Supination and cavus deformity of forefoot. *(Courtesy of Jay Cummings, MD; from Canale ST and Beaty JH: Campbell's Operative Orthopaedics, 11th ed. St. Louis, Mosby, 2007.)*

History: Amputation has been practiced since Neolithic times for punitive, therapeutic, and ritualistic reasons. Until the development and adoption of general anesthesia, it was the most major operation to which a surgeon could aspire, and a speedy technique was essential.

Prevalence: Amputation of the lower limb accounts for 85% of all amputations.

Indications: Peripheral vascular disease, with or without diabetes, is the major cause of lower limb amputations (approximately 85% of patients). Nonischemic indications for lower limb amputation include tumor, trauma, infection, or congenital anomaly.

Prognosis: Success of rehabilitation after amputation is related to the level of limb loss, with a more distal amputation corresponding to a better success rate. At least 90% of patients with transtibial amputations will achieve success with a prosthesis, as opposed to 25% of geriatric vasculopathic patients with transfemoral amputations. The primary underlying reason for increased success with more distal amputations is the marked increase in energy requirements with more proximal amputations. The self-selected walking velocity decreases as the amputation progresses proximally from Syme to transtibial to transfemoral. The slower rates reflect a compensatory mechanism to conserve energy expenditure per unit time (power). Malnourished or immunocompromised patients have increased rates of perioperative complications, although this is less evident with more proximal amputations.

Level of Amputation: Determining the ideal level of amputation is a balance between increased function of a more distal amputation and decreased complication rate of a more proximal one. To determine the level of the amputation, it is first necessary to determine the lowest level at which an amputation will heal. Clinical assessment of skin color, hair growth, and skin temperature are cues to level of viability. Clinical judgment is needed, but can be aided with tests such as transcutaneous measurement of oxygen tension. This method is accurate, easy, and relatively inexpensive. Vascular surgery consult is always appropriate. Revascularization may allow for a more distal amputation; however, peripheral bypass may compromise wound healing of a future amputation.

Stump Configuration: The location of the scar is not very important, because modern prostheses have increased surface area contact with the stump. It is important that the scar not be adherent to bone, because this type of scar often breaks down with use. Redundant soft tissue and dog-ears should be avoided. Muscles should be divided at least 5 cm distal to intended bone resection. Bony prominences at the margin should be resected and the bony stump rasped to form a smooth contour.

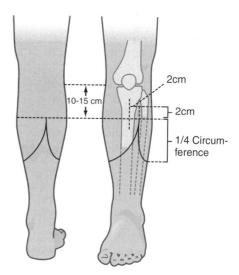

Fig. 9-1   Transtibial amputation: Skew flap incisions. *(Redrawn from Ruckley CV, Stonebridge PA, Prescott RJ: Skewflap versus long posterior flap in below-knee amputations: Multicenter trial. J Vasc Surg 13:423–427, 1991; from Rutherford RB: Vascular Surgery, 6th ed. Philadelphia, Saunders, 2005.)*

2cm

2cm

10-15 cm

1/4 Circumference

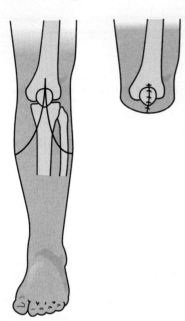

Fig. 9-2 Through-knee amputation. Equal sagittal skin flaps for a through-knee amputation. *(Redrawn from Robinson KP: Amputations in vascular patients. In Bell PRF, et al [eds]: Surgical Management of Vascular Disease. London, WB Saunders, 1992, pp 609–635.) (From Rutherford RB: Vascular Surgery, 6th ed. Philadelphia, Saunders, 2005.)*

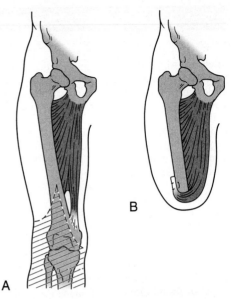

Fig. 9-3 **A**, Surgical incision for medial-based flap technique of transfemoral amputation. **B**, Adductor myodesis is accomplished to control the position of the residual femur in order to optimize weight bearing. *(Modified from Gottschalk F. In Bowker JH, Michael JW [eds]: Atlas of Limb Prosthetics. St. Louis, Mosby-Year Book, 1992; from Browner BD: Skeletal Trauma: Basic Science, Management, and Reconstruction, 3rd ed. Philadelphia, Saunders, 2003.)*

Hemostasis: The use of a tourniquet after exsanguinations with an Esmarch is indicated except during amputations for infection, malignancy, or in severely ischemic limbs. A drain is generally recommended for 48 to 72 hours.

Nerves: A neuroma forms after a nerve is divided, and it becomes painful if it is in a location subjected to repeated trauma. Nerves should be isolated at the amputation margin, pulled distally, and divided sharply so the cut end retracts proximal to the level of the bone stump. Large nerves should be ligated because they often contain relatively large arteries.

Types of Leg Amputations

Amputations About the Foot: Amputation of a single toe seldom causes disturbance of stance or gait. Even amputation of the great toe does not greatly affect standing or walking at a normal gait, but will cause a limp when running. Amputation of the second toe frequently causes severe hallux valgus, with the great toe tending to drift toward the midline. The fifth toe is the most commonly amputated, indicated due to overriding of the fourth toe. This usually requires no prosthesis other than a shoe filler. Amputation through the metatarsals impairs gait by loss of the fulcrum of the ball of the foot. This is disabling in loss of push-off.

Midfoot Amputation: Amputations more proximal than transmetatarsal result in more pronounced gait disturbance due to loss of support and push-off; consequently, it is generally preferred to amputate at the hindfoot. The Lisfranc amputation is done at the tarsometatarsal joints, and often results in an equinus deformity due to loss of dorsiflexor attachments. Chopart amputations are done through the midtarsal joints and may result in severe equinovarus deformities. In the Pirigoff amputation, the calcaneus is rotated forward to be fused to the tibia after vertical section through its middle. Salvage of midfoot amputations that have developed equinus deformity can be done by dividing the Achilles tendon.

Hindfoot and Ankle Amputations: Amputations about the ankle must not only bear weight but must also allow for space between the stump and ground for a prosthetic ankle joint mechanism. The Syme amputation is the most effective of these procedures. The bone is cut at the level of the distal tibia and fibula, 0.6 cm proximal to the ankle joint and passing through the dome of the ankle centrally. The durable skin of the heel flap provides normal weight-bearing skin. The two most common reasons for failure are posterior migration of the heel pad and skin slough. The Boyd amputation involves talectomy, forward shift of calcaneus, and calcaneotibial arthrodesis.

Below-Knee Amputation (Transtibial): Transtibial amputation is the most common type of amputation and has reported success rates of more than 85%. Different techniques are indicated depending on whether the procedure is done on an ischemic or nonischemic limb. The variation is in the construction of the skin flap and muscle stabilization technique. In nonischemic limbs, most often equal anterior-posterior flaps are used. Tension myodesis and myoplasty can be used as muscle stabilization techniques. Tension myodesis is a procedure in which transected muscle groups are sutured to bone under physiologic tension. Myoplasty is a procedure in which muscle is sutured to soft tissue, such as opposing muscle groups or fascia. In most instances, myoplasty is performed, but myodesis is argued to be indicated for younger, more active patients. In ischemic limbs, tension myodesis is contraindicated because it may further compromise an already marginal blood supply. In ischemic patients, there should be a long posterior myocutaneous flap and a short anterior flap because the anterior blood supply is less robust. Complications of this type of amputation include knee flexion contractures and distal ulcers. The ideal level of amputation in nonischemic limbs is at the musculotendinous junction of the gastrocnemius muscle. The leg distal to this level is unsatisfactory because the vascular supply is weaker and soft tissue padding for flap development is less. In adults, the ideal bone length for the stump is 12.5 to 17.5 cm, depending on body height. A rule of thumb is to allow 2.5 cm of bone length for each 30 cm of body height. Usually this is about 15 cm distal to the medial tibial articular surface. Shorter stumps are less mechanically efficient. Amputations performed in ischemic limbs are customarily at a higher level, 10 to 12.5 cm distal to joint line.

Through-Knee Amputation (Disarticulation of the Knee): Disarticulation of the knee results in an excellent end-bearing stump. Newer socket designs provide swing phase control that have improved prosthesis function. This type of amputation is not indicated in older patients or in those with peripheral vascular disease, because the long flaps required are subject to necrosis in ischemic limbs. Benefits include large end-bearing surface of distal femur naturally suited for weight bearing, long lever arm controlled by strong muscles, and stable prosthesis. Some of the bulk of the bone at the end of the stump can be removed for cosmesis. This type of amputation is ideal for the nonambulating patient because the additional length of the extremity provides increased sitting support and balance.

Above-Knee Amputation (Transfemoral): Amputation through the thigh is the second most common type of amputation. It is extremely important for the stump to be as long as possible to provide a strong lever arm for control of the prosthesis. The conventional constant-friction knee joint is used in most AKA prostheses and extends 9 to 10 cm distal to the end of the prosthetic socket, and so bone must be resected to allow room for this joint. Amputation stumps that extend less than 5 cm distal to the lesser trochanter are essentially functionless and are prosthetically fitted as hip disarticulations. Complications due to the division of musculature include muscle atrophy and contraction over the femur.

Prostheses: The stump and prosthesis assume walking and weight-bearing functions of the amputated limb, with the stump functioning like a foot and the prosthesis functioning like a shoe. Early prosthesis designs varied, but by the late eighteenth century designs using metal with stump-fitting sockets, some lined with shortly trimmed dog hair for adhesion purposes, were being used. Current prostheses are of varying designs, with some created for cosmetic purposes and others for athletic performance.

Knee Joint:
- Mainly acts as a hinge joint
- Motions: Flexion, extension, internal rotation, and external rotation
- Composed of three different joints:
  - Patellofemoral joint—between patella and femur
  - Lateral tibiofemoral joint—between lateral femoral condyle and lateral meniscus of tibia
  - Medial tibiofemoral joint—between medial femoral condyle and medial meniscus of the tibia

Bony Anatomy: Composed of four bones.

Muscular Anatomy:
Flexors: Primarily biceps femoris, semitendinosus, and semimembranosus, also known as hamstrings. Sartorius, gracilis, gastrocnemius, plantaris, and popliteus muscles also assist in flexion.
Extensors: Rectus femoris, vastus medialis, vastus lateralis, and vastus intermedius. All four are collectively known as the *quadriceps* or the *quadriceps femoris*. They form a common tendon called the quadriceps tendon, which inserts into the patella. Below the patella, the quadriceps tendon becomes the patellar tendon and inserts into the tibial tuberosity.
Internal Rotators: When the knee is flexed, the semitendinosus, semimembranosus, sartorius, gracilis, and popliteus muscles internally rotate the leg.
External Rotators: When the knee is extended, the biceps femoris externally rotates the leg.

Menisci: Medial and lateral:
Fibrocartilaginous Rings: Located on the proximal surface of the tibial condyles. These are basically shock absorbers that deepen the shallow concave articular surface of the tibia and help prevent side-to-side rocking of the femur.

Ligaments:
Extracapsular Ligaments:
- Lateral collateral ligament (LCL)—helps to resist varus forces placed on the knee and helps prevent internal and external rotation of the tibia
- Medial collateral ligament (MCL)—helps to resist valgus forces and external rotation of the tibia
- Oblique popliteal ligament
- Arcuate popliteal ligament

Intracapsular Ligaments:
- Anterior cruciate ligament (ACL)—prevents anterior displacement of the tibia on the femur when the leg is flexed, prevents excessive internal rotation, stabilizes the fully extended knee, and checks for hyperextension of the knee

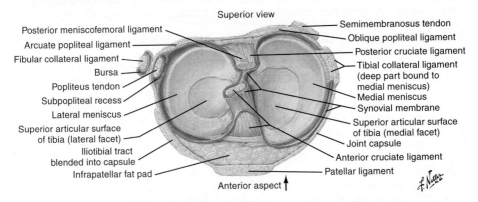

Fig. 10-1 *From Netter F: Atlas of Human Anatomy, 4th ed. Philadelphia, Saunders, 2006.*

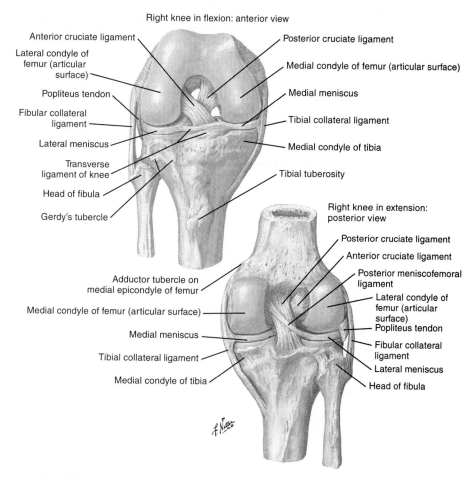

Right knee in flexion: anterior view

Anterior cruciate ligament

Lateral condyle of femur (articular surface)

Popliteus tendon

Fibular collateral ligament

Lateral meniscus

Transverse ligament of knee

Head of fibula

Gerdy's tubercle

Posterior cruciate ligament

Medial condyle of femur (articular surface)

Medial meniscus

Tibial collateral ligament

Medial condyle of tibia

Tibial tuberosity

Right knee in extension: posterior view

Posterior cruciate ligament

Anterior cruciate ligament

Posterior meniscofemoral ligament

Lateral condyle of femur (articular surface)

Popliteus tendon

Fibular collateral ligament

Lateral meniscus

Head of fibula

Adductor tubercle on medial epicondyle of femur

Medial condyle of femur (articular surface)

Medial meniscus

Tibial collateral ligament

Medial condyle of tibia

Fig. 10-2 *From Netter F: Atlas of Human Anatomy, 4th ed. Philadelphia, Saunders, 2006.*

- Posterior cruciate ligament (PCL)—prevents posterior sliding of the tibia or anterior sliding of the femur, therefore helping to prevent hyperflexion of the knee; also stops excessive internal rotation
- Posterior meniscofemoral ligament (ligament of Wrisberg)

Arteries and Nerves:

- Blood supply—predominantly via the popliteal artery
- Nervous supply—innervation of the anterior and anteromedial sides of the knee via the femoral and obturator nerves, which originate from the lumbosacral plexus

The sciatic nerve innervates the posterior side of the thigh, which divides to form the common peroneal and tibial nerves.

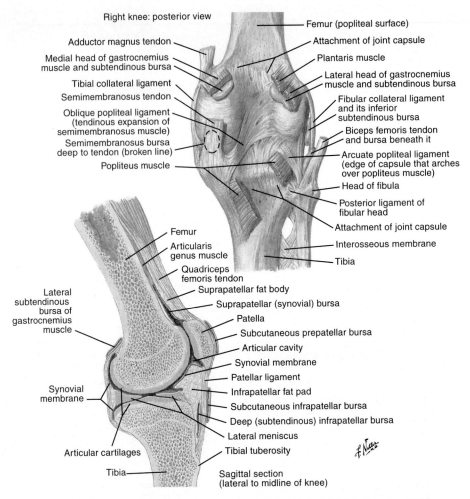

Right knee: posterior view

Adductor magnus tendon
Medial head of gastrocnemius muscle and subtendinous bursa
Tibial collateral ligament
Semimembranosus tendon
Oblique popliteal ligament (tendinous expansion of semimembranosus muscle)
Semimembranosus bursa deep to tendon (broken line)
Popliteus muscle

Femur (popliteal surface)
Attachment of joint capsule
Plantaris muscle
Lateral head of gastrocnemius muscle and subtendinous bursa
Fibular collateral ligament and its inferior subtendinous bursa
Biceps femoris tendon and bursa beneath it
Arcuate popliteal ligament (edge of capsule that arches over popliteus muscle)
Head of fibula
Posterior ligament of fibular head
Attachment of joint capsule
Interosseous membrane
Tibia

Femur
Articularis genus muscle
Quadriceps femoris tendon
Suprapatellar fat body
Suprapatellar (synovial) bursa
Patella
Subcutaneous prepatellar bursa
Articular cavity
Synovial membrane
Patellar ligament
Infrapatellar fat pad
Subcutaneous infrapatellar bursa
Deep (subtendinous) infrapatellar bursa
Lateral meniscus
Tibial tuberosity

Lateral subtendinous bursa of gastrocnemius muscle

Synovial membrane

Articular cartilages
Tibia

Sagittal section (lateral to midline of knee)

Fig. 10-3 *From Netter F: Atlas of Human Anatomy, 4th ed. Philadelphia, Saunders, 2006.*

Definition: The aneurysmal bone cyst (ABC) is an expansile cystic lesion that most often affects persons during their second decade of life.

Etiology/Pathophysiology: Tumor-like lesion of uncertain etiology. These are considered to be the result of a vascular malformation within the bone. Frequently found in diaphyses of long bones and vertebral neural arches. Also found in short tubular bones and pelvic and facial bones. In 30% to 40% of cases, ABCs may be caused by a reaction secondary to another bony lesion (Table 11-1)

Clinical: Pain, swelling, and tenderness are the common presenting features. Occasionally, there is limited range of motion due to joint obstruction. Spinal lesions can cause neurologic symptoms secondary to cord compression. Pathologic fractures are rare (8%) due to the eccentric location of the lesion, but can be as high as 21% if the spine is involved.

Pathology: The gross appearance of the ABC is that of a blood-soaked sponge. A thin subperiosteal shell of new bone surrounds the structure and contains cystic blood-filled cavities. The tissue within shows brownish intertwining septa. The stroma contains proliferative fibroblasts, spindle cells, areas of osteoid formation, and an uneven distribution of multinucleated giant cells. The tissue within the septations includes cavernous channels that do not contain a muscular or elastic layer in their walls. Areas of new and reactive bone formation also can be found in the ABC. Mitotic figures are common to the ABC, but no atypical figures should be evident.

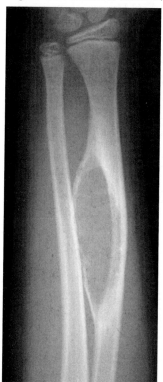

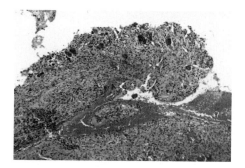

Fig. 11-1 AP radiograph of the forearm showing a subperiosteal aneurysmal bone cyst of the radius. *(From Adam A, et al: Grainger & Allison's Diagnostic Radiology, 5th ed. Philadelphia, Churchill Livingstone, 2008.)*

Fig. 11-2 Aneurysmal bone cyst lining composed of connective tissue and scattered multinucleated giant cells. *(From Regezi JA, et al: Oral Pathology: Clinical Pathologic Correlations, 5th ed. Philadelphia, Saunders, 2008.)*

Table 11-1. INCIDENCE AND CLASSIFICATION OF ABC

Incidence	Classification (Campanacci)
1% to 5% of benign bone tumors Age: 10 to 30 years Male:Female 1:2 50% occur in long bones 30% occur in the spine 20% occur in flat or short bones	Type I: Cyst in center of bone, little or no expansion—intralesional curettage Type II: Lesion substitutes whole bone segment—intralesional excision Type III: Eccentric interosseous lesion with little or no expansion—en bloc or wide excision Type IV: Subperiosteal cyst and superficial erosion of cortex Type V: Periosteum eroded, expansion into soft tissues

Differential Diagnosis: Unicameral bone cyst, chondroblastoma, chondromyxoid fibroma, eosinophilic granuloma, osteomyelitis.

Diagnostic Studies: Pathognomonic findings on radiographs, computed tomography scans, and magnetic resonance imaging scans may be used to confirm a diagnosis of ABC. However, if any doubt exists, an open biopsy must be performed because there is a high frequency of accompanying tumors.

Treatment: Curettage and bone graft 20% recurrence. For older patients with lesions in an inaccessible site, radiotherapy is the treatment. Investigate to exclude other pathology.

Definition: Ankle arthroscopy is a relatively new method of investigating and treating ankle conditions, using fiberoptic camera and small surgical tools that are inserted into the ankle joint through multiple small incisions. There are five portals through which the arthroscope can be positioned. Anterior approaches include the anteromedial, anterolateral, and anterocentral portals. Posterior approaches include the posterolateral and posteromedial portals, with the latter rarely being used.

Indications:

Diagnostic Ankle Arthroscopy:
- Joint evaluation before some ligamentous reconstruction procedures
- Remove loose intra-articular fragments
- Joint evaluation in cases of arthritis
- Nonspecific synovitis of the ankle
- Visual assessment of articular cartilage in osteochondritis desiccans and osteonecrosis of the talus
- Evaluation of cases of persistent post-traumatic disorders

Operative Ankle Arthroscopy:
- Osteoarthritis
- Rheumatoid synovitis
- Impingement exostosis
- Septic arthritis
- Post-traumatic synovial impingement
- Chondral lesions
- Meniscoid lesions of the ankle
- Chronic lateral instability of the lateral collateral ligaments

Risks:
- Infection (superficial, deep)
- Bleeding
- Local nerve damage
- Risks related to anesthesia, depending on the type that is chosen
- Breakage of an instrument

Benefits:
- Fewer complications than open surgery
- Less blood loss
- Less scarring
- Faster recovery
- Less postoperative pain

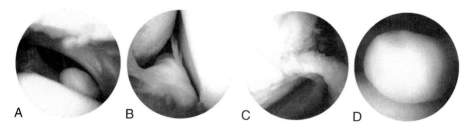

A   B   C   D

Fig. 12-1 A, Loose body in posterolateral gutter of ankle joint has been expressed from behind posteroinferior tibiofibular ligament. Transverse ligament can be seen inferior to loose body. **B,** Area of soft tissue impingement in lateral gutter after recurrent ankle sprains. **C,** After previous open repair of ankle ligaments. Calcaneofibular ligament is evident, as is extensive synovitis. **D,** Stage IV osteochondritis desiccans of ankle with loose osteochondral fragment. *(From Canale ST: Campbell's Operative Orthopaedics, 10th ed. St. Louis, Mosby, 2002.)*

- Very common— more than 250,000 per year in the United States
- Highest incidence in elderly women
- Increased body mass and smoking associated with increase in ankle fracture rate
- Isolated malleolar (66%), bimalleolar (25%), trimalleolar (7%), open (2%)

Anatomy:
- Dorsiflexed (weight-bearing) ankle primarily stabilized by bony anatomy
- Plantarflexed ankle primarily stabilized by ligamentous structures
- *Medial Stabilization:*
- Superficial and deep deltoid ligaments (deep is first degree stabilizer)
- *Lateral Stabilization:*
  - Anterior talofibular ligament (ATFL)—weakest, injured in sprains
  - Calcaneofibular ligament (CFL)—limits inversion
  - Posterior talofibular ligament (PTFL)—strongest, rarely ruptured
- *Syndesmotic Stabilization:*
  - Anterior tibiofibular ligament—weaker, prone to rupture
  - Interosseous ligament—blends with interosseous membrane
- *Posterior Tibiofibular Ligament:*
- Inferior portion stronger, more likely to cause avulsion fractures (posterior malleolus)

Radiographic Criteria: Standard series, anteroposterior, lateral, mortise (15-degree internal rotation). Ninety-five percent of fractures identified with lateral and mortise views.

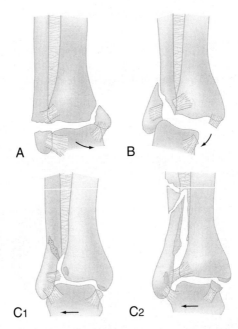

Fig. 13-1 The Danis-Weber classification of ankle fractures focuses on the location of the fibular fracture in relation to the tibiotalar joint. *(From Wilson FC: The pathogenesis and treatment of ankle fractures: Classification. In Green WB (ed): Instructional Course Lectures, vol 39, III. Easton, PA, American Academy of Orthopedic Surgeons, 1990, pp 79-83.)*

	Normal	Abnormal
Talocrural angle—angle formed by parallel line to distal tibial articular surface and line connecting malleolar tips	**8 to 15 degrees** (or 83 degrees ± 4 degrees if perpendicular used)	> 2 to 3 degrees difference from contralateral = **fibular shortening**
Medial clear space—distance between lateral border of medial malleolus and lateral border of talus	< **4 mm** and equal to superior clear space	> 4 mm = lateral talar shift and **instability**
Tibiofibular clear space—distance between medial wall of fibula and tibial incisura	< **6 mm** on AP and mortise views	> 6 mm = **syndesmotic disruption (instability)**
Talar tilt—difference between medial and lateral superior clear space measurements	< **2 mm**	> 2 mm = **instability**

Classification:

1. **Danis-Weber**—based on location of fibular fracture	2. **Lauge-Hansen**—based on position of foot and deforming force
A. Below syndesmosis	Supination external rotation—most common
B. At level of syndesmosis	Supination adduction
C. Above syndesmosis	Pronation external rotation
	Pronation abduction

Treatment: Surgical decisions mostly based on stability.

Stable	Unstable
Isolated lateral malleolar fractures if:	**Lateral malleolus fractures** if:
Below syndesmosis	Medial injury/tenderness (bimalleolar equivalent)
No medial ligament injury or talar shift	Talar shift
Displacement < 5 mm	Above syndesmosis
No shortening	Shortened or displaced > 5 mm
Isolated medial malleolus fractures (although 5% to 15% nonunion rates have been reported)	**Bimalleolar fractures**
	Trimalleolar fractures (fix posterior if > 25% of articular surface)
	Maisonneuve fractures

Complications:
- Osteochondral fractures/defects (2% to 6% of ankle sprains)
- Wound complications—marginal skin edge necrosis occurs in 3% (greatly decreased if surgery delayed in setting of significant swelling or soft tissue damage)
- Deep infection—<2%
- Malunion—usually a shortened and/or externally rotated fibula; nonunion more common at medial malleolus
- Arthrosis—correlated with quality of reduction and initial fracture displacement

Definition: Lateral-sided ligamentous laxity resulting in recurrent ankle sprains during activities of daily living.

Etiology: Weakness/tear of the anterior talofibular ligament (ATFL)/calcaneal fibular ligament (CFL) and inadequate strength and proprioceptive properties of the dynamic stabilizers of the lateral ankle, namely, the peroneal muscles.

Incidence: Symptomatic in 20% of all patients who suffer inversion sprains of the lateral ankle ligaments.

Symptoms: Recurrent ankle sprains with activities of daily living, walking on uneven terrain, or playing sports.

Clinical Findings: Injury to the superficial peroneal nerve results in altered sensation and sensitivity in the anterolateral foot. Palpable tenderness posterior to the lateral malleolus may be indicative of injury to the peroneal tendons. Combined motion of the ankle and subtalar joints is estimated clinically by measuring the angle between the hindfoot and the leg during maximal inversion stress. Always compare one side with the other. The diagnosis is made based on history and physical examination in combination with radiographic evidence of ligamentous laxity.

Diagnostic Studies: Mortise and lateral x-ray studies, as well as anteroposterior and lateral stress radiographs, should be obtained to quantify the degree of laxity and confirm the clinical diagnosis of ankle instability. Again, always compare one side with the other. Anterior translation is measured on lateral stress radiographs as the perpendicular distance between the posterior edge

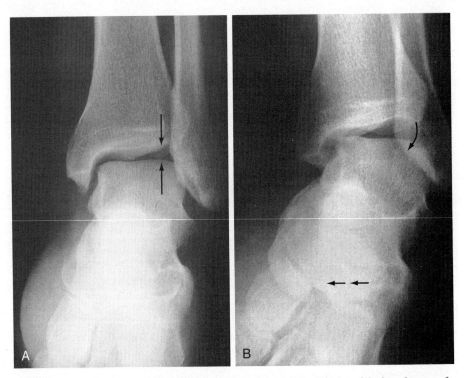

Fig. 14-1 **A,** An anteroposterior view of the ankle demonstrates slight widening of the lateral aspect of the ankle mortise *(arrows)*. **B,** A stress view was obtained by inverting the foot (in the direction of the *arrows*). This makes the ligamentous injury much more obvious by opening the ankle mortise even farther *(curved arrow)*. *(From Mettler F: Essentials of Radiology, 2nd ed. Philadelphia, Saunders, 2004.)*

of the tibial articular surface and the talus. Anterior translation 5 mm greater than that of the uninvolved side or an absolute of 9 mm is indicative of instability. Talar tilt 5 degrees greater than the uninvolved side or an absolute of 10 degrees is indicative of pathologic laxity. The talar tilt angle is measured on the mortise view as the angle between the talar and tibial articular surfaces.

Treatment:

Nonoperative: Initially, rest, ice, compression, and elevation, followed by controlled motion with use of a functional brace, allowing limited dorsiflexion and plantar flexion while preventing inversion. If recurrent ankle sprains occur, most patients become less symptomatic with a supervised rehabilitation program aimed at improving proprioception and strengthening peroneal muscles. Bracing is also effective in improving functional symptoms of instability.

Operative: Patients who continue to sustain multiple recurrent inversion sprains despite bracing and rehabilitation are candidates for surgical repair/reconstruction of the lateral ankle ligaments. Most reconstructive procedures involve either direct late repair with or without augmentation or indirect stabilization with the use of tendon grafts. In 1966, Brostrom was the first to report on his series of direct lateral tendon repairs. Karlsson modified Brostrom's procedure by attaching the shortened CFL and ATFL to the fibula through drill holes using suture. Sjolin added local fibular periosteal flaps to augment the repair. Evans, Watson-Jones, Colville, and Chrisman and Snook all have developed procedures involving tenodesis of the peroneus brevis tendon to control excessive ankle and subtalar motion.

Complications: Loss of subtalar motion and wound infection are the most frequently cited complications.

Definition: An inflammatory and erosive arthritis affecting primarily the spine and sacroiliac joints (spondyloarthropathies).

Incidence and Etiology: Prevalence in the United States is 129 per 100,000. Strong genetic association with HLA B27 (90%) and familial element.

Age and Gender: Generally men ages 17 to 35 years, but does occur in women and can be particularly hard to diagnose.

Symptoms and Associations: Chronic low back pain and stiffness, especially in the early morning, which gets better as the day progresses; groin pain; decreased respiratory reserve. Inflammatory bowel disease, iritis, cardiac involvement that includes aortic valve incompetence, conduction blocks, and pericarditis.

Clinical Findings: Loss of mobility and pain in the lumbar and cervical spine. Occiput to wall test is reduced if the cervical spine is involved. Shoulder and hip pain if the peripheral joints are affected. Eye involvement, such as uveitis, is the most common extra-articular manifestation.

Investigations: Associated with HLA-B27, elevated erythrocyte sedimentation rate, chronic anemia, and negative rheumatoid factor. Radiologic exams show sacroiliitis and eventual fusion of the vertebral columns showing the characteristic "bamboo spine."

Pathology: Inflammation, fibrosis, ossification, and ultimately loss of joint space at sites of attachment of ligaments, tendons, and joint capsules. Chronic synovitis exists within synovial joints.

Treatment: Physical therapy, control of posture, and retention of mobility where possible.

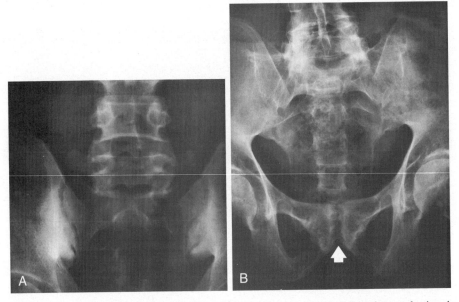

Fig. 15-1 Ankylosing spondylitis. **A,** Bilateral symmetrical reactive sclerosis and erosions predominantly involving the iliac wing aspect of the sacroiliac joint. **B,** Late changes include bony ankylosis and obliteration of sacroiliac joint. Note symphysis pubis erosions *(white arrow)*. *(From Noble J: Textbook of Primary Care Medicine, 3rd ed. St. Louis, Mosby, 2001.)*

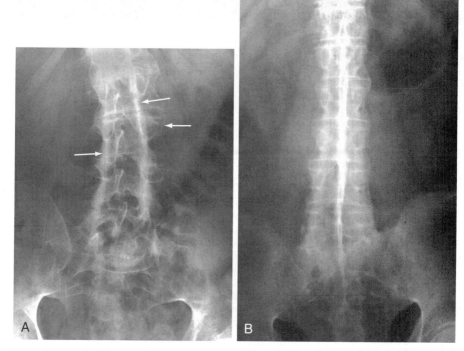

Fig. 15-2 Ankylosing spondylitis. **A,** Fusion of the facet joints and ossification of the adjacent soft tissue has produced a "trolley track" appearance *(arrows).* The sacroiliac joints are fused. Syndesmophytes *(open arrow)* are present. **B,** In another patient, there is a prominent fusion of the interspinous ligaments producing a saber sheath appearance. *(From Harris ED: Kelley's Textbook of Rheumatology, 7th ed. Philadelphia, Saunders, 2005.)*

Medical Care: Nonsteroidal anti-inflammatory drugs, sulfasalazine, methotrexate.
Surgical Care: Surgery of spine is considered when the spine is fixed in a flexed position, the spine is compromised, or neurologic deficits exist. Arthroplasty of large joints is often indicated.
Complications: Progressive kyphosis, reduced lung capacity, cardiac failure, spinal injury, unstable injury status post fusion, chalk stick fractures most common at cervicothoracic and thoracolumbar junctions. Heterotopic ossification is common following total joint replacement.

β-Lactam Antibiotics: Lead to bacterial cell death by inhibiting synthesis, export, assembly, and cross-linking of peptidoglycan, which confers bacterial cell wall rigidity and resistance to osmotic rupture.

- *Penicillinase-Sensitive Penicillins (Penicillin G, Ampicillin):* Spectrum includes streptococci groups A and B, *Streptococcus viridans*, and *Streptococcus pneumoniae*, most *Neisseria* species, and some isolates of *Salmonella, Shigella,* and *Escherichia coli.*
- *Penicillinase-Resistant Penicillins (Methicillin, Oxacillin):* Used solely for the treatment of *Staphylococcus aureus* infections.
- *First-Generation Cephalosporins (Cefazolin, Cephalexin):* Spectrum includes methicillin-sensitive *S. aureus* (MSSA) and streptococci with some *E. coli* and *Klebsiella pneumoniae* coverage.
- *Second-Generation Cephalosporins (Cefuroxime, Cefamandole, Cefaclor):* Extend the gram-negative spectrum of the first-generation cephalosporins.
- *Third-Generation Cephalosporins (Ceftriaxone, Ceftazidime):* Broad coverage against enteric gram-negative rods and hospital-acquired multiresistant organisms including *Pseudomonas.*
- *Carbapenem (Imipenem):* Excellent activity against all organisms except methicillin-resistant *Staphylococcus aureus* (MRSA) and *Enterococcus faecium.*
- *Monobactam (Aztreonam):* Has excellent gram-negative spectrum, including *Pseudomonas,* but poor coverage against gram-positive organisms and anaerobes.

Vancomycin: Interferes with the addition of new cell wall subunits (muramyl pentapeptides) to the peptidoglycan layer. Spectrum is limited to enterococci, streptococci, and staphylococci, including MRSA.

Macrolides: Binds specifically to the 50S ribosomal subunit and prevents protein chain elongation (e.g., erythromycin, clarithromycin, azithromycin). Has broad-spectrum activity against gram-positive organisms, including atypical bacteria such as *Mycoplasma, Legionella,* and *Chlamydia.*

Lincosamides: Although structurally unrelated to macrolides, they bind to a site on the 50S ribosome nearly identical to the binding site of macrolides, and therefore inhibit protein chain elongation (e.g., clindamycin, lincomycin). It has broad-spectrum, gram-positive coverage including staphylococci.

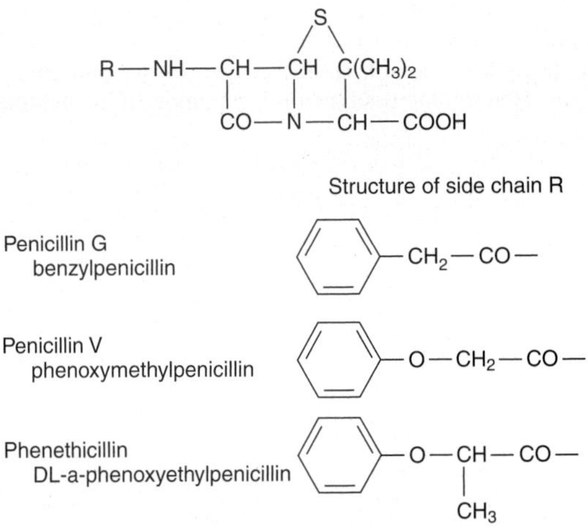

Fig. 16-1 The structures of penicillin G and penicillin V. *(From Mandell GL, Bennett JF, and Dolin R: [eds]: Principles and Practice of Infectious Diseases, 6th ed. Philadelphia, Churchill Livingstone, 2005.)*

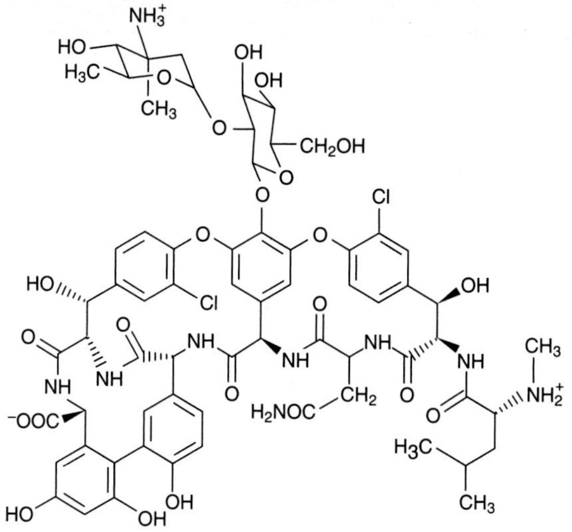

Fig. 16-2 Structural formula of vancomycin. *(From Schafer M, Schneider TR, Shieldrick GM: Crystal structure of vancomycin. Structure 4(12):1509–1515, 1996.)*

Chloramphenicol: The bacteriostatic effect is due to binding reversibly to the 50S portion of ribosomal subunit at a site close to but not identical with the binding sites of the macrolides and lincosamides. Covers both gram-positive and gram-negative bacteria, but is rarely used due to irreversible bone marrow aplasia.

Tetracyclines: The bacteriostatic mechanism of action is through the reversible binding to the 30S ribosomal subunit, blocking the binding of aminoacyl tRNA to the mRNA ribosomal complex (e.g., tetracycline, doxycycline). Covers gram-positive and gram-negative bacteria involved in non–hospital-acquired infections.

Aminoglycosides: Although it binds irreversibly to the 30S subunit and blocks initiation of protein synthesis, its effect is lethal against bacteria, contrary to the bacteriostatic effect of macrolides, lincosamides, chloramphenicol, and the tetracyclines (gentamycin, tobramycin, streptomycin, neomycin, and amikacin). Activity is limited to gram-negative bacteria that are not anaerobes and staphylococci.

Sulfonamides/Trimethoprim: They are structural analogues that competitively inhibit enzymes involved in the two steps of folic acid synthesis. In combination, they can be bactericidal against gram-negative bacteria and staphylococci.

Rifampin: Binds tightly to the bacterial DNA-dependent RNA polymerase, thus inhibiting transcription of DNA to RNA. It can be used in combinations with other antibiotics against MRSA.

Metronidazole: In the presence of an anaerobic electron transport system, it is reduced to reactive intermediates that cause DNA damage. The spectrum is limited to anaerobes only.

Quinolones: Inhibits the activity of DNA gyrase that is responsible for negative DNA supercoiling (e.g., ciprofloxacin, ofloxacin, levofloxacin, moxifloxacin, gatifloxacin). They have excellent activity against gram-negative rods and staphylococci but variable activity against streptococci, and no activity against anaerobes.

Oxazolidinones: Disrupts bacterial growth by inhibiting the initiation process of protein synthesis (e.g., linezolid) rather than affecting the elongation process as aminoglycosides, macrolides, and lincosamides. It is indicated for treatment of certain gram-positive infections as *S. pneumoniae,* MSSA, MRSA, vancomycin-sensitive *Enterococcus faecalis,* and vancomycin-resistant *E. faecalis* but has limited gram-negative coverage.

Introduction: Prophylactic anticoagulation in some orthopedic procedures is advisable, in that the Virchow's triad (venous stasis, endothelial damage, and a hypercoagulable state) can be established, increasing the possibility of developing a deep vein thrombosis (DVT) and eventually a pulmonary embolism (PE).

Venous thrombi form in regions where there is stasis. Venous thrombi are composed of red blood cells surrounded by a mesh of fibrin strands and aggregated platelets, usually in the presence of

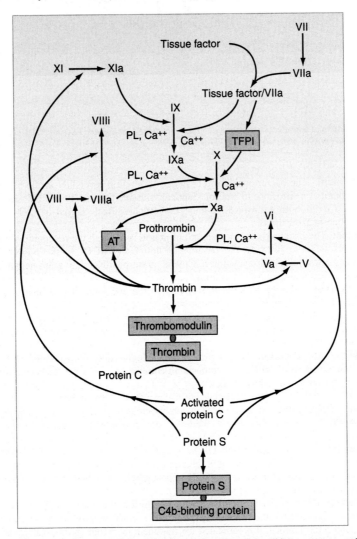

Fig. 17-1 Natural inhibitors of coagulation: AT (antithrombin III, antithrombin); components of the protein C pathway (thrombomodulin, protein C, protein S); TFPI (tissue factor pathway inhibitor). For details of inhibitory mechanisms, see text. *(From McPherson RA and Pincus MR: Henry's Clinical Diagnosis and Management by Laboratory Methods, 21st ed. Philadelphia, Saunders, 2006.)*

a hypercoagulable state. Arterial thrombi, on the other hand, occur in high-pressure vessels with a fast flow rate; these thrombi are composed mainly of platelet aggregates and few fibrin strands, usually the result of platelet reaction to damage of the intimal vessel. When a thrombus is established, usually at the proximal veins of the lower extremities, it may break loose and travel up to the pulmonary vasculature, where, if large enough, can cause a fatal PE.

Coagulation Cascade: Coagulation consists of a series of self-regulating steps that give rise to a fibrin clot. The steps are controlled by a few relatively inactive cofactors called *zymogens*. When these cofactors are activated, they promote the clotting process. The reaction takes place at the phospholipid surface of platelets, endothelial cells, and macrophages.

The coagulation process can be divided into two distinct pathways: intrinsic and extrinsic. The intrinsic system involves plasma factors; the extrinsic system starts with activation by tissue lipoprotein that is released at injury or trauma. Both pathways come to a common pathway at the level of inactivated factor X, which, once activated, forms factor Xa.

Anticoagulant and Antithrombotic Drugs

ASA and Cyclooxygenase-1 (COX-1) Inhibitors: These are platelet-active drugs that have been used to prevent thrombosis. Aspirin is effective as a platelet inhibitor, preventing aggregation at very low doses (50 to 100 mg/day). This dose is not enough for anti-inflammatory purposes.

Coumadin (Warfarin): Coumadin is an oral anticoagulant drug, whose mechanism of action is to interfere with the interaction between vitamin K and coagulation factors II, VII, IX, and X by inhibiting the carboxylation necessary for its biologic activity. Warfarin is made from two isomers: the R and S forms in similar proportions. Warfarin requires 36 to 72 hours to reach a stable loading dose. The dose response is variable, being influenced by various genetic and environmental factors.

The effectiveness of warfarin is measured by the prothrombin, or *protime*, against a standard control. The use of international normalized ratio (INR) is now the standard in hospital use. INR uses a standardized protime, which allows for comparisons between hospitals and laboratories.

As prophylaxis after joint arthroplasties, warfarin reduces total DVT by 60% and proximal DVT by 70%.

Disadvantages of warfarin use include its long onset of action, the need for frequent INR monitoring, a long half-life, and the eventual requirement of vitamin K for reversal of effect on drug and dietary interaction.

Hemorrhagic complications are reported in 3% to 5% of patients on warfarin prophylaxis.

Heparin: Unfractionated heparin (UFH) acts in conjunction with a circulating plasma cofactor, ATIII, catalyzing the inactivation of factors IIa, Xa, IXa, and XIIa.

As thrombin IIa is inactivated, fibrin formation is prevented and activation of factor V and factor VIII through thrombin is inhibited, making heparin both an anticoagulant and an antithrombotic.

Therapeutic levels of UFH are measured by the activated partial thromboplastin time (aPTT).

Postoperative prophylaxis after joint arthroplasties using heparin reduces DVT and PE up to 60% to 70%.

Disadvantages of UFH therapy include requirement for aPTT monitoring, short half-life and low bioavailability, lack of oral dosage form (an oral form is currently in clinical trials), and susceptibility to development of heparin-induced thrombocytopenia (HIT) in 2% to 4% of patients.

Hemorrhagic complications range between 8% and 15%.

Low-Molecular-Weight Heparins (LMWHs) LMWHs share the same mechanisms with heparin. The ability of the molecule to prolong the aPTT is lost, but it keeps the ability to couple with ATIII. LMWHs have more bioavailability (approximately 90%, compared with 29% for UFH); half-life is 4 hours compared with 1 hour for UFH. The activity ratio of anti-Xa to anti-IIa is greater, resulting in increased antithrombotic activity.

LMWHs produced a 70% to 80% risk reduction for DVT.

Hemorrhagic complications, despite its greater activity, are similar to those of heparin.

Pentasaccharide Fondaparinux: Fondaparinux is a new antithrombotic agent that selectively inhibits factor Xa. It acts indirectly on Xa by binding to antithrombin III potentiating its antifactor Xa activity. Unlike other anticoagulants, fondaparinux has no effect on thrombin or platelet aggregation but rather on the generation of thrombin. Studies to date suggest it has a half-life of approximately 17 hours and a dose response that is predictable independent of age or gender, which allow for a fixed dosing regimen.

Definition: Apophyseal injuries are unique to patients with skeletal immaturity. Apophyseal injuries involve inflammation at the site of a major tendinous insertion onto a bony prominence that is undergoing active growth.

Etiology: Several theories have been postulated:
- Injury develops from a major traumatic event to the apophysis, such as a violent contraction that avulses a portion of the apophysis and is followed by inflammation.
- Repetitive microtrauma to the apophyseal area causes multiple tiny avulsion fractures. This process is followed by an inflammatory cycle, which is believed to develop from repetitive running and jumping in such sports as soccer, basketball, and distance running.
- A macrotraumatic event is either preceded or followed by multiple episodes of repetitive microtrauma to the apophysis.

In athletes with skeletal immaturity who are going through a growth spurt, significant muscle-tendon imbalance commonly develops. Muscle growth lags behind bony development, resulting in tight and inflexible muscles. This relative inflexibility can increase the traction forces on the apophysis, causing a predisposition for injury.

Incidence: Unknown. Variable by specific apophyseal location.

Age: Typically occurs in active adolescents between the ages of 8 and 15 years.

Gender: No preponderance.

Symptoms: Periarticular pain, warmth, tenderness, and local swelling and prominence at the area of tendon insertion. Symptoms are usually exacerbated by flexion of muscles involved in putting traction on the apophysis.

Clinical Findings: Pain with active flexion of muscles applying traction to apophysis; local swelling; occasionally, bony prominence on physical examination.

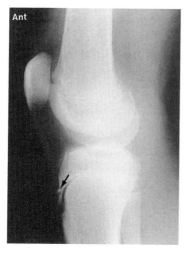

Fig. 18-1 Osgood-Schlatter disease. A lateral view of the knee demonstrates a tiny avulsion fracture of the anterior tibial tuberosity in this young male athlete. This disease is quite common and usually is self-limiting. *(From Mettler FA Jr: Essentials of Radiology, 2nd ed. Philadelphia, Saunders 2005.)*

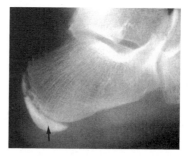

Fig. 18-2 Lateral view of hindfoot demonstrates a relative increase in density of the apophysis *(arrow)* compared with the rest of the calcaneus. This normal apophyseal hyperdensity will resolve by skeletal maturity. *(From DeLee D, Drez D (eds): DeLee and Drez's Orthopaedic Sports Medicine, 2nd ed. Philadelphia, Saunders 2003.)*

Diagnostic Studies: Mostly a clinical diagnosis. X-ray, magnetic resonance imaging, and ultrasound may demonstrate soft tissue swelling around the apophysis, elevation of the apophysis away from bone, fragmentation or increased density of the apophysis, superficial ossicles in tendons, and calcification within or thickening of the tendon. These changes in the surrounding soft tissues are reliable diagnostic features. Severe cases may show avulsion fracture.

Treatment: Goal of treatment is to reduce pain and inflammation

Nonoperative: Often benign and self-limited. Resolution is common with skeletal maturity. Reduction of stress at the apophysis can usually be achieved through activity restriction. Stretching and strengthening exercises, ice, nonsteroidal anti-inflammatory drugs, and protective padding are commonly used. In severe cases, immobilization of the muscle connecting to the apophysis has been shown to be effective.

Operative: Rarely necessary. Involves excision of intratendinous ossicles or bony prominence at tendon insertion.

Complications: Rare. Condition usually resolves within 1 to 2 years depending on the injury. Possible increased risk of fracture at apophyseal site. Persistent pain due to development of ossicles at injury site. Complete avulsion fracture.

Definition: A congenital, nonprogressive abnormality featuring multiple joint contractures; also known as *arthrogryposis multiplex congenita (AMC).*

Etiology: Numerous factors, such as environmental agents, single gene defects (autosomal dominant, autosomal recessive, X-linked recessive), chromosomal abnormalities, known syndromes, or unknown conditions may be contributory to this manifestation.

Incidence: Approximately 1 in every 3000 live births. Most cases of arthrogryposis are caused by a lack of normal joint movement during fetal development. Therefore, cases of nongenetic arthrogryposis are more frequent in multiple birth pregnancies than in single birth pregnancies.

Age: Identified in utero via ultrasonography or at birth.

Gender: 1:1 male-to-female ratio for nongenetic etiology; however, males are primarily affected by X-lined recessive disorders.

Race: No predilection.

Associations: Infants born to mothers affected with myotonic dystrophy, myasthenia gravis, or multiple sclerosis are at risk of developing AMC. Bowen-Conradi syndrome, FG syndrome, Marden-Walker syndrome, and faciocardiomelic syndrome comprise a partial list of associated maladies.

Signs and Symptoms: Contractures, malformations, deformities, and connective tissue abnormalities may be present. Distal joints are more commonly involved than proximal joints.

Diagnostic Studies: Laboratory studies to identify the pathogen or genetic defect may pinpoint the etiology. Radiographs, computed tomography, magnetic resonance imaging, and ultrasound provide bone and tissue depictions before treatment.

Pathology: Fetal akinesia due to muscular, neurogenic, or tissue abnormalities. Additionally, maternal influences include drug use, infection, and trauma. At least 21 recognized forms of AMC exist, 10 of which are characterized as distal arthrogryposes. Four of these are syndromes that include AMC as a set of symptoms. Each involves at least two joint contractures evident from birth.

Treatment: Limited medical treatment exists. Physical therapy goals are to increase range of motion and decrease contractures. Surgical interventions are patient and joint specific.

Complications: Surgical obstacles may be present, particularly with anesthesia administration due to restricted vascular access and intubation due to limited movement of the temporomandibular joint. Additionally, fracture may occur following interventions.

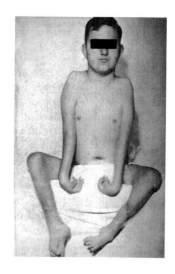

Fig. 19-1 Joint contractures, lack of creases in skin, and deep dimples at joints are characteristic of arthrogryposis. *(From Hosalkar HS, Moroz L, Drummond DS, Finkel R: Neuromuscular disorders of infancy and childhood and arthrogryposis. In Dormans JP [ed]: Pediatric Orthopedics: Core Knowledge in Orthopedics. Philadelphia, Mosby, 2005.)*

Definition: Highly organized viscoelastic material that provides a low friction surface for repetitive gliding motion of joints and distributes loads onto subchondral bone.

Composition: Large extracellular matrix (ECM) and small amount of chondrocytes. No blood vessels, lymphatics, or nerves. Chondrocytes synthesize collagen, proteoglycans, and other matrix components. Obtain nutrition via diffusion and sense mechanical changes through intracytoplasmic filaments and cilia. ECM consists of water (65% to 80% of wet weight), collagen (10% to 20%), proteoglycans (10% to 15%), and smaller amounts of other molecules (lipids and proteins). Water content increases with osteoarthritis and decreases with age. Collagen is mainly type II (90% to 95%), with smaller amounts of types V, VI, IX, X, and XI. Major structural molecules provide tensile strength. Proteoglycans are macromolecules containing a protein core and glycosaminoglycan chains (chondroitin sulfate 4- and 6-isomers, keratin sulfate, and dermatan sulfate). Keratin sulfate concentration increases with age, chondroitin 4-sulfate decreases with age and chondroitin 6-sulfate remains essentially constant. These proteoglycans provide compressive strength.

Structure: Four zones from the surface to subchondral bone of varying cellular morphology, biomechanical composition, and structural properties.
- Superficial zone contains collagen oriented parallel to surface, elongated chondrocytes, low proteoglycan content, and high water content.
- Middle (transition) zone has randomly arranged collagen fibrils and rounded chondrocytes.
- Deep zone contains collagen organized perpendicular to surface, highest concentration of proteoglycans, and lowest water content. Chondrocytes are spherical and arranged in columns. The tidemark separates deep zone from calcified zone.
- Calcified zone is deepest layer (divides hyaline cartilage from subchondral bone), consisting of small chondrocytes mixed with hydroxyapatite crystals.

Growth Factors: Involved in regulation of normal cartilage synthesis and may contribute to the development of osteoarthritis.
- Platelet-derived growth factor (PDGF)—healing of cartilage lacerations
- Basic fibroblast growth factor (bFGF)
- Insulin and insulin-like growth factors (IGF-I and IGF-II)
- Transforming growth factor-beta (TGF-beta)—stimulates proteoglycan synthesis and suppresses type II collagen synthesis.

Normal   Osteoarthritis

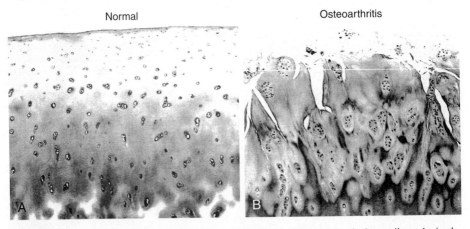

Fig. 20-1 Histologic sections of normal (*left*) and osteoarthritic (OA) (*right*) articular cartilage obtained from the femoral head. The OA cartilage demonstrates surface irregularities, with clefts to the radial zone and cloning of chondrocytes. (*From Harris ED Jr: Kelley's Textbook of Rheumatology, 7th ed. Philadelphia, Saunders, 2005.*)

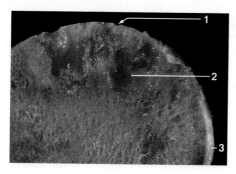

Fig. 20-2 Severe osteoarthritis with small islands of residual articular cartilage next to exposed subchondral bone. *1*, Eburnated articular surface; *2*, subchondral cyst; *3*, residual articular cartilage. *(From Kumar V et al: Robbins and Cotran Pathologic Basis of Disease, 7th ed. Philadelphia, Saunders, 2005.)*

Healing: Depends on depth of lesion; may be improved by passive motion. Deep lacerations that extend below tidemark into subchondral bone cause inflammatory response, formation of fibrin clot, and undifferentiated mesenchymal stem cell production of fibrocartilage. Superficial lacerations do not cross tidemark. Cartilage is associated with poor healing because cartilage is avascular.

Treatment: Nonoperative treatment includes viscosupplementation with intra-articular hyaluronic acid injection and use of oral chondroprotective agents like chondroitin sulfate and glucosamine.

Surgical Treatment: Arthroscopic débridement, abrasion arthroplasty, microfracture, autologous chondrocyte cell implantation, and mosaicplasty (autograft or allograft), or injection of growth factors (current research).

Shoulder:
- "Burners" or "Stingers"
  - Minor traction and compression injuries commonly seen in football players
  - Serious if recurrent or persist for more than a short time; if recurrent, player should be removed from competition until cervical spine radiographs are obtained
  - Complete resolution of symptoms is necessary before return to play
- Little Leaguer's Shoulder
  - Salter-Harris type I fracture of the proximal humeral physis
  - X-rays may reveal physeal widening; responds to rest and activity modification

Elbow:
- Osteochondritis Dissecans
  - Cracks forming in the articular cartilage and underlying subchondral bone typically occurring in the capitulum of adolescent athlete
  - Seen in repetitive overhead or upper extremity weight-bearing activities
  - Related to vascular insufficiency and repetitive microtrauma
  - If stable fragment, activity modification and supportive measures
  - If unstable fragment, arthroscopic reduction and stabilization versus excision and drilling of the defect
  - Osteochondrosis of the capitulum (Panner's disease) is associated with a more benign course
- Little Leaguer's Elbow
  - Stress fracture of the medial epicondyle
  - Seen in adolescents due to repetitive valgus loading with throwing
  - Avoid complete or displaced fracture by rest and limiting pitching/throwing
- Lateral Epicondylitis (Tennis Elbow)
  - Microtear at extensor carpi radialis brevis (ECRB)
  - Caused by activities involving repetitive pronation and supination of forearm with elbow extended (backhand in tennis)

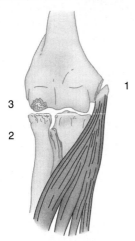

Fig. 21-1 Little leaguer's elbow. 1, Avulsion fracture of medial epicondyle; 2, compression fractures of the radial head; and 3, compression fracture of the capitellum. *(From Connolly JF: DePalma's Management of Fractures and Dislocations. Philadelphia, Saunders, 1981.)*

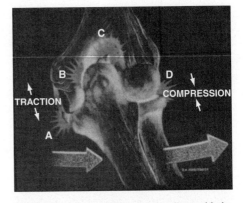

Fig. 21-2 Forces occurring on the elbow with the throwing motion. *A* to *D* are sites of possible injury. *(From DeLee J, Drez D [eds]: DeLee and Drez's Orthopaedic Sports Medicine, 3rd ed. Philadelphia, Saunders, 2009.)*

- Angiofibroblastic hyperplasia seen in microscopic evaluation of tissue
- Treatment: Activity modification, physical therapy, nonsteroidal anti-inflammatory drugs, counterforce bracing, and corticosteroid injections (95% success rate)
- Medial Epicondylitis (Golfer's Elbow)
  - Overuse syndrome of flexor/pronator mass
  - Less common and more difficult to treat than tennis elbow
  - Similar treatment as tennis elbow
- Ulnar Collateral Ligament (UCL) Injury
  - Repetitive, high-velocity, valgus load to medial aspect of the elbow (late cocking and acceleration)
  - Attenuation or rupture of the anterior band
  - Surgery/ligament reconstruction is favored over direct repair; only indicated for high-level athletes

Hand/Wrist:
- "Jersey Finger"
  - Avulsion injury of flexor digitorum profundus tendon from base of P3
  - Requires retrieval of retracted tendon and reattachment to base of phalanx
  - Arthrodesis is favored over late repair due to finger stiffness following tendon grafting
- "Mallet Finger"
  - Avulsion of the terminal extensor tendon
  - Forced flexion of the extended distal interphalangeal joint
  - Treated with prolonged extension splinting (>6 weeks); chronic injuries may result in swan neck deformities

Hip:
- Hip Pointer
  - Iliac crest contusion due to direct trauma in contact sports
  - Avulsion of iliac apophysis should be ruled out in adolescent athletes
  - Treatment consists of ice, compression, pain control, and placing affected leg in maximum stretch

Knee:
- Meniscal Tears
  - Medial torn three times more commonly than lateral meniscus
  - Gold standard for meniscal repair remains the inside-out technique with vertical mattress sutures
  - Protect saphenous nerve medially and peroneal nerve laterally!
- Meniscal Cysts
  - Commonly seen with horizontal cleavage tears of lateral meniscus
- Anterior Cruciate Ligament (ACL) Injury
  - Lachman test (anterior drawer test at 30 degrees (flexion) is the most sensitive examination for acute injuries
  - Early surgery can result in arthrofibrosis if full range of motion is not achieved preoperatively
- Posterior Cruciate Ligament (PCL) Injury
  - Hyperflexion of knee with plantar flexed foot or direct blow to anterior tibia with knee flexed
  - Key test is the posterior drawer test; nonoperative treatment favored for isolated injuries
  - Chronic injury can result in late chondrosis of patellofemoral compartment and/or medial femoral condyle
- Collateral Ligament Injury
  - *Medial Collateral Ligament:* Instability with valgus stress at 30 degrees flexion; nonoperative treatment with brace highly successful; chronic injuries—Pellegrini-Stieda sign (calcification at meniscofemoral complex insertion)
  - *Lateral Collateral Ligament:* Varus instability at 30 degrees flexion; isolated injuries uncommon; nonoperative treatment if mild laxity

Foot/Ankle:

- Jones Fracture
  - Fracture of the metaphyseal-diaphyseal junction of the fifth metatarsal
  - Treated more aggressively in athletes with open reduction and internal fixation to allow an earlier return to sport with less chance of a nonunion or delayed union

Achilles Rupture

- Complete tendon rupture caused by maximum plantar flexion with foot planted
- Patients felt as if they were "shot" or "kicked" at the site of the rupture
- Thompson test helps confirm the diagnosis (squeezing calf results in poor/asymmetrical plantar flexion)
- Treatment controversial—recurrence reduced with primary repair; higher rate of wound complications.

Definition: Avascular necrosis (AVN) is ischemic death of bone due to insufficient blood supply.

Incidence: Avascular necrosis is most commonly associated with the hip. AVN accounts for 10% of total hip replacement surgeries per year in the United States.

Age: Onset of avascular necrosis depends on the underlying cause. AVN usually occurs in middle age unless predisposing conditions place different age groups at risk (see Associations).

Gender: Avascular necrosis is 4 times more frequent in males than in females.

Race: More common in Far East (genetic etiology).

Etiology and Pathophysiology: The pathophysiology of avascular necrosis is not fully understood. However, the etiology of AVN falls under two broad categories of anatomic regions: extravascular and intravascular factors. Intravascular pathology is considered the primary etiology of osteonecrosis. Arterial factors are considered the most common source of AVN. AVN affects bones with a terminal blood supply, such as the femoral head and humerus. Limited collateral circulation in these regions results in increased susceptibility to necrosis of marrow, medullary bone, and cortex. Extravascular pathology includes vasoconstriction by external factors, such as through the encroachment of fat cells or other abnormal cells, which restrict normal circulation to the bone.

Associations: Trauma is the most common cause of AVN, which can occur as soon as 8 hours after disruption to the blood supply. Alcoholism is also commonly associated with AVN, in that alcohol can be toxic to osteogenic cells. Other associations include hemoglobinopathies, caisson disease (decompression sickness), corticosteroids, pancreatitis, chronic renal failure, lupus, and cancer treatments, including chemotherapy and radiation treatments.

Signs and Symptoms: AVN is often asymptomatic in early stages. Later stages of AVN manifest as pain or limited range of motion in the affected joint. This pain can develop gradually or appear suddenly in great intensity.

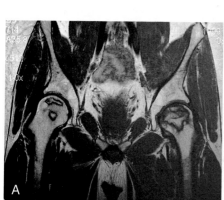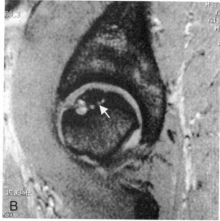

Fig. 22-1   Avascular necrosis of the hip. (**A**) Coronal T1-weighted MR image through both hips confirms the presence of geographic areas of abnormality in both femoral heads, which are well demarcated from the adjacent normal bone by a thin rim of low signal material. High signal within each abnormal area indicates viable fat. (**B**) Gradient-echo sagittal image demonstrates the osteochondral fragment, with fluid between the fragment and the parent bone (*arrow*), suggesting that the fragment itself is loose. (*From Adam A, et al: Grainger & Allison's Diagnostic Radiology, 5th ed. Philadelphia, Churchill Livingstone, 2008.*)

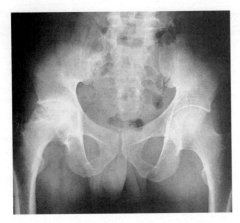

Fig. 22-2   Avascular necrosis due to long-term corticosteroid use. *(From Ford M: Clinical Toxicology. Philadelphia, Saunders, 2001.)*

Diagnostic Studies: AVN occurs in stages.
Stage 0: preclinical and pre-radiologic. Can only be suggested if it has occurred in the contralateral hip.
Stage 1: normal radiographic findings, but abnormal magnetic resonance imaging (MRI) and histologic findings. Symptoms may or may not be present.
Stage 2: abnormal radiographs, however the femoral head still appears spherical, and there is no subchondral lucency.
Stage 3: mechanical failure of the femoral head.
Stage 4: all or part of the femoral head is collapsed.
Stage 5: indicates a loss of joint space and can include presentation of degenerative joint disease.
Stage 6: extensive bone destruction.

MRI is the most sensitive and effective method to diagnose AVN. While radiographs and single-photon emission computed tomography (SPECT) are useful in detecting late stage AVN, MRI scans clearly show the size of the lesion and changes in the bone that best indicate early stages of AVN. Bone scans reveal increased uptake of the necrotic regions in early stages of AVN.
Micropathology: Histologic changes are observed in both cortical bone and bone marrow. Following necrosis of cortical bone, a regenerative process begins in the surrounding tissues. Increased osteoclastic activity occurs to remove necrotic bone while increased osteoblastic activity serves to rebuild the boney tissue.
Macropathology: AVN arises most often in the femoral head, leading to hip pain. AVN affects bones with a single terminal blood supply, which also includes the carpals, talus, and humerus.
Treatment: If detected in early stages, AVN can be treated with core decompression. However, it is difficult to identify in the early stages, and late-stage AVN is most often treated by total joint arthroplasty.

Mechanical Axis

The mechanical axis of a bone is defined as the straight line connecting the center of the proximal and distal joints. The lower limb itself has a mechanical axis line between center of hip joint and center of ankle joint, just as the femur or tibia would have its own mechanical axis. The mechanical axis of femur is a straight line drawn between the center of the femoral head and the center of the knee. The mechanical axis is always a straight line, either in the sagittal or frontal plane, connecting the center of two joints

Anatomic Axis

The anatomic axis of a bone is the mid diaphyseal line. It may be straight or curved. For example, the anatomic axis of femur is straight in the anteroposterior plane but curved in the sagittal plane. It is drawn as follows: two sets of two parallel points are drawn in the diaphysis of the long bone, one at the proximal diaphysis and one at the distal diaphysis. Two new points are derived from bisecting the line that joins the respective pairs (proximal and distal). A line is then drawn that connects the bisector points and this line is the anatomic axis. It is roughly a line that runs the length of the diaphysis.

The anatomic axis and mechanical axis are not the same. In the tibia, they closely approximate each other but are not exactly equal.

These are important concepts to understand for proper fracture fixation, deformity correction, and joint replacement techniques in the lower extremity. For example, intramedullary rods are designed to follow the anatomic axis of the long bone of the lower extremity.

Mechanical axis deviations can place greater than normal stresses across joints and can lead to ligamentous laxity and/or arthritis

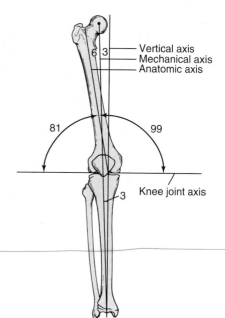

Fig. 23-1 Lower extremity axes. *(From Browner BD: Skeletal Trauma: Basic Science, Management, and Reconstruction, 3rd ed. Philadelphia, Saunders, 2003.)*

47

Definition: There are multiple types of benign bone tumors, including bone-forming tumors, cartilage-forming tumors, giant cell tumors, connective tissue tumors, and vascular tumors. These tumors are considered benign because they do not metastasize. Osteoid osteoma and osteoblastoma are bone-forming tumors. Osteochondroma, chondroblastoma, and chondroma are cartilage-forming tumors. Nonossifying fibroma is a fibrous tumor.

Incidence: Osteoblastomas and chondroblastomas each account for approximately 1% of all bone tumors where as giant cell tumors account for 4% to 5% of all bone tumors. Of all benign

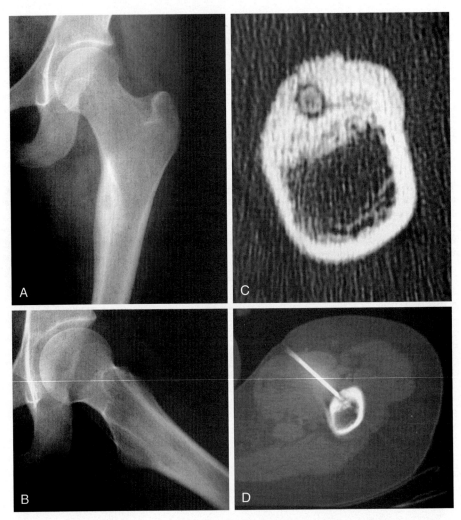

Fig. 24-1   This 17-year-old girl complained of left thigh pain for several months. **A** and **B,** Anteroposterior and lateral views of the left hip show a small radiolucent lesion with thick sclerotic rims of reactive bone. **C,** CT clearly shows nidus and confirms the diagnosis. **D,** A radiofrequency ablation probe placed into nidus under CT guidance. *(From Canale ST, & Beaty JH: Campbell's Operative Orthopaedics, 11th ed. Philadelphia, Mosby, 2007.)*

bone tumors, 10% to 13% are osteoid osteoma, 35% to 50% are osteochondroma, 25% are chondroma, and approximately 5% are nonossifying fibroma. Osteochondromas are the most common type of benign bone tumor.

Age: Most benign bone tumors occur in patients younger than 30 years old. However, osteoid osteomas and giant cell tumors usually occur in patients younger than the age of 40. Chondromas may occur in people of all ages.

Sex: Benign bone tumors are typically more common in males. Two exceptions are giant cell tumors, which occur slightly more often in females, and chondromas, which occur equally in males and females.

Etiology: The etiology of many benign bone tumors is unknown. Chondroblastoma may have a genetic association. Osteochondroma may possibly have a traumatic or idiopathic cause. Nonossifying fibroma may be formed due to vascular disturbance or hemorrhage. Stage I tumors are latent, noninvasive, and usually self-limited. Stage II tumors are active; they deform the bone but do not extend into the soft tissue. Stage III tumors are aggressive; they extend into the soft tissue near the bone.

Clinical Presentation: Benign bone tumors are often asymptomatic but may manifest with pain, swelling, limp, limb bowing, decreased range of motion, and/or fractures, depending on the type of tumor. Osteoid osteoma, osteoblastoma, chondroblastoma, and giant cell tumor may manifest with pain. In osteoid osteoma, the pain increases at night. Osteochondromas often manifest as a painless lump.

Pathology: Osteoid osteomas tend to occur in long bones within the diaphysis or metaphysis. In osteoid osteoma, the bone-forming lesion, called the nidus, is surrounded by reactive bone. Osteoblastomas, which produce osteoid and woven bone, tend to occur in the spine. Osteochondromas consist of a bony protrusion of cartilage capped and adjacent to the physis. They usually occur around the knee and the humerus. Chondroblastomas usually occur in the epiphysis of long bones and consist of immature cartilage with thin calcified precipitates and multinucleated giant cells. Giant cell tumors tend to occur in the long bone metaphysis of children and in the long bone epiphysis of adults. Giant cell tumors have irregular margins. Nonossifying fibroma consists of a well-defined lesion of fibrous tissue and usually occurs in the metaphysis of long bones.

Diagnostic Procedures: Radiography, magnetic resonance imaging, and computed tomography may be useful for diagnosis. It may be difficult to distinguish similar types of tumors; for example, osteoid osteomas may be easily confused with osteoblastomas. Osteoid osteomas are usually smaller than 1.5 cm, whereas osteoblastomas are often larger than 1.5 cm.

Treatment: Nonsteroidal anti-inflammatory drugs may help relieve the pain associated with some types of benign bone tumors. Osteoid osteoma, osteoblastoma, osteochondroma, and giant cell tumor may be treated with excision or resection. Chondroblastoma, chondroma, giant cell tumor, and nonossifying fibroma may be treated by curettage and bone graft. After curettage, adjuvants such as cryotherapy, phenol, and/or polymethyl methacrylate may be used.

Osteochondroma

- Most common benign bone tumor. Originates within the periosteum as small cartilaginous nodules.
- Perichondrial proliferation with transformation to bone. May be single or multiple—90% of patients have only a single lesion. Most often seen on the distal femur, proximal tibia, and proximal humerus. Growth generally parallels that of the patient and usually stops with skeletal maturity
- Radiographic appearance—either stalked or sessile lesion. Gross appearance lesion covered by a cartilaginous cap that is typically only a few millimeters thick—lesions with thicker caps or any growth of the cap should be carefully assessed for chondrosarcoma.
- Histology—cartilaginous lesion on a bony stalk. Bone marrow is incorporated into the lesion.
- Malignant transformation is rare.
- Surgical excision is indicated if the lesion causes cosmetic deformity or produces symptoms from pressure on surrounding tissues or if there is concern for malignancy.
- *Osteochondromatosis*: May cause growth disturbances—bowing of radius, shortening of ulna. Gross and histologic appearance similar to solitary osteochondroma. Rate of sarcomatous change 1%—biopsy any mass that is enlarging or painful.

Enchondroma

- Benign hyaline cartilage tumor. Generally located centrally in bone but may be subperiosteal—50% located in the small bones of the hand. Generally painless, but may expand the bone and break the cortex. Pain suggests growth of mass or malignancy.
- Histology—normal-appearing hyaline cartilage with large lacunar spaces and a rim of trabecular bone.
- Treatment—curettage and bone grafting. Periosteal lesions should be excised en bloc with an intact rim of normal bone.

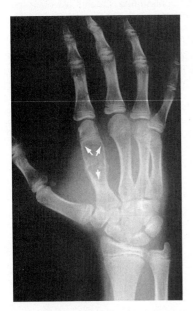

Fig. 25-1 Enchondroma. A lucent lesion in a metacarpal or phalanx is most likely to be an enchondroma. It may be some-what expansile *(arrows)*, and a fracture may be noted through the area of weakened bone. A healing fracture with some periosteal reaction is seen in the midportion of this lesion. *(From Mettler FA: Essentials of Radiology, 2nd ed. Philadelphia, Saunders, 2005.)*

- *Ollier's Disease:* Disseminated enchondromas. The malignant transformation rate has been found to be as high as 50%.
- *Maffucci's Syndrome:* Disseminated enchondromas and hemangiomas. Malignant transformation rate of 25% to 50%.

Chondromyxoid Fibroma

- Less than 0.5% of all bone tumors.
- Most occur in patients between 10 and 30 years of age.
- Radiographic appearance—metaphyseal lesion that is eccentric and sharply circumscribed.
- Histology—myxoid cartilaginous ground substance with numerous spindle cells. Must differentiate from a myxoid chondrosarcoma; myxoid chondrosarcoma is generally more pleomorphic with foci of cartilaginous differentiation.
- Treatment—wide resection/extended curettage with bone grafting.

Chondroblastoma

- 1% of all bone tumors.
- Occurs in patients 10 to 25 years of age; 2:1 male-to-female ratio.
- Presenting symptom—usually progressive pain.
- Distal femur, proximal humerus, proximal tibia are the most common sites of occurrence.
- Radiographic appearance—well-circumscribed lesion centered in epiphysis of long bone, may have sclerotic rim or intralesional calcification.
- Histology—sheets of chondroblasts with stippled calcification, that is, "chicken-wire calcification."
- Treatment—curettage and bone grafting or bone cement. Follow-up x-ray studies of site and chest every 6 months for at least 3 years and then annually thereafter.

Scalar Quantity: Magnitude but no direction (mass, distance).
Vector Quantity: Quantified by magnitude and direction (velocity, acceleration, force).
Newton's Laws:
1st Law (Law of Inertia): Any body in a state of uniform motion tends to stay in that state unless an external force is applied.
2nd Law: A body subjected to a net force will accelerate. F = ma
3rd Law: For every action there is an equal and opposite reaction.

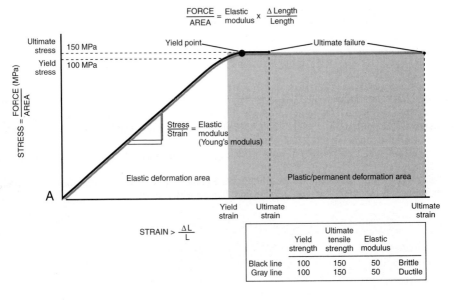

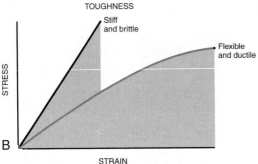

Fig. 26-1 A, Stress-strain curve. The red line is an example of a ductile material; it can be stressed beyond the yield point. If a stress lower than the yield point is applied and released, the object will return to its original shape. The plastic or permanent deformation area is the portion of the curve between the amount of stress needed to reach the yield point and the amount of stress needed to reach the ultimate failure point. **B,** Toughness is defined as the area underneath the stress-strain curve. The two materials illustrated in this diagram have vastly different characteristics; however, they both have the same toughness because of equivalent areas under their respective curves. *(From Browner B, et al: Skeletal Trauma: Basic Science, Management, and Reconstruction, 3rd ed. Philadelphia, Saunders, 2003.)*

Moment: A force applied to a body at a distance about which that body is constrained to rotate (torque).

Work: Force × distance (product of force and displacement it causes).

Energy:

Kinetic energy = ½ mv² (energy due to an object's motion)

Potential energy = stored energy

Stress: Force applied to a body divided by the cross-sectional area over which it acts. (N/m^2)

Strain: The change in length of a material divided by its original length.

Toughness: Energy expended in deforming a material; corresponds to area under the stress-strain curve.

Ductility: The amount of deformation that a material undergoes before failure.

Creep: Increased elongation (strain) associated with a constant load over time.

Stress Relaxation: Decrease in stress associated with a constent strain over time.

Viscoelasticity: A viscolelastic material exhibits different properties when loaded at different strain rates; its mechanical properties are time-dependent.

Isotropic Materials: Same mechanical properties in all directions.

Anisotropic Materials: Mechanical properties vary with the direction of applied load.

• Bending rigidity of a rectangular structure (plate) proportional to (base) × (height)³/12

• Bending rigidity of a cylinder proportional to $(\pi)r^4/4$

Brittle: A material that can undergo elastic deformation but very little plastic deformation before failure (e.g., a rubber band).

Ductile: A material that can undergo a large amount of plastic deformation before failure.

Definition: A biopsy is undertaken to provide tissue from any region for histologic examination or culture. It may be undertaken via open or closed means to diagnose inflammatory, infected, metabolic, or neoplastic conditions of the musculoskeletal system. Musculoskeletal tumors should only be biopsied by a surgeon with experience in this field and when possible, following discussion with the local musculoskeletal tumor group. This prevents patients who may potentially have resectable lesions being rendered nonresectable by a poorly placed biopsy contaminating tissue fields.

Planning: Make certain all appropriate investigations and staging have been completed to prevent problems with artifact on scans. Collaboration with pathologists and radiologist should be undertaken to ensure maximal chance of diagnostic information, anatomic safe region, and the tract with which the sample can potentially be excised. Arrangements should be made for the appropriate storage and collection method. The use of ultrasound, computed tomography, or fluoroscopic guidance should be considered to accurately collect the tissue sample.

Operation:
- Meticulous hemostasis throughout.
- Avoid large flaps, multiple compartments, or exposure of neurovascular bundles.
- *No* transverse incisions.
- *Always* send samples for microbiology!
- Ensure that the sample does not simply represent necrotic material but also the margins of the lesion with viable cellular material, to ensure proper sections.
- For bony tumors, cortical section and marrow should be sent and assessed for any risk of pathologic fracture.
- Protect weight bearing before definitive procedure.
- Thoroughly lavage the wound to prevent seeding of malignant cells.
- *Complications:* Hematoma, pathologic fracture, nondiagnostic or nonrepresentative biopsy.

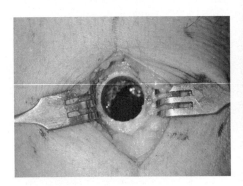

Fig. 27-1 If hole must be made in bone during biopsy, defect should be round to minimize stress concentration, which otherwise could lead to pathologic fracture. *(From Canale ST, Beaty JH: Campbell's Operative Orthopaedics, 11th ed. Philadelphia, Mosby 2007.)*

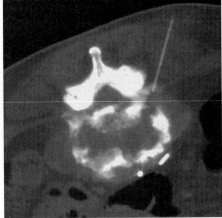

Fig. 27-2 CT guidance for biopsy of infected diskitis. *(From Adam A, et al: Grainger & Allison's Diagnostic Radiology, 5th ed. Philadelphia, Churchill Livingstone, 2008.)*

Brachial Plexus Palsy

Definition: Stretching or contusion of the brachial plexus during the birth.

Etiology: Occurs most commonly with large babies, shoulder dystocia, forceps delivery, breech position, and prolonged labor.

Incidence: Two per 1000 births.

Symptoms and Clinical Findings: A broad spectrum of weakness and sensory deficits involving the C5-T1 nerve roots. Erb Duchenne palsy involving the C5 and C6 roots portend the best prognosis, and a total plexus injury portends the worst.

Diagnostic Studies: Although magnetic resonance imaging and electromyography are often employed to evaluate return of neuromuscular function, they provide little value above the physical examination.

Prognosis and Treatment: Infants showing improvement in brachial plexopathy symptoms in the first 2 months generally go on to a full recovery. Vital in all cases is passive range of motion exercise. Failure to show symptomatic improvement beyond 6 months usually results in poorer outcomes. The timing of microsurgical reconstruction is debated; however, with microsurgical reconstruction, there is improvement in outcome in a high percentage of patients. Shoulder, forearm, and hand corrective operations have been described to improve functional outcome.

Congenital Muscular Torticollis

Definition: Torticollis is any deformity in which the head is tilted and abnormally rotated. In this case, the injury occurs in utero, not during the birth.

Etiology: Unilateral contracture of the sternocleidomastoid of unclear etiology. It is thought to be related to intrauterine compartment syndrome involving the sternocleidomastoid muscle compartment. It is associated with a difficult labor and delivery, as a well as metatarsus adductus, and hip dysplasia.

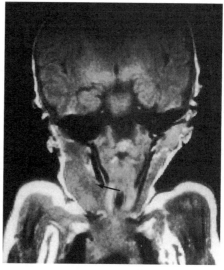

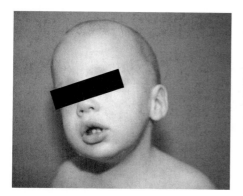

Fig. 28-1   Congenital torticollis in a 14-month-old boy. *(From Canale ST, Beaty JH: Campbell's Operative Orthopaedics, 11th ed. Philadelphia, Mosby, 2007.)*

Fig. 28-2   Magnetic resonance imaging of an infant with congenital torticollis shows enlargement of the sternocleidomastoid muscle *(arrow)*. *(From Cummings C: Otolaryngology: Head & Neck Surgery, 4th ed. Philadelphia, Mosby, 2005.)*

Incidence: Accounts for 80% of all cases of infant torticollis.

Symptoms and Clinical Findings: Unilateral lateral flexion of the neck. Fibrosis of the muscle with a palpable mass is present within the first 4 weeks of life.

Diagnostic Studies: Imaging of the brain and cervical spine should be done to evaluate for other etiologies of torticollis, which include atlanto-occipital abnormalities, posterior fossa tumors, and Klippel-Feil syndrome.

Prognosis and Treatment: Ninety percent of patients respond to passive stretching within the first year; however, Z-plasty of the sternocleidomastoid may be required if torticollis persists beyond the first year.

Blood Transfusions

Transmission of Disease:
- HIV: Risk estimated as 1 in 2 million.
- Hepatitis B: Risk estimated as 1 in 200,000.
- Hepatitis C: Now that second-generation screening tests are available, estimated transfusion risk is 1 in 2 million. Probably 2% to 3% of U.S. population has hepatitis C antibodies, and hepatitis C–related cirrhosis is the leading cause of liver transplantation in the United States.
  - Combination of interferon and ribavirin has been approved by the Food and Drug Administration for treatment of hepatitis C.
  - With needlestick injury, consider interferon treatment (50% effective); with no treatment, risk of infection is about 3.5%.

Predicting the Need for Transfusion in Orthopedic Patients

- Preoperative hemoglobin (Hgb) is main indicator for need of postoperative transfusion.
- Preoperative Hgb less than 11 g/dL is strong indicator for need for transfusion in joint replacement.
- Salido and colleagues (2002) studied risk factors for transfusion in patients undergoing joint replacement:
  - Patients with a preoperative hemoglobin level of less than 13.0 g/dL had a 4 times greater risk of having a transfusion than those with a hemoglobin level between 13.0 and 15.0 g/dL and a 15.3 times greater risk than those with a hemoglobin level greater than 150 g/L.
  - Preoperative hemoglobin level ($P = 0.0001$) and low BMI ($P = 0.011$) were shown to predict the need for blood transfusion after hip and knee replacement.

Hematopoietic Disorders

Gaucher's Disease: Aberrant autosomal recessive lysosomal storage disease. Deficiency of the enzyme beta-glucocerebrosidase leads to accumulation of cerebroside in cells of the reticuloendothelial system.

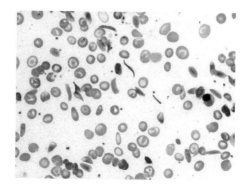

Fig. 29-1 Blood film, sickle cell anemia. The erythrocytes are far from one another, suggesting a severe anemia. Numerous pointed sickle cells and target cells are present. Close to the nucleated red blood cell, elliptical cells are seen. These cells have a dense center instead of the usual central pallor, suggesting that they are incipient sickle cells. (×500) *(From McPherson RA, Pincus MR: Henry's Clinical Diagnosis and Management by Laboratory Methods, 21st ed. Philadelphia, Saunders, 2006.)*

Niemann-Pick Disease: Autosomal recessive disorder caused by accumulation of sphingomyelin in cells of the reticuloendothelial system.
• Common in Eastern European Jews.
• Marrow expansion and cortical thinning common in long bones; coxa valga seen as well.

Sickle Cell Anemia: Sickle Cell Disease is a blood disorder caused from a point mutation in the β-globin chain of hemoglobin. This causes the amino acid glutamate to be replaced by valine rendering the red blood cell to assume a rigid sickle shape. Sickle cell disease is more severe but less common than sickle cell trait.
• Crises usually begin at age 2 to 3; caused by substance P; may lead to characteristic bone infarcts.
• Clinical Findings: Growth retardation/skeletal immaturity, osteonecrosis of femoral and humeral heads, osteomyelitis, biconcave "fish" vertebrae, dactylitis, and septic arthritis. (*Salmonella* is more common in the population; however, *Staphylococcus aureus* is still the most common cause of osteomyelitis in sickle cell patients.)
• Hydroxyurea has produced dramatic relief of pain from bone crises.

Thalassemia: Thalassemia is an autosomal recessive blood disease caused from the underproduction of globin chains. Similar to sickle cell anemia in presentation; common in people of Mediterranean descent.
• Bone pain and leg ulceration.
• X-ray Findings: Long-bone thinning, metaphyseal expansion, osteopenia, and premature physeal closure.

Hemophilia: X-linked disorder with decreased factor VIII (hemophilia A), abnormal factor VIII with platelet dysfunction (von Willebrand's disease), or factor IX (hemophilia B—Christmas disease); characterized as mild, moderate, or severe based on amount of factor present.
• Associated with bleeding episodes (hemarthrosis) and skeletal/joint sequelae; knee most commonly affected; pseudotumor or blood cyst can form in soft tissue or bone due to deep intramuscular bleeding.
• Other Findings: Squaring of patellae/condyles, epiphyseal overgrowth with LLD, and osteopenia.
• Treatment: Desmopressin increases amount of factor VIII; helps blood to clot; used for mild to moderate von Willebrand's disease. IgG antibody inhibitors (present in 4% to 20% of hemophiliacs) are a relative contraindication to surgery. Factor levels should be increased for prophylaxis preoperatively.

Leukemia: Most common malignancy of childhood; acute lymphocytic leukemia represents 80% of cases.
• Peak incidence is 4 years of age; one fourth to one third of patients have pain complaints.
• Causes demineralization of bones, periostitis, occasional lytic lesions.
• Treatment: Chemotherapy.

Definition: A growth disturbance of the medial tibial physis that results in varus deformity, medial tibial rotation, and limb shortening in severe cases.

Etiology: Abnormal forces across the physis; familial element varus deformity may be initiator.

Differential: Physiologic bow legs, rickets, hypophosphatasia, osteogenesis, dysplasias, enchondromas, neuromuscular.

Associations: Obesity, African American race, familial element, early walking children.

Age and Gender: Males are especially more likely to have the disease; divided into infantile (2 to 3 years) and juvenile/adolescent (4 to 14 years).

Clinical Findings: Must be aware of the normal evolution of limb alignment and the broad spectrum of variation of normal. Normally, infants born with genu varum transition to genu valgum by 2½ years, which then returns to physiologic valgus by 4 years old. Varus alignment may be symmetrical (generally infantile) or asymmetrical (juvenile/adolescent). Gait may additionally have a varus thrust with medial collateral ligament laxity. Generally toward top of height/weight; dysplasias generally lower centile. May have a tender "beak" over the medial tibial metaphysic.

Staging:

I: Irregular metaphyseal ossification combined with medial and distal protrusion of the metaphysis.

II, III, IV: Evolves from a mild depression of the medial metaphysis to a step-off of the medial metaphysis.

V: Increased slope of medial articular surface and a cleft separating the medial and lateral epicondyle.

VI: Bony bridge across the physis.

Drennan's angle (metaphyseal-diaphyseal angle) should be less than 11 degrees. Angle formed between a line perpendicular to the long axis of the shaft and a line drawn through the metaphyseal beaks. Radiology differentiates those likely to progress; can be assisted by measuring the contribution of tibial deformity to the total deformity; all patients with a greater than 50% contribution from the tibia and metaphyseal-diaphyseal angle of more than 16 degrees progressed in one study.

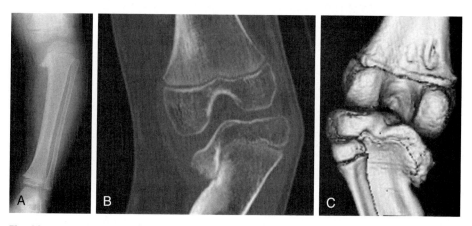

Fig. 30-1 Blount's disease. Plain radiograph (**A**), coronal CT (**B**), and 3D CT reconstruction (**C**, posterior view). *(From Adam A, et al: Grainger & Allison's Diagnostic Radiology, 5th ed. Philadelphia, Churchill Livingstone, 2008.)*

Table 30-1   DIFFERENTIATING PHYSIOLOGIC VARUS FROM BLOUNT'S

Physiologic Varus	Blount's Disease
Minimal asymmetry	Unilateral or bilateral asymmetry
Gentle curve	Sharp angulation
Lateral thrust absent	Lateral thrust often
Metaphyseal diaphyseal angle < 11 degrees	Metaphyseal diaphyseal angle > 11 degrees
Upper tibial metaphysis normal	Upper tibial metaphysis fragmentation
Upper tibial epiphysis normal slope medially	Upper tibial epiphysis narrows medially
Upper tibial physis normal	Upper tibial physis widening laterally

Treatment: The majority can be managed conservatively with observation to detect the small numbers that have progressive deformity. Computed tomography scan can be of use in determining the prognosis in severe cases, when surgery might be considered. Generally there is a high rate of spontaneous resolution in stages I and II; however, after age 6 years, there is little if any resolution.

Surgical Care: Generally limited to adolescents and depends on degree of deformity, limb shortening, and residual growth. Care ranges from osteotomy, which can be metaphyseal or epiphyseal to hemiepiphysiodesis.

Complications: Growth disturbance, limb shortening, progressive deformity.

Definition: Bone, also called *osseous tissue,* is a type of hard endoskeletal connective tissue found in many vertebrate animals. Bones support body structures, protect internal organs (in conjunction with muscles), facilitate movement, and are involved with cell formation, calcium metabolism, and mineral storage.

Classification:

Compact: Cortical (outer layer) bone is compact. Cortical bone makes up a large portion of skeletal mass, but because of its density, it has a low surface area.

Cancellous (Spongy): Cancellous bone is *trabecular* (has an open, meshwork, or honeycomb-like structure). It has a relatively high surface area but forms a smaller portion of the skeleton.

Woven: Woven bone is put down rapidly during growth or repair. It is so called because its fibers are aligned at random and as a result it has low strength.

Lamellar: Lamellar bone has parallel fibers and is much stronger. Woven bone is often replaced by lamellar bone as growth continues.

Structure: Bone is a relatively hard and lightweight composite material, formed mostly of calcium phosphate in the chemical arrangement termed *calcium hydroxyapatite* ($Ca_{10} [Po_4]_6(OH)_2$). It has relatively high compressive strength but poor tensile strength. Even though bone is essentially brittle, it has a degree of significant elasticity contributed by its organic components (collagen). Bone has an internal meshlike structure, the density of which may vary at different points. This matrix comprises a major constituent of bone.

Cytal Architecture:

Osteoblasts: Osteoblasts are typically viewed as bone-forming cells. They are located near to the surface of bone and their functions are to make osteoid and manufacture hormones. Osteoblasts are mononucleate.

Bone-lining cells (BLCs): BLCs share a common lineage with osteogenic (bone-forming) cells. They are flattened, mononucleate cells that line bone and function as a barrier for certain ions.

Osteocytes: Osteocytes originate from osteoblasts, which have migrated into and become trapped and surrounded by bone matrix, which they themselves produce.

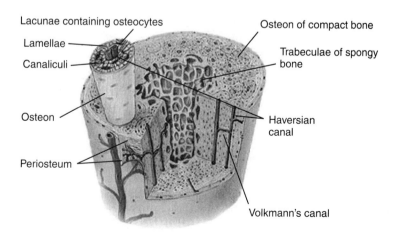

Fig. 31-1 Compact and spongy (cancellous).

LONG BONE

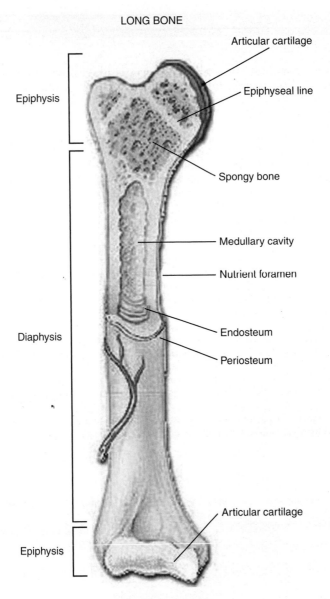

Articular cartilage

Epiphyseal line

Epiphysis

Spongy bone

Medullary cavity

Nutrient foramen

Diaphysis

Endosteum

Periosteum

Articular cartilage

Epiphysis

Fig. 31-2   Long bone.

Osteoclasts: Osteoclasts are the cells responsible for bone resorption. Osteoclasts are large, multinucleated cells located on bone surfaces.

Pathologies: One of the most common bone illnesses is a bone fracture. Bones heal by natural processes, but left untended or unsupported, can lead to misgrown bone. Other illnesses are, for example, osteoporosis and bone cancer (osteosarcoma). The joints can be affected by arthritis.

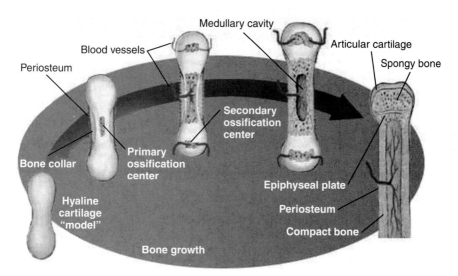

Fig. 31-3 Bone formation.

Definition: The use of bone in reconstructive orthopaedics is to repair skeletal defects and accelerate bone healing. Bone grafts serve a combined mechanical and biologic function.

Incidence: Reports in the literature suggest that more than 1.5 million bone grafts occur in the United States annually.

Background: The standard in bone grafting consists of tissue harvested from the patient, or *autograft*, usually at the iliac crest and less commonly at the distal femur or proximal tibia. *Allografts*, from donors or cadavers, serve as alternatives to autograft in the reconstruction of bone.

Osteogenic: Graft contains cells, such as osteoblasts, which promote osteogenesis, or the synthesis of new bone by cells derived from either the graft or the host. Examples include autologous bone and bone marrow, and allogeneic bone and blood concentrates such as autologist growth facter (AGF) concentrate.

Osteoconduction: Ingrowth of capillaries, mesenchymal tissues, and osteoprogenitor cells, or osteoblasts, from the recipient host bed into the implant or graft. Fibroblast growth factor (FGF), prostaglandin agonist, thrombin peptides, and a class of others including PDGF and VEGF are further examples.

Osteoinduction: Mitogenesis of undifferentiated mesenchymal cells leading to the formation of osteoprogenitor cells, which form new bone such as osteogenic protein-1 and bone morphogenetic protein-2.

Summary: See Tables 32-1 and 32-2.

Complications: Autograft complications include infection and pain at the site of harvest as well as a limited quantity of available donor bone. While allografts eliminate donor site morbidity and issues of limited supply, they are not without complications. These include disease transmission, despite the use of freezing, gamma irradiation, electron beam irradiation, and the use of ethylene oxide, as well as host rejection and failed osteointegration.

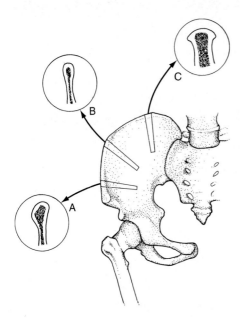

Fig. 32-1   Use of iliac bone as a source of cortical or cancellous bone. Note the amount of cancellous bone available in the anterior ilium (**A** and **B**) vs. the amount available in the posterior ilium (**C**). *(From Cummings CW: Otolaryngology: Head & Neck Surgery, 4th ed. Philadelphia, Mosby, 2005.)*

Table 32-1. BONE GRAFT SUBSTITUTES

Class	Description
Allograft based	Allograft bone used alone or in combination with other materials
Factor based	Natural and recombinant growth factors used alone or in combination with other materials
Cell based	Cells used to generate new tissue alone or seeded onto a support matrix
Ceramic based	Includes calcium phosphate, calcium sulfate, and bioglass used alone or in combination
Polymer based	Both degradable and nondegradable polymers used alone and in combination with other materials

Table 32-2. BONE GRAFT PROPERTIES

Type	Osteoconduction	Osteoinduction	Osteogenic Cells	Structural Integrity
Autograft				
Cancellous	Excellent	Good	Excellent	Poor
Cortical	Fair	Fair	Fair	Excellent
Allograft	Fair	Fair	None	Good
Ceramic	Fair	None	None	Fair
DBM*	Fair	Good	None	Poor
Marrow	Poor	Poor	Good	Poor

*DBM, demineralized bone matrix.

Definition: A bone scan is a radionuclide scanning test designed to detect areas of increased or decreased bone metabolism. A compound that is attracted to areas of high metabolic bone activity has an attached radioactive label and is injected into the bloodstream through a vein. As it decays, the radiotracer emits gamma radiation, which is detected by a camera. The more active the bone turnover, the more radioactive material will be seen emitting in that region (so-called "hot spots"). The test is performed to detect fractures, infections, tumors, and other conditions that may increase the rate of bone turnover. The three most commonly used radioisotopes are technetium-99m phosphate, gallium-67 citrate, and indium-111–labeled leukocytes. The most common is technetium-99m phosphate. The uptake of this compound is related primarily to osteoblastic activity, although regional blood flow also plays a role in skeletal uptake. After intravenous injection, the technetium is rapidly distributed throughout the extracellular compartment. Bone uptake is rapid, with more than 50% of the administered dose being delivered to bone within an hour. The remainder of the dye is excreted by the kidneys into the urine. An alternative technique is the indium-111–labeled white blood cell scan. Although this examination is sensitive to the presence of infection, image resolution is poor and often fails to distinguish whether the infection is in bone, soft tissue, or both.

Technique: The standard technique of technetium-99m phosphate imaging is to perform a three-phase study. Although this does not significantly increase the sensitivity of the test, it does increase specificity. In the diagnosis of osteomyelitis, the reported sensitivity and specificity is 70% to 90% and 38% to 79%, respectively. The three phases consist of images taken in (1) the flow phase, (2) the immediate or equilibrium phase, and (3) the delayed phase. The flow-phase

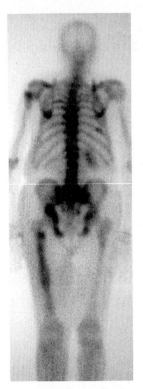

Fig. 33-1 Whole body[99m] Tc-MDP (methylene diphosphonate) bone scintigram (posterior view) showing multiple regions of increased uptake due to prostatic carcinoma metastases. Involvement typically occurs in the spine, pelvis, and ribs. *(From Adam A, et al: Grainger & Allison's Diagnostic Radiology, 5th ed. Philadelphia, Churchill Livingstone, 2008.)*

image is similar to a radionuclide angiogram in that it demonstrates blood flow to a potential lesion immediately after injection of the radioisotope. The equilibrium or blood pool image is taken within 5 minutes after injection and shows relative vascular flow and distribution of the radioisotope into the extracellular space. The first phase characterizes the blood flow to the area, whereas the second visualizes the blood pool. These two early phases act to characterize degree of inflammation and hyperemia that may be present. The delayed-phase image generally is obtained 2 to 4 hours after injection when renal excretion has eliminated most of the isotope except that taken up by osteoblastic activity. This image shows osteoblastic activity and is positive in a number of disease states, including osteomyelitis, tumors, degenerative joint disease, trauma, and postsurgical changes.

Disadvantages: A major disadvantage of a bone scan is that the increased uptake caused by osteomyelitis is difficult to distinguish from that caused by degenerative joint disease or post-traumatic or postsurgical changes. The relative activity in each of the three phases may be helpful in differentiating other causes of increased uptake. Cellulitis causes increased activity during the flow and equilibrium phases and a decreased or normal uptake in the delayed phase. Osteomyelitis causes increased uptake in all three phases. Increased uptake in the delayed phase but not in the flow or equilibrium phase suggests degenerative joint disease. Technetium bone scans are unreliable in neonates (younger than 6 weeks of age) and usually are negative in 60% of those patients with bone or joint infections.

Definition: A preganglionic brachial plexus injury occurs when the spinal roots are avulsed directly from the spinal cord or the rootlets rupture proximal to the dorsal root ganglion. An injury distal to the dorsal root ganglion is called *postganglionic* (Fig. 34-1).

Etiology: Adult brachial plexus injury can result from penetrating injuries, falls, and motor vehicle accidents, causing fracture or compression. Obstetric brachial plexus injury is associated with shoulder dystocia, which occurs more frequently with fetal macrosomia.

Incidence: The true incidence of adult brachial plexus injuries is undetermined due to significant underreporting, but they account for 5% of peripheral injuries. However, obstetric palsies complicate 1% of all births.

Age and Gender: Most adult traumatic brachial plexus injuries occur in males aged 15 to 25 years. Obstetric brachial plexus palsy occurs more frequently in males due to their greater mean birth weight.

Signs and Symptoms: Acute pain over a nerve suggests a rupture, whereas lack of percussion tenderness indicates an avulsion. The classic Erb's palsy occurs at C5-6, producing a classic "waiters tip" with the forearm adducted, internally rotated, and the elbow extended (Fig. 34-2). Total brachial palsy is characterized by complete arm paralysis, decreased sensation, and a pale extremity. The suprascapular nerve supplies the supraspinatus and infraspinatus muscles, so injury can be assessed by lack of shoulder external rotation and abduction and the presence of infraspinatus atrophy. Loss of shoulder flexion, internal rotation, and abduction may be caused by injury to the axillary nerve that supplies the deltoid. Horner's syndrome suggests C8-T1 root avulsion. Injury to the long thoracic nerve that innervates the serratus anterior causes scapular winging on arm flexion. The dorsal scapular nerve is derived from C4-5 roots and innervates the rhomboids; studies indicate that injury to this nerve causes rhomboid atrophy.

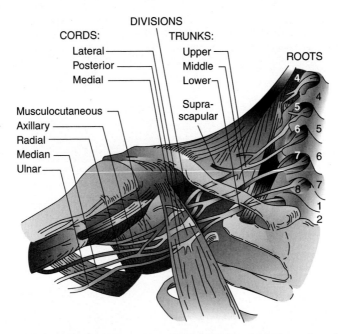

Fig. 34-1   Detailed view of brachial plexus. *(From Urschel HC, Razzuk M: Upper plexus thoracic outlet syndrome: Optimal therapy. Ann Thorac Surg 63:935-939, 1997. Reprinted with permission from the Society of Thoracic Surgeons.)*

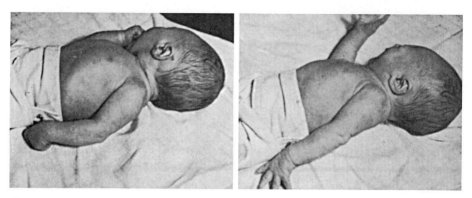

Fig. 34-2 Brachial palsy of the left arm (asymmetrical Moro reflex). *(From Kliegman: Nelson Textbook of Pediatrics, 18th ed. Philadelphia, Saunders, 2007.)*

Diagnostic: Plain radiographs of the cervical spine, shoulder, and chest should be done after a traumatic injury. Transverse process fractures suggest root avulsion at that level. Clavicle or first and second rib fracture may indicate brachial plexus injury. With avulsion of a cervical root, the dural sheath heals with development of a pseudomeningocele that is evident on CT myelogram at 3 to 4 weeks. MRI can visualize much of the brachial plexus, large neuromas, and inflammation or edema. Electromyogram and nerve conduction velocity studies help confirm a diagnosis, localizing lesions, defining the severity of axon loss, and revealing subclinical recovery.

Treatment: Surgery should be performed in the absence of clinical or electrical evidence of recovery or when spontaneous recovery is impossible. Nerve grafting using interpositional grafts such as the sural nerve and other cutaneous nerves can be performed with rupture or postganglionic neuromas that do not conduct across the lesion. Neurotization or nerve transfer in which a nerve of lesser importance such as the spinal accessory nerve, intercostal nerves, or medial pectoral nerves can be transferred to the denervated distal nerve. Free functioning muscle transfer is the transplantation of a muscle and its neurovascular pedicle to a new location. The latissimus dorsi, rectus femoris, and the gracilis are most commonly used to provide reliable elbow flexion.

Definition/Characteristics:
- Painful prominence on the lateral aspect of the fifth metatarsal head
- Not as common as a medial bunion (hallux valgus)
- Cause of chronic pain and shoe-fitting problems in feet characterized by a widened forefoot or in those who have a lateral splaying/prominence over the fifth metatarsal

Incidence:
- Related to narrow footwear or predisposed foot anatomy
- Commonly seen in patients who present with hallux valgus 2/2 splaying of the forefoot
- 90% female

Etiology:
- *Extrinsic:* Traumatic, either acute or more commonly chronic (tailors' working posture, footwear)
- *Intrinsic:* Related to structural abnormalities (congenital lateral bowing of the metatarsal shaft, abnormal intermetatarsal ligament insertion with prominence of the fifth metatarsal, brachymetatarsia, or primary hypertrophy of the metatarsal head)

Pathophysiology:
- Inflamed bursa overlying the lateral aspect of the metatarsal head
- Bony enlargement of the head itself
- Increased intermetatarsal angle (IMA) between the fourth and fifth metatarsals with secondary medial angulation of the phalanx and abnormal curvature of the fifth metatarsal

Signs and Symptoms:
- Classically, painful keratoses over the lateral aspect of the metatarsal head
- Medial deviation of the fifth phalanx with some rotation frequently seen

Imaging:
- Erect weight-bearing views of both feet

Classification (Based on X-Ray Measurements):
- *Type 1:* Enlarged head as an isolated lesion
- *Type 2:* Abnormal lateral bowing of the fifth metatarsal
- *Type 3:* 4/5 IMA in excess of the normal 6 to 8 degrees

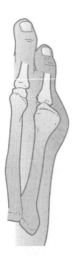

Fig. 35-1   Type 1. *(From http://www. emedicine.com/orthoped/topic468.htm.)*

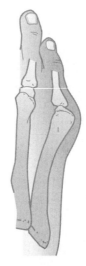

Fig. 35-2   Type 2. *(From http://www. emedicine.com/orthoped/topic468.htm.)*

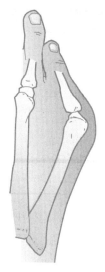

Fig. 35-3   Type 3. *(From http://www.emedicine.com/orthoped/topic468.htm.)*

Treatment:
- *Nonoperative:* Padding, shoe modification with arch supports or orthotic devices, anti-inflammatory medications, and occasionally corticosteroid injections into the bursae
- *Surgery (When Conservative Treatments Fail):*
  - *Type 1*: Condylectomy and capsular plication (if no evidence of increased IMA), may be associated with bursectomy or with nodule removal in patients with arthropathy
  - *Type 2*: Midshaft rotational osteotomy with or without lateral distal condylectomy
  - *Type 3*: Lateral condylectomy and distal metatarsal osteotomy (Chevron); large deformities require a midshaft or proximal osteotomy

Definition: Fractures of the calcaneus, or *os calcis*, have been observed and documented for centuries. Axial loading, which occurs due to falls from a height or from high-energy trauma such as motor vehicle accidents, accounts for the vast majority of intra-articular calcaneal fractures, where the talus is driven downward into the calcaneus.

Incidence: Calcaneal injuries represent 2% of all fractures seen in adults. The os calcis is the most frequently fractured tarsal bone, accounting for more than 60% of tarsal fractures.

Age: Patients 30 to 50 years of age.

Gender: Five times more often in males than in females.

Signs and Symptoms: Tenderness, excessive swelling, ecchymosis, and possible tarsal tunnel neural compromise.

Classifications:

Essex Lopresti: Most commonly used; separates fractures into intra-articular (75%) and extra-articular (25%).

Extra-articular Fracture Types: Anterior process, tuberosity, medial calcaneal process, sustentaculum tali, and body not involving the subtalar joint; often avulsion/direct blow.

Intra-articular Fracture Types:

- Joint Depression: More frequent, secondary fracture line begins at the angle of Gissane, extends posteriorly, but deviates dorsally to exit just posterior to the posterior articular facet. This fragment contains most of the posterior facet.
- Tongue Type: The secondary fracture line directly extends in a posterior direction, producing a large superior, posterior, and lateral fragment, with the remainder of the calcaneal body forming the inferior fragment.
- Sanders: A computed tomography (CT) classification system that carries prognostic implication. Choose the coronal CT image that shows the posterior facet in the widest profile to determine the primary fracture line; mark two vertical lines to divide the posterior facet into three equal sections.
  - Type I Fractures: Nondisplaced
  - Type II Fractures: Two part
  - Type III Fractures: Three-part fracture with depression of posterior facet
  - Type IV Fracture: Severely comminuted
- Treatment: Type I—nonoperative treatment; types II and III—open reduction and internal fixation (ORIF); type IV—ORIF with possible fusion of the subtalar joint.

Diagnostic Studies: Plain lateral and axial x-ray studies usually demonstrate shortening and widening of the calcaneus, usually with varus orientation and medial displacement of tuberosity. CT scanning (with 3-mm cuts) helps assess posterior facet and comminution and helps evaluate calcaneocuboid joint.

Treatment: No formal indications or agreement on approach or outcome criteria. ORIF, closed reduction, nonreduction, and primary arthrodesis are used.

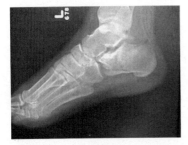

Fig. 36-1 Calcaneus fracture, sustained as a result of a fall from a height. *(From Auerbach PS: Wilderness Medicine, 5th ed. Philadelphia, Mosby, 2007.)*

Nondisplaced Articular Fractures: Bulky, Robert-Jones dressing, active subtalar range of motion with subsidence of swelling. Weight bearing usually starts 8 to 12 weeks postoperatively, depending on the extent of comminution.

Displaced Intra-articular Fractures with Large Fragments: ORIF when soft tissue allows. Lateral extensile approach is most popular, whereas modified subtalar approach, medial approach, or combined approaches are also acceptable.

Displaced Intra-articular Fractures, with Severe Comminution: Increasing intra-articular comminution leads to less satisfactory results; initial attempt at ORIF may be reasonable. With an unreconstructable joint, the surface is associated with a high rate of post-traumatic subtalar arthritis. Arthrodesis should be considered in this type of fracture. Nonsteroidal anti-inflammatory drugs are the preferred pharmacologic treatment.

Complications: Soft tissue breakdown is most common at the apex of the incision. Anterior ankle impingement following malreduction after the talus settles and lateral impingement of the fibula on the peroneals can occur. Cutaneous neuromas, especially the sural nerve, have been reported. The surgeon should also be alert for tendon incarceration (flexor hallucis longus medially, peroneals laterally), compartment syndrome, local infection, and subtalar arthrosis.

Note: Ten percent are associated with compression fractures of the dorsal or lumbar spine, 26% are associated with other injuries of the lower extremities, and 10% are bilateral. Articular reduction using the sustentacular fragment is the key to maintaining a normal relationship to the talus in displaced fractures.

Carpal Instability

Definition: Misalignment of the carpal ligaments leading to abnormal carpal kinematics. Carpal instability is not always painful and therefore is considered clinically unstable only when symptomatic. It is a significant finding because, when left untreated, it can lead to cartilage degeneration, erosion, and ultimately exposure and damage of bone.

Carpal Bones

There are eight carpal bones divided into distal and proximal rows. Beginning proximally, these are the scaphoid, lunate, triquetrum, and pisiform, with the pisiform not participating in wrist kinematics. The distal row—trapezium, trapezoid, capitate, and hamate—has metacarpals fixed to it. In comparison with the distal row, the proximal row has no muscle or tendon insertions and therefore relies on the capsular and the interosseous ligaments between the triquetrum, scaphoid, and lunate for stability.

Carpal Ligaments

Divided into intrinsic (interosseous) and extrinsic components. The main intrinsic ligaments include the lunotriquetral and scapholunate ligaments, each with its own palmar, dorsal, and proximal segments. Intrinsic ligaments are always damaged in carpal instability. The extrinsic ligaments span the radiocarpal joint and are distinguished by location, either palmar or dorsal. The palmar extrinsic ligaments play a larger role in joint stability and include the radioscaphocapitate, long radiolunate, and short radiolunate. The space of Poirier is an area of capsular weakness situated between the long radiolunate and radioscaphocapitate ligaments. The ulnolunate and ulnotriquetral ligaments are also located on the palmar aspect.

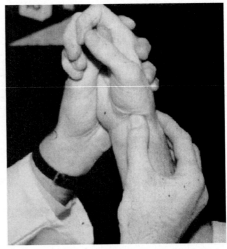

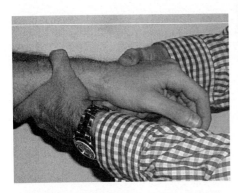

Fig. 37-1   Pseudoinstability test. *(From Trail IA, et al: Twenty questions on carpal instability. J Hand Surg 32:240-255, 2007.)*

Fig. 37-2   Watson's maneuver. *(From Trail IA, et al: Twenty questions on carpal instability. J Hand Surg 32:240-255, 2007.)*

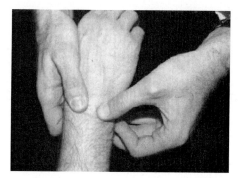

Fig. 37-3 Reagan's test for lunotriquetral instability.*(From Trail IA, et al: Twenty questions on carpal instability. J Hand Surg 32:240-255, 2007.)*

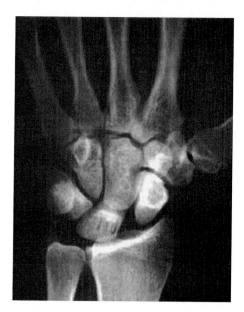

Fig. 37-4 The rupture of the scapholunate ligament generates two signs, which are visible on x-ray posteroanterior view. The Terry-Thomas sign is the widening of the gap between scaphoid and lunate, which under normal conditions does not exceed 2 mm; it is best seen with the wrist in ulnar deviation. The name *signet ring sign* derives from a cortical shadow that is not usually present at scaphoid level and that is generated by the rotatory dislocation of the bone, leading to the overlapping of the distal pole and the body. Failure to observe these signs does not, however, guarantee that the scapholunate ligament is intact. *(From De Filippo M, et al: Pathogenesis and evolution of carpal instability: Imaging and topography. Acta Bio Med 77:168-180, 2006.)*

Etiology: Multiple pathogeneses can be differentiated into acute traumatic events, chronic repetitive stress, or microcrystal deposits secondary to underlying disease. Acute traumatic events are most common and include falling on an outstretched hand, distal radius fracture, and scaphoid fracture. Chronic repetitive stress may occur in paraplegics who are weight bearing with their extremities. Microcrystal deposits can occur from congenital diseases (ulna minus variance) or metabolic diseases, such as rheumatoid, gout, and pseudogout. Most agree that intrinsic and extrinsic ligaments must be damaged for instability to occur. Although joint laxity appears to play a role in increasing the chances of becoming symptomatic after carpal trauma, congenital joint laxity does not appear to cause instability.

Incidence: Studies have shown the incidence as 10% to 40% for acute traumatic events. For patients with chronic repetitive stress, the incidence increases to around 20%. For patients with rheumatoid, incidence may be as high as 40%.

Classification: Several classifications have been established. Linscheid (1972) and Dobyns (1975) classified according to clinical-radiologic presentations: dorsal intercalated segment instability (DISI), volar intercalated segment instability (VISI), and ulnar translocation and dorsal subluxation. Taleisnik (1984) extended the classification by defining instability as static versus dynamic. Static describes total rupture of the intrinsic ligaments, whereas dynamic describes partial ligamentous injury that lacks radiographic changes on plain films. Dobyn and Gabel (1990) identified additional groups including dissociative carpal instability (CID), nondissociative carpal instability (CIND), complex carpal instability (CIC), and adaptive carpal instability (CIA).

Diagnosis: History and physical examination are of utmost importance—timing of injury, wrist position at injury, location and duration of pain, weakness, evidence of inflammation, range of motion, grip strength, and history of underlying disorder. Other specific tests include pseudoinstability test, Watson's maneuver (scaphoid shift test), and Reagan's shuck test (see Figs. 37-1, 37-2, and 37-3).

Radiographic Studies: First line studies includes x-ray examination with standard posterolateral (PA) and lateral views, in addition to ulnar deviation PA view, to completely evaluate the scaphoid. Second line includes computed tomography and/or magnetic resonance imaging to better evaluate bones, ligaments, and cartilage. Gold standard is arthroscopy via an intra-articular injection of contrast medium and video recording. Dynamic instability requires recording via arthroscopy for its diagnosis (see Fig. 37-4).

Treatment: Controversial among hand surgeons. Various nonsurgical and surgical means are available to treat carpal instability. Regardless, some means to promote healing of a torn ligament is crucial to avoid severe functional deficit via carpal collapse.

Nonoperative: Lifestyle modifications and immobilization via splinting or casting. Most agree nonoperative treatment is appropriate for minor disability when greater than 80% of normal range of motion and grip strength is maintained.

Operative: Soft tissue and bony reconstructive surgery, including capsulodesis, tenodesis, and arthrodesis. Reported problems include decrease in range of motion, and nonunion.

Complications: Long-term complications from untreated instability appear to be degenerative joint changes leading to osteoarthritis. However, debate remains as to whether or not sufficient evidence has shown a causal relationship.

Definition: Compression of the median nerve in the carpal tunnel at the wrist.

Etiology: Occupational pathogenesis seems to be the most frequent cause of carpal tunnel syndrome (CTS). An association with repetitive tasks, both with (higher risk) and without the application of elevated force have been shown.

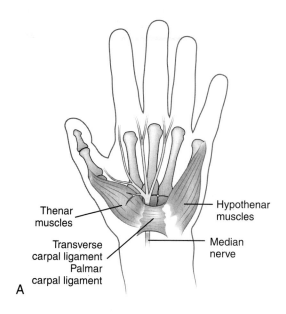

Thenar muscles
Hypothenar muscles
Transverse carpal ligament
Median nerve
Palmar carpal ligament
A

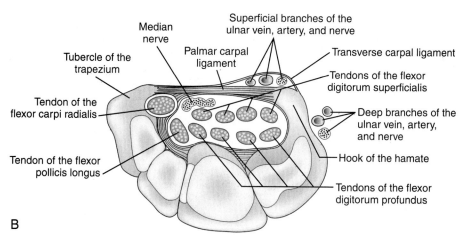

Median nerve
Superficial branches of the ulnar vein, artery, and nerve
Palmar carpal ligament
Transverse carpal ligament
Tubercle of the trapezium
Tendons of the flexor digitorum superficialis
Tendon of the flexor carpi radialis
Deep branches of the ulnar vein, artery, and nerve
Tendon of the flexor pollicis longus
Hook of the hamate
Tendons of the flexor digitorum profundus
B

Fig. 38-1   Anatomic basis of carpal tunnel syndrome. **A,** General view of the relationship between the median nerve and the flexor retinaculum. **B,** Cross-section at the distal carpal row, showing the structures in the carpal tunnel. *(Redrawing based on an illustration by Li-Guo Liang, in Yu HL, Chase RA, Strauch B: Atlas of Hand Anatomy and Clinical Implications. Philadelphia, Mosby, 2004, p 513.From Auerbach: Wilderness Medicine, 5th ed. Philadelphia, Mosby, 2007.)*

Fig. 38-2 Phalen's test. Patients maximally flex both wrists and hold the position for 1 to 2 minutes. If symptoms of numbness or paresthesia within the median nerve distribution are reproduced, the test result is positive. *(Reprinted with permission from Concannon M. Common Hand Problems in Primary Care. Philadelphia, Hanley & Belfus, 1999.)*

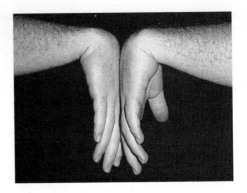

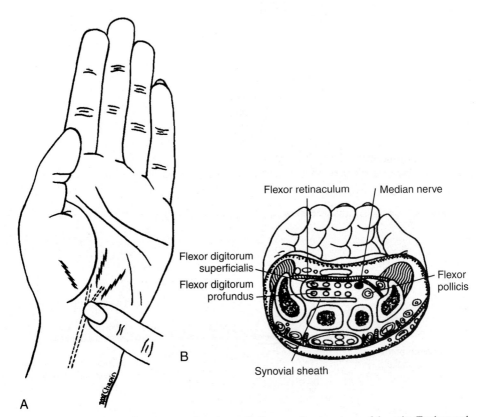

Fig. 38-3 A, Tinel's sign in carpal tunnel syndrome. **B,** Cross-sectional anatomy of the wrist. Tendons and median nerve may be compressed by inflammation or infection because they are encompassed by synovial sheath and flexor retinaculum. *(From Noble: Textbook of Primary Care Medicine, 3rd ed. Philadelphia, Mosby, 2001.)*

Incidence: Incidence is 1 to 3 cases per 1000 subjects per year.

Predisposing Factors: Other systemic illnesses can be associated with CTS (e.g., diabetes mellitus, rheumatoid arthritis, myxedema, and amyloidosis) as can physiologic situations (e.g., pregnancy, use of oral contraceptives, menopause), traumas (wrist fractures with articular deformation), arthritis, and deforming arthrosis.

Age and Gender: The peak age of development of CTS is between 45 and 60 years. Only 10% of CTS patients are younger than 31 years. The female-to-male ratio is 3-10:1.

Clinical Findings: Numbness, not pain, is the hallmark of CTS (Semmes-Weinstein monofilament test). The classic complaint is awakening at night or in the morning with numbness in the fingers.

Symptoms: Aching and paresthesia in the thumb, index, middle, and one half of the ring finger, which is worse at night, forearm pain, dropping things.

Signs: Usually normal on examination. If CTS is severe thenar wasting and trophic ulcers may be seen; weakness of thumb abduction may be seen in later stages.

Special Tests: Hoffmann-Tinel sign, Tinel's sign, Phalen's sign, median nerve compression test, the square wrist sign, and Durkan's test may be useful in confirming CTS. Electromyography and nerve conduction velocity testing (EMG/NCV) is an excellent test for carpal tunnel syndrome (accuracy = 85% to 90%). Not only can EMG/NCV detect the presence or absence of nerve dysfunction, it can quantify it.

Pathology: The median nerve is compressed within the rigid confines of the carpal tunnel, initially undergoing demyelination followed by axonal degeneration. Sensory fibers often are affected first, followed by motor fibers. Autonomic nerve fibers carried in the median nerve also may be affected.

Treatment:

Medical Care: Futura splint, injection (75% to 81% achieve short-term relief).

Surgical Care: Patients whose condition does not improve following conservative treatment and patients who initially are in the severe CTS category (as defined by EMG) should be considered for surgery. Surgical release of the transverse ligament provides high initial success rates (greater than 90%) with low rates of complication. Success rates also are considerably lower for individuals with normal EMG studies.

Complications: The condition may continue to increase median nerve damage leading to permanent impairment and disability.

Definition: Cartilage is a tough, semitransparent, elastic, flexible connective tissue consisting of cartilage cells scattered through a glycoprotein material that is strengthened by collagen fibers. There are no nerves or blood vessels in cartilage, which is found in the joints, the rib cage, the ear, the nose, the throat, and between vertebral disks.

Function: The main purpose of cartilage is to provide a framework on which bone deposition may begin. Another important purpose of cartilage is to cover the surfaces of joints, allowing bones to slide over one another, thus reducing friction and preventing damage; it also acts as a shock absorber

Clasification:

Hyaline Cartilage: Hyaline cartilage is the most abundant type of cartilage. Hyaline cartilage is found lining bones in joints (articular cartilage). It is also present inside bones, serving as a center of ossification or bone growth. In addition, hyaline cartilage forms the embryonic skeleton.

Elastic Cartilage: Elastic cartilage (also called *yellow cartilage*) is found in the pinna of the ear and several tubes, such as the walls of the auditory and eustachian canals and larynx. Elastic cartilage is similar to hyaline cartilage but contains elastic bundles (elastin) scattered throughout the matrix. This provides a tissue that is stiff yet elastic.

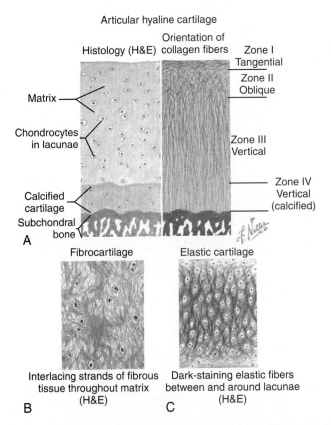

Structure of three types of cartilage.

Articular hyaline cartilage

Histology (H&E) | Orientation of collagen fibers

Matrix

Chondrocytes in lacunae

Calcified cartilage

Subchondral bone

A

Zone I Tangential
Zone II Oblique
Zone III Vertical
Zone IV Vertical (calcified)

Fibrocartilage

Elastic cartilage

Interlacing strands of fibrous tissue throughout matrix (H&E)

B

Dark-staining elastic fibers between and around lacunae (H&E)

C

Fig. 39-1 *(From Ovale WK, Nahirey PC: Netter's Essential Histology. Philadelphia, Saunders, 2008.)*

Fibrocartilage: Fibrocartilage (also called *white cartilage*) is a specialized type of cartilage found in areas requiring tough support or great tensile strength, such as between intervertebral disks, at the pubic and other symphyses, and at sites connecting tendons or ligaments to bones.

Composition:

Cells: Chondrocytes and the precusor forms of chondrocytes known as *chondroblasts* are the only cells found in cartilage. Chondrocytes make up "cell nests," groups of chondrocytes within lacunae. Chondroblasts are responsible for the secretion and maintenance of the matrix.

Fibers: Cartilage is composed of collagen and elastic fibers. In hyaline cartilage, type II collagen makes up 40% of its dry weight. Elastic cartilage also contains elastic fibers, and fibrocartilage contains more collagen than hyaline cartilage.

Matrix: The matrix is mainly composed of proteoglycans, which are large molecules with a protein backbone and glycosaminoglycan (GAG) side chains.

Diseases: Chondrodystrophies are a group of diseases characterized by disturbance of growth and subsequent ossification of cartilage. Some common diseases affecting/involving the cartilage are arthritis, achondroplasia, costochondritis, and herniated disk.

Four decades ago, John Charnley, Ken McKee, and Maurice Mueller pioneered the use of cement in total hip arthroplasty procedures. Polymethylmethacrylate (PMMA) bone cement is an agent intended for use in arthroplasty procedures for the fixation of the metallic or polymer prosthetic components to living bone. Bone cements that are currently available commercially are all based on the chemical substance methylmethacrylate. Bone cement usually comes in two-component parts, a liquid monomer and a granular powder component. PMMA bone cement is the gold standard for stabilization of total joint prostheses.

The mechanical properties of bone cement include mobility of polymeric chains, grafting between polymerizing monomer and prepolymerized beads, additive matrix bond strength, linear versus branched polymer chains, and gamma sterilization of powder components.

Although bone cement has been used successfully for the past 40 years, risks and failures are associated with application. PMMA is generally well tolerated. However, complications such as inflammation potential, tissue necrosis, systemic and cardiovascular reactions (drop in systolic, pressure), sensitization, implant loosening, wear, and osteolysis may occur. The cement surrounding the joint prosthesis has been demonstrated to crack, and investigations are ongoing aimed at improving longevity and performance of the material. Recent efforts toward improvement in outcomes have focused on intraoperative preparation and handling of the cement. Variables including the manufacturer, clinical technique, and patient parameters (weight, activity, bone quality) influence the success/failure rates of bone cement use in procedures.

Laboratory investigations are focused on improving the cement performance with the introduction of reinforcement fibers and other materials to withstand the demands in vivo. Metallic, polymeric, and carbon fibers have demonstrated mechanical performance; however, their influence on bone adherence remains unresolved. Laboratory studies are also in progress investigating issues raised regarding shrinkage of the materials during polymerization in the traditional methylmethacrylate. One method to reduce voids in the internal composition is centrifugation or vacuum mixing, yet caution must be used to ensure the vacuum is not set too high during mixing to prevent excessive evaporation. Although controlled laboratory results have shown improvements, questions arise regarding the practicality of such results in the operating room due to variances in handling and application technique. Lastly, recent studies have demonstrated that the mechanical properties of bone cement can be severely compromised by hand-mixing antibiotics into bone cement at the time of surgery.

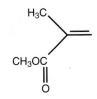

Fig. 40-1   Medical cement.

Definition: Central slip extensor tendon injury occurs when the proximal interphalangeal (PIP) joint is forcibly flexed while actively extended.

Basics: The bony anatomy of the PIP joint consists of medial and lateral condyles on the proximal phalanx, with matching concavities on the distal phalanx. This allows for a wide range of motion in flexion and extension, but is relatively rigid in abduction and adduction, making it a functional hinge joint.

The extrinsic flexors across the PIP and distal interphalangeal (DIP) joints are at least four times stronger than the extensors, allowing flexor contractures to develop rapidly, especially with immobilization in flexion.

Etiology: Laceration, closed trauma, elongation secondary to synovitis of the PIP joint, volar PIP dislocation.

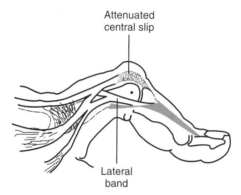

Fig. 41-1 Diagram of the boutonnière deformity. Stretching of the dorsal capsule and central slip allows the lateral bands to slip toward the palmar surface, producing flexion at the proximal interphalangeal (PIP) joint and hyperextension at the distal interphalangeal (DIP) joint. *(From Harris ED: Kelley's Textbook of Rheumatology, 7th ed. Philadelphia, Saunders, 2005.)*

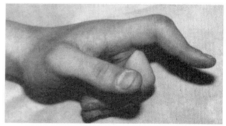

Fig. 41-2 The boutonniére deformity, involving hyperextension of the DIP joint with flexion of the PIP joint, also is caused by a derangement of the extensor mechanism—typically a rupture of the central extensor tendon at its insertion in the middle phalanx. Early diagnosis and prolonged splinting of the PIP joint in extension are necessary for successful treatment of this difficult injury. *(From Frontera WR: Essentials of Physical Medicine and Rehabilitation, 2nd ed. Philadephia, Saunders, 2008.)*

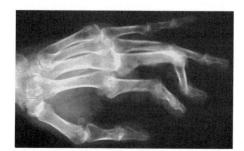

Fig. 41-3 Radiographic image of central slip extensor tendon injury.

Incidence: Related to etiology.
Age: None.
Gender: None.
Signs and Symptoms: Tender at dorsal aspect of the PIP joint, inability to actively extend the PIP joint, PIP flexed, and DIP extended.
Associations: Hand trauma, rheumatoid arthritis.
Imaging: Radiographs may show dorsal chip fracture from the base of the middle phalanx, which represents an avulsion of bone by the central slip of extensor tendon.
Treatment: When the central slip is acutely lacerated, it should be directly repaired and the joint pinned in full extension for 3 to 6 weeks to protect the repair. Acute closed rupture should be treated with weeks of splinting of the PIP joint in full extension. Surgical indications include failure of nonoperative treatment, central slip injury with avulsion fracture, open central slip injuries, and volar PIP dislocation.

If there is a large displaced avulsion fracture, open reduction and internal fixation are required.

Definition: Cerebral palsy is a static encephalopathy that causes disordered movement and posture.

Incidence: Moderate to severe cerebral palsy is estimated to affect 1.5 to 2.5 per 1000 people born in the United States. Premature babies are at higher risk. The rates of cerebral palsy per live births have been rising. One possibility for the increased rate of this disease is the increased survival of children with very low birth weights.

Age: The brain abnormalities may be prenatal, perinatal, or postnatal. Cerebral palsy is usually diagnosed at approximately 1 year of age.

Race: Cerebral palsy affects all races.

Etiology: Cerebral palsy has many prenatal, perinatal, and postnatal causes. The causes may be due to trauma, toxins, radiation, infections, genetics, vascular insufficiency, or anoxia. Several causes often contribute to the development of cerebral palsy.

Clinical Presentation: There are several common presentations of cerebral palsy. Spastic hemiplegia affects one side of the body more than the other and frequently includes learning disabilities and seizures. Spastic diplegia mostly affects the lower extremities. Dyskinesia mostly affects the upper extremities. Spastic quadriplegia affects all of the limbs and is associated with many medical complications. Clinical signs of cerebral palsy include an asymmetrical posture or gait, abnormal coordination, growth disturbances, and abnormal muscle tone. Patients may be either hypotonic or hypertonic with joint contractures due to spastic muscles. The hip is often flexed and adducted. The knee is often flexed and extended. Both the knee and the hindfoot may be in varus or valgus. Patients with cerebral palsy often retain primitive reflexes that are normally lost during normal development.

Pathology: In cerebral palsy, the muscles have shortened muscle fibers and the brain has defects or lesions.

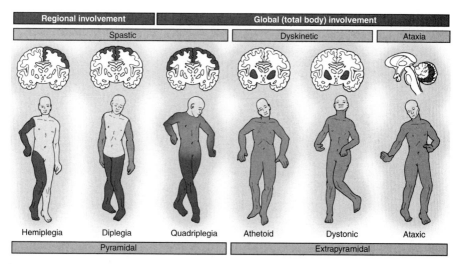

Fig. 42-1   Classification of cerebral palsy. Although overlaps in terminology exist, cerebral palsy can be classified according to distribution (regional versus global involvement, hemiplegic, diplegic, quadriplegic), physiologic type (spastic, dyskinetic/dystonic, dyskinetic/athetoid, ataxic), or presumed neurologic substrate (pyramidal, extrapyramidal). *(From Canale ST, Beaty JH: Campbell's Operative Orthopaedics, 11th ed. Philadelphia, Mosby, 2007.)*

85

Diagnostic Procedures: Neuroimaging studies are useful in determining brain damage. Neonatal sonography, magnetic resonance imaging, and computed tomography may all be used to check for white matter disease, periventricular leukomalacia, injury, hemorrhage, and malformation. Laboratory studies are also useful, and endpoints include lactate and pyruvate levels, thyroid functioning, amino acids, cerebrospinal protein, and chromosome studies.

Treatment: Several surgical interventions can treat cerebral palsy. Spastic muscles may be treated by tendon lengthening, or posterior rhizotomy, which treats velocity dependent spasticity, or an intrathecal baclofen pump, which targets the lower extremities. Hip dislocations, most often posterior, may be treated with hip relocation surgery. Furthermore, scoliosis repair and/or an osteotomy may be necessary.

Definition: Loss of the spine's ability to limit displacement under physiologic loads, leading to damage or irritation of the spinal cord and nerve roots causing structural changes, deformity, and pain.

Mechanisms: Trauma, inflammatory disease, tumor, infection, degenerative disease, post surgery.

3-Column Theory for Thoracolumbar Spine (Fig. 43-1): Mechanical instability occurs with injury of at least two of the following three columns:
- Anterior column is anterior longitudinal ligament and anterior half vertebral body and disk
- Middle column is posterior longitudinal ligament and posterior half vertebral body and disk
- Posterior column is pedicles, facets, spinous processes, interspinous ligaments

Trauma: Most common mechanism for cervical spine instability; four types of injury:
- Compression Fracture—flexion with axial loading, stable (anterior column only)
- Burst Fracture—axial loading, unstable (anterior and middle columns), stable in brace
- Flexion-Distraction Injury—"lap belt," bending with posterior column elongation, unstable (anterior and posterior columns involved, middle is center of rotation)
- Fracture and Dislocation—translation/rotation with flexion/axial loading/distraction, all three columns involved

Chronic Instability: Infections and tumors destroy bone and ligament. This instability can lead to pathologic fractures and deformity, Kostuik and Errico developed a 6 column system where destruction of 2 or fewer columns is stable, 3 and 4 columns is unstable, and 5 and 6 column destruction is markedly unstable.

Assessment: Clinical diagnosis and assessment of need for surgery.
- Intractable pain (usually with axial loading)
- Neurologic dysfunction
- Significant or progressive deformity
- Sepsis

Occipital-Atlanto-Axial Complex Instability:
- C0-C1 has respiratory center, dislocation is fatal, usually anterior
  - Dens-Basion distance (normal 4 to 5 mm in adults, 10 mm in children)
  - Powers Ratio (Fig. 43-2)—ratio > 1 indicates anterior dislocation
  - Surgical stabilization indicated for dislocation
- C1-C2 stabilized by transverse ligament (TL); if disrupted, is unstable and requires surgery
  - TL disrupted if C1 lateral masses overhang lateral C2 more than 7 mm on open mouth
  - Atlantodens interval should be less than 3 mm in adults, less than 5 mm in children on lateral
  - In rheumatoid arthritis atlantodens, interval greater than 9 mm on flex-ex is unstable

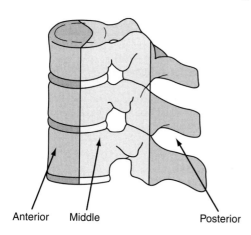

Fig. 43-1 3-columns: Spinal Cord (2003) 41, 385–396 Classification of spinal injuries based on the essential traumatic spinal mechanisms S M Iencean1.

Anterior   Middle   Posterior

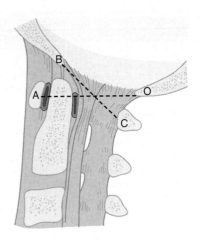

Fig. 43-2 Powers Ratio uses four points of reference in the midsagittal section through the craniocervical junction. B, basion; O, opisthion; A, anterior arch of atlas; C, posterior arch of atlas. The ratio of BCOA should always equal one or less. If it is greater than one, the patient most likely has an anterior occipitocervical sublaxation dislocation. *(From Powers B, Miller MD, Kramer RS, et al: Traumatic anterior atlanto-occipital dislocation. Neurosurgery 1979, 4:12-17.)*

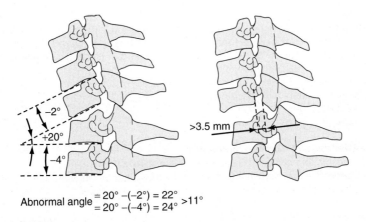

$$\text{Abnormal angle} \begin{array}{l} = 20° - (-2°) = 22° \\ = 20° - (-4°) = 24° \end{array} > 11°$$

Fig. 43-3 Metastatic Instability: Measurement of regional instability includes angular displacement: 11 degrees greater than those of the adjacent vertebral segments and translation greater than 3.5 mm. *(From White AA, Panjabi M: Clinical Biomechanics of the Spine 2nd ed. Philadelphia: Lippincott: 1990.)*

Dvorak: Unstable if axial rotation between C0-C1 is greater than 8 degrees or C1-C2 is greater than 56 degrees.

White and Panjabi's Checklist (Table 43-1) **for Subaxial C-Spine (C2-7):** Radiographic criteria most reliable:
- Sagittal plane translation greater than 3.5 mm or 20% on flexion-extension on resting x-ray
- Sagittal plane rotation greater than 20 degrees on flexion-extension or 11 degrees on resting x-ray
- Unilateral facet fractures usually stable

Table 43-1. CHECKLIST FOR THE DIAGNOSIS OF CLINICAL INSTABILITY IN THE MIDDLE AND LOWER CERVICAL SPINE

Element	Point Value
Anterior elements destroyed or unable to function	2
Posterior elements destroyed or unable to function	2
Positive stretch test	2
Radiographic criteria	4
A. Flexion-extension X-rays	
1. Sagittal plane translation >3.5 mm or 20% (2 points)	
2. Sagittal plane rotation >20 degrees (2 points)	
OR	
B. Resting X-rays	
1. Sagittal plane displacement >35 mm or 20% (2 points)	
2. Relative sagittal plane angulation >11 degrees (2 points)	
Developmentally narrow spinal canal (sagittal diameter <13 mm or Pavlov's Ratio <0.8)	1
Abnormal disk narrowing	1
Spinal cord damage	2
Nerve root damage	1
Dangerous loading anticipated	1

Total of 5 or more — unstable. From White AA, Panjabi MM. Clinical Biomechanics of the Spine, 2nd ed. Philadelphia: Lippincott: 1990.

Definition: A subset of the flexion-distraction injuries of the thoracolumbar spine, Chance fractures are bony injuries with a fracture line extending posterior to anterior from the spinous process through the pedicles and body.

Background: First described by Chance in 1948 and then further by Smith and Kaufer, Chance fractures are commonly the result of the forward flexion over a lap seatbelt during deceleration in a motor vehicle accident, or a "seatbelt injury."

Incidence: Rare. Flexion-distraction injuries account for less than 10% of all thoracolumbar fracture patterns, and Chance fractures are a subset thereof.

Mechanism: A force whose fulcrum lies anterior to the vertebral bodies causes failure of the anterior and middle columns or of all three columns of the spine through tension. Forces occur predominantly through bony structures as opposed to ligamentous structures but may include both. Contrast Chance fractures with ligamentous flexion distraction injuries in which tensioning at the posterior and middle column with compression at the anterior column is the rule; ligamentous flexion distraction injuries typically result in different injury patterns such as facet dislocation and compression fracture.

Anatomy: Distracting forces often disrupt posterior elements: interspinous ligaments, ligamentum flavum, facet capsules. Anterior longitudinal ligament may remain intact and act as a hinge. Chance fracture stability depends upon the integrity of the posterior column.

Associated Injuries: Chance fracture is commonly associated with intra-abdominal injuries. Neurologic injury is relatively uncommon. Chance fracture can occur in combination with shear injuries of the thoracolumbar spine: very rare, requires bidirectional translation forces.

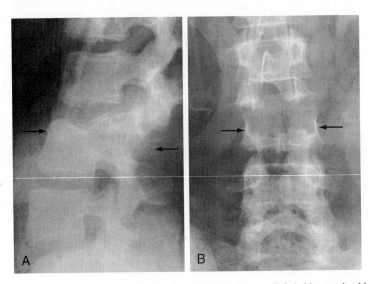

Fig. 44-1 An 11-year-old boy was a passenger restrained by only a seat belt (without a shoulder harness) in a motor vehicle accident. He sustained a flexion-distraction injury with paraplegia at the T12 level. *A,* A lateral radiograph demonstrates a Chance fracture with the fracture line proceeding through the pedicles and the vertebral body in a line between the *arrows. B,* An anteroposterior radiograph shows both the transverse processes and the pedicle to be split in a coronal plane as marked by the *arrows.* Because this injury is strictly a bony injury, adequate bone-bone contact can be maintained and healing achieved without ligamentous instability. *(From Browner BD: Skeletal Trauma: Basic Science, Management, and Reconstruction, 3rd ed. Philadelphia, Saunders, 2003.)*

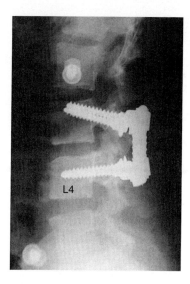

L4

Fig. 44-2 A 17-year-old girl sustained a Chance fracture of L4 and had flexion instability after nonoperative treatment. A posterior compression construct was able to reduce the kyphosis and eliminate the instability. One-level compression instrumentation can be used acutely in flexion-distraction injuries with posterior instability, but the purchase in the fractured body must be carefully assessed if a two-level/one-interspace construct is chosen. *(From Browner BD: Skeletal Trauma: Basic Science, Management, and Reconstruction, 3rd ed. Philadelphia, Saunders, 2003.)*

Treatment: Dictated by degree of injury of associated ligamentous structures and associated neurologic compromise. Well-reduced fractures with little posterior column compromise can be treated conservatively in a hyperextension orthosis. High degree of cancellous bone in vertebral body may predispose to good healing. Otherwise posterior spinal stabilization with rods and pedicle screws provides sound fixation.

Definition: Charcot-Marie-Tooth (CMT) disease is the most common progressive hereditary neurologic disease, characterized by degeneration of the peroneal muscles, resulting in club foot, cavus, drop foot, and ataxia.

Etiology: Genetic familiar predisposition with different degrees of penetrance. There have also been reported spontaneous mutations.

Prevalence: The prevalence of CMT is approximately 1 person per 2500 population, or about 125,000 patients in the United States.

Age: The age of onset depends on the type of CMT that is diagnosed. Usually, most have an age of onset within the first 2 decades of life.

Gender: There is no tendency to either gender known.

Race: There is no racial tendency recognized.

Signs and Symptoms: Physically, weakness and muscle atrophy affect the lower extremities more severely than the upper extremities. Foot deformities include either high arched (cavus) or flat feet (pes planus).

Etiology/Pathophysiology: Inherited hypertrophic neuropathies are the most common.

Pathology: Demyelination of nerves, proliferation of Schwann cells, and a thick layer of abnormal myelin around the peripheral axons. These changes cause an "onion bulb" appearance.

Treatment: Surgically, depending on the degree of the foot/feet deformities, the patient may benefit from Achilles hammertoe correction and the release of the plantar fascia. Often, boots can delay CMT and help patients resume certain activities of daily living.

Sequelae: Patients may have a limp and have an impaired gait.

Complications: Patients are susceptible to foot ulcers, and in severe cases, bony deformities, because of the loss of protective sensation in all four limbs. In general, CMT causes deformities because of the slow progressive neuropathy, although it does not shorten the patient's life span.

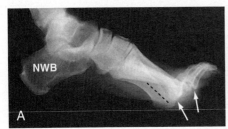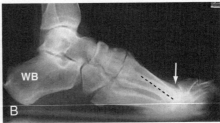

Fig. 45-1 **A,** Non–weight bearing view of cavus and claw toe deformities in a patient with Charcot-Marie-Tooth disease. **B,** On weight bearing view, plantar flexion of first ray is less noticeable, but clawed hallux remains, indicating fixed extension contracture at first metatarsophalangeal joint. *(From Canale ST, Beaty JH: Campbell's Operative Orthopaedics, 11th ed. Philadelphia, Mosby, 2007.)*

Definition: Charcot's neuropathic arthropathy is a progressive degenerative arthropathy characterized by joint dislocations, pathologic fractures, and debilitating deformities as a result of bone and soft tissue destruction.

Etiology: Charcot's joint disease (CJD) occurs as a complication of any condition that causes sensory or autonomic neuropathy, including diabetes, syphilis, chronic alcoholism, meningomyelocele, syringomyelia, renal dialysis, and Charcot-Marie-Tooth disease. Diabetes with peripheral neuropathy is the most common cause of CJD.

Incidence: The incidence of acute Charcot's arthropathy in diabetic patients ranges from 0.1% to 7% and in tabes dorsalis is from 5% to 10%; whereas in syringomyelia, 20% to 40% of patients can be affected.

Age: Most diabetic patients aged 40 to 59 years are affected, whereas those with tabes dorsalis present later at approximately age 60 years. It is rare in children.

Gender: Few studies indicate that the male-to-female ratio is 1:1, whereas others have reported a 3:1 predilection for males.

Race: Among diabetics, CJD is more prevalent among African Americans, Native Americans, Hispanic Americans, and Asian Americans.

Signs and Symptoms: The initial signs of CJD are subtle but include foot swelling and difficulty in shoe fitting. The typical acute presentation includes a painless, warm, erythematous, edematous foot in the presence of intact skin and loss of sensation. Structural changes in the foot such as a depressed arch or a total dislocation of the tarsometatarsal joint may manifest as a "rocker-bottom" foot deformity (Fig. 46-1). Approximately 40% of patients have concomitant ulceration, raising the concern for osteomyelitis.

Diagnostic Studies: Definitive diagnosis of CJD is by synovial tissue biopsy. Plain radiographs may show disruption of the articular surfaces, fragmentation, osteopenia, and dislocation of the joint. However, plain radiographs and computed tomography scans lack sensitivity and specificity, especially during the acute phase. Magnetic resonance imaging of CJD demonstrates low signal

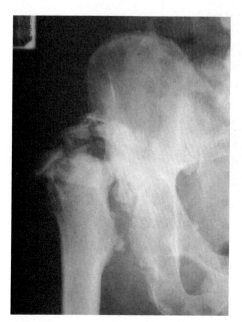

Fig. 46-1 Neuropathic arthropathy of the right hip. There are destruction and fragmentation of the right femoral head leading to bony dislocation and disorganization of the joint. The underlying cause in this patient was syphilis. *(From Adam A, et al: Grainger & Allison's Diagnostic Radiology, 5th ed. Philadelphia, Churchill Livingstone, 2008.)*

intensity of the marrow space on both T1- and T2-weighted images, whereas there is high signal intensity on T2-weighted images in the presence of osteomyelitis. Three-phase bone scans are sensitive for CJD but are nonspecific for osteomyelitis. White blood cell (WBC)-labeled scans using indium-111 or technetium-99m (HMPAO) when used in conjunction with a three-phase scan have a greater specificity for infection in cases of acute CJD.

Macropathology: CJD most commonly affects the tarsometatarsal joint, knees, and hips. The hypertrophic osseous stages are described in three stages:

Acute Stage: Characterized by joint effusion, intraarticular fracture, fragmentation, and joint subluxation.

Coalescent Stage: Fracture healing begins.

Reconstructive Phase: Remodeling and bony ankylosis become apparent (Fig. 46-2).

Micropathology: Synovial tissue biopsy contains shards of bone and cartilage embedded in the synovium similarly found in ochronosis and degenerative arthritis.

Treatment: The goals of treatment include control of foot position and shape to achieve a stable and plantigrade foot. Off-loading modalities include the use of total contact casts, custom-molded shoes, a cam-walker, and a Charcot-restraint orthotic walker, as well as wearing a patellar tendon brace. The indications for surgery in CJD are the following: acute dislocation, recurrent ulceration secondary to instability or bony prominence that cannot be managed nonsurgically, or severe deformity that may make it impossible to fit a brace or footwear. Approaches vary from simple exostectomy, ulcer excision with or without flap or graft, to arthrodesis with internal or external fixators or Achilles tendon lengthening due to the presence of equinus deformity.

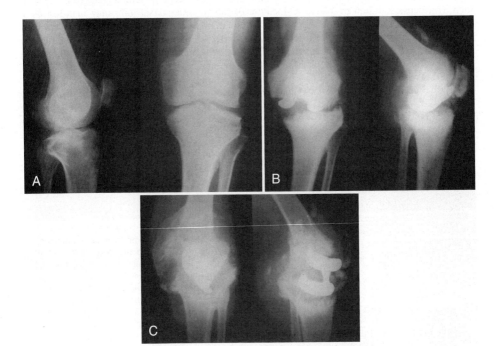

Fig 46-2 Fourteen years after total knee arthroplasty, radiographs show almost vertical rotation of femoral component and complete destruction of polyethylene tibial component. (Courtesy of Andrew H. Crenshaw, Jr., MD.) *(From Canale ST & Beaty JH: Campbell's Operative Orthopaedics, 11th ed. Philadelphia, Mosby, 2007.)*

Definition: Injury to the thoracic cage, which may be associated with underlying organ injury and dysfunction. Some injuries are imminently lethal or life-threatening and must be diagnosed and treated without delay.

Tension Pneumothorax

Clinical Presentation: Characterized by chest pain, air hunger, respiratory distress, tachycardia, tracheal deviation, unilateral absence of breath sounds, and neck vein distention.
Pathophysiology/Mechanism:
- Air enters the pleural space, either from the lung or external environment, where it is trapped secondary to the presence of a flap valve mechanism.
- Results in increased ipsilateral intrapleural pressure and shift of the mediastinum, with cardiovascular compromise.

Treatment: Immediate decompression with insertion of a large-bore needle into the second intercostal space in the midclavicular line. Usually followed by a rush of air, and chest tube.

Open Pneumothorax

Clinical Presentation: Variable depending on interval between injury and treatment. Patients may present in extremis if tension pneumothorax has developed.
Pathophysiology/Mechanism: Equilibration between atmospheric and intrathoracic pressure is immediate, and if open wound is two thirds the diameter of the trachea, air flows down the path of least resistance through the defect, impairing adequate ventilation and ultimately leading to respiratory collapse.
Treatment:
- Placement of sterile occlusive dressing over defect and taping it on three sides to allow air out with expiration. No air can enter during inspiration, because negative intrathoracic pressure sucks the occlusive dressing into the defect.
- Distant placement of a chest tube is necessary and surgical closure of the defect is frequently required.

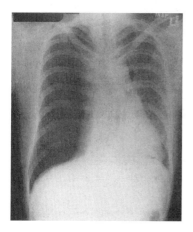

Fig. 47-1   Radiograph of tension pneumothorax with mediastinal shift to left. *(From Marx J: Rosen's Emergency Medicine: Concepts and Clinical Practice, 6th ed. Philadelphia, Mosby, 2006.)*

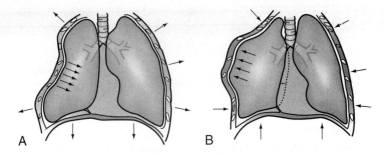

Fig. 47-2 Forces producing disordered chest wall motion in flail chest. **A,** During inspiration, the lowering of pleural pressure produces inward motion of the flail segment. **B,** During expiration, the increase in pleural pressure produces an outward displacement of the flail segment. *(From Mason RJ: Murray & Nadel's Textbook of Respiratory Medicine, 4th ed. Philadelphia, Saunders, 2005.)*

Flail Chest

Clinical Presentation: Mechanism of injury suspicious for rib fractures, respiratory splinting, crepitus over segment of thoracic cage, pain with palpation, and x-rays showing multiple segmental rib fractures.

Pathophysiology/Mechanism:
- Multiple segmental rib fractures cause a portion of the chest wall to lose continuity with the rest of the thoracic cage, resulting in deficient chest wall mechanics.
- Pain, splinting, abnormal respiratory mechanics, and the presence of severe underlying lung injury all contribute to respiratory distress.

Treatment: Follow advanced trauma life support protocol, which may require supplemental oxygen, intubation, analgesia, and careful fluid management.

Incidence: Twenty-five percent of individuals in the United States will be sexually or physically abused during their lifetime. Child abuse may kill 14,000 U.S. children each year and hurt thousands more.

Age: Affects children usually younger than 3 years of age.

Gender: Boys and girls

Geography: Compounded by various stressful environmental circumstances, such as inadequate physical and emotional support within the family and any major life change or crisis, especially those crises arising from marital strife.

Symptoms: The result of multiple and complex factors involving both the parents and the child, compounded by various stressful environmental circumstances such as inadequate physical and emotional support within the family and any major life change or crisis, especially those crises arising from marital strife. Parents at high risk for abuse are characterized as having unsatisfied needs, difficulty in forming adequate interpersonal relationships, unrealistic expectations of the child, and a lack of nurturing experience, often involving neglect or abuse in their own childhoods.

Signs: Obvious physical marks on a child's body, such as burns, welts, or bruises, and signs of emotional distress, including symptoms of failure to thrive, are common indications of some degree of neglect or abuse. Often, radiograph films are used to detect healed or new fractures of the extremities, or diagnostic tests identify sexual molestation.

Macropathology: Physical marks on a child's body, such as burns, welts, or bruises, fractures of the extremities, or diagnostic tests that identify sexual molestation.

Sequelae and Prognosis: Any person who has been reared in an environment of violence may be more likely to inflict violence on others. These behaviors in young children continue as they get older and can transform into other personality or mental disorders that can be difficult or impossible to treat.

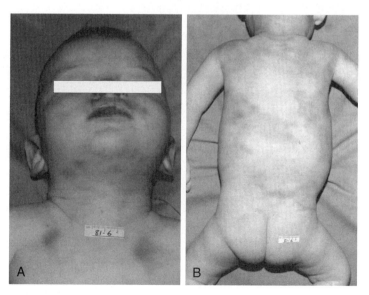

Fig. 48-1   A and B, Shaken baby syndrome is often recognizable by external bruising about the chest, shoulders, and neck caused by the fingers and hands. *(From Grosfeld JL et al: Pediatric Surgery, 6th ed. Philadelphia, Mosby, 2006.)*

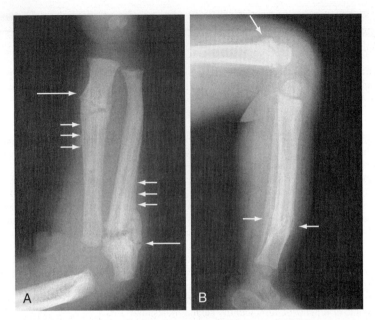

Fig. 48-2 Child abuse. **A,** A view of the forearm in this child shows extensive periosteal reaction (*small arrows*) and transverse fracture lines (*large arrows*). Fractures of long bones in children, particularly with different stages of healing, are very suggestive of a battered child. **B,** A lateral view of the lower extremity in the same child also reveals fractures of the distal fibula and tibia (*small arrows*) as well as a metaphyseal corner fracture (*large arrow*) of the distal femur. This latter fracture also is typical of child abuse. (*From Mettler EA, Jr: Essentials of Radiology, 2nd ed. Philadelphia, Saunders, 2005.*)

Table 48-1. RADIOGRAPHIC SERIES FOR SUSPECTED CHILD ABUSE

AP skull	AP humeri
Lateral skull	AP forearms
Lateral cervical spine	Oblique hands
AP thorax	AP femora
Lateral thorax	AP tibias
AP pelvis	AP feet
Lateral lumbar spine	

From Manaster BJ: Musculoskeletal Imaging—The Requisites, 3rd ed. Philadelphia, Mosby, 2006.

Table 48-2. SPECIFICITY OF RADIOLOGIC FINDINGS FOR CHILD ABUSE

High Specificity

Classic metaphyseal lesions

Rib fractures, especially posterior

Scapular fractures

Spinous process fractures

Sternal fractures

Moderate Specificity

Multiple fractures, especially bilateral

Fractures of different ages

Epiphyseal separations

Vertebral body fractures and subluxations

Digital fractures

Complex skull fractures

Common but Low Specificity

Subperiosteal new bone formation

Clavicular fractures

Long bone shaft fractures

Linear skull fractures

From Manaster BJ: Musculoskeletal Imaging—The Requisites, 3rd ed. Philadelphia, Mosby, 2006.

Definition: Chondrosarcoma is a malignant cartilaginous group of tumors with highly diverse features and behavior patterns that characteristically produce cartilage matrix from neoplastic tissue devoid of osteoid in which ossification, calcification, and myxoid changes can occur.

Incidence: Accounts for approximately 20% of all malignant bone tumors and is second only to osteosarcoma in frequency as a primary malignant bone tumor. Peak incidence for primary or central chondrosarcomas arising de novo are between 40 and 60 years of age and between 25 and 45 years of age for secondary or peripheral chondrosarcomas, most often from preexisting benign cartilage lesions such as solitary osteochondromas, enchondromatosis syndromes (Ollier's disease, Maffucci's syndrome, metachondromatosis), or multiple hereditary exostoses. About 90% of all chondrosarcomas are conventional chondrosarcomas and 10% are subtypes: de-differentiated, clear-cell, mesenchymal, and myxoid. The tumors are predominantly axial, most commonly involving the pelvis, proximal femur, and proximal humerus, with the metaphysis being the most common location of long bones. There is a slight male predominance but no racial predilection.

Clinical: The most common symptom at presentation is pain, which is often dull in character and present for months. Rarely, a palpable mass is present.

Diagnostic Studies: Radiography is essential for the initial diagnosis with the radiographic appearance of the chondrosarcoma frequently being diagnostic. X-ray findings demonstrate a lucent lesion frequently containing a pattern of calcification described as punctuate, popcorn, or comma-shaped. There is often an aggressive appearance with cortical destruction, periosteal reaction, and an occasional soft tissue mass. Computed tomography can be helpful in identifying matrix calcifications, endosteal scalloping, and cortical destruction and as a guide in percutaneous biopsies. Magnetic resonance imaging is best for clarifying extraosseous and intramedullary tumor extension.

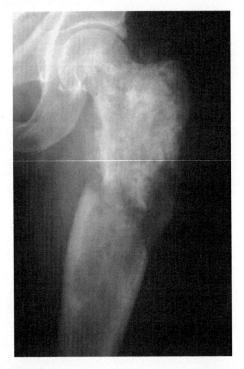

Fig. 49-1 De-differentiated chondrosarcoma. AP radiograph of the left femur showing a proximal femoral chondrosarcoma with an adjacent area of lytic destruction and pathologic fracture, due to associated de-differentiation to malignant fibrous histiocytoma. *(From Adam A, et al: Grainger & Allison's Diagnostic Radiology, 5th ed. Churchill Livingstone, 2008.)*

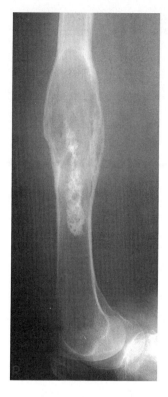

Fig. 49-2 Myxoid chondrosarcoma. Lateral radiograph of the femur showing a grade II myxoid chondrosarcoma. Bone expansion indicates a more aggressive behavior. *(From Adam A, et al: Grainger & Allison's Diagnostic Radiology, Philadelphia, Churchill Livingstone, 2008.)*

Histology: On gross examination, conventional chondrosarcomas appear smooth, hard, and lobulated. Microscopically, they are again lobulated, showing increased cellularity with hyperchromatic and pleomorphic binucleated or multinucleated malignant chondrocytes. Microscopic grading of conventional chondrosarcoma has prognostic value and is differentiated as follows:

- *Grade I (Well Differentiated):* Lesions have chondrocytes with small, round nuclei and occasional binucleated cells. Mitoses are absent.
- *Grade II (Moderately Differentiated):* Lesions are more cellular and have less matrix than grade I tumors. Chondrocyte nuclei are enlarged and hyperchromatic, and often demonstrate greater than one cell in a lacuna.
- *Grade III (Poorly Differentiated):* Chondrocytes are arranged in chords or clumps with less matrix, irregular vesicular or spindle-shaped nuclei, and diffuse mitoses.

About 10% of chondrosarcomas include de-differentiated (high-grade sarcoma adjacent to typical low-grade chondrosarcoma), clear-cell (low-grade malignancy with round cells with abundant clear cytoplasm), mesenchymal (high-grade malignancy with small round blue cells with islands of benign-appearing cartilage), and myxoid chondrosarcoma.

Treatment: Wide or radical resection is the mainstay of treatment. Due to cartilage being relatively avascular, cells survive transplantation easily allowing for local recurrence after intraoperative tumor contamination. Thus, care must be taken with resection. Wide resection without biopsy may be indicated to decrease the chance of tumor contamination. Chemotherapy has no role in the treatment of conventional chondrosarcoma. Radiotherapy efficacy is limited and is used only as a palliative measure for unresectable lesions.

Prognosis: The prognosis of patients with chondrosarcoma depends on the size, location, and histologic grade of the lesion. Low-grade lesions have an approximately 90% 10-year survival rate, compared with a 20% to 40% 10-year survival rate with a high-grade conventional chondrosarcoma.

Definition and Anatomy: The clavicle is an S-shaped bone that serves as an osseous strut to maintain shoulder width. Distally it is firmly attached to the scapula by the acromioclavicular (AC) and coracoclavicular (CC) ligaments. The supraclavicular nerve crosses over the clavicle and the ulnar nerve runs beneath the proximal third.

Incidence: Clavicular fractures account for approximately 5% of emergency department visits for fractures and are common fractures. They account for approximately 4% to 10% of all adult fractures and about 35% to 45% of all fractures that occur in the shoulder area.

Etiology: Direct blow—91%; indirect mechanisms (fall on outstretched arm)—9%.

Signs and Symptoms: Presentations include crepitus motion, ecchymosis, edema, tenderness, and perhaps deformity.

Clinical Findings: Neurovascular examination (proximity to brachial plexus/subclavian artery/vein) must be documented; skin examination shows tenting/severe swelling. Examination of sternoclavicular (SC) and AC joints should be performed; pneumothorax occurs in 3% of cases.

Diagnostic Studies: Radiographs in anteroposterior and 45-degree cephalic tilt are obtained. Computed tomography scans are helpful if the SC joint is involved.

Classification:
- *Group I:* 80%; middle third fractures
- *Group II:* 15%; distal third fractures
  - *Type I:* Nondisplaced between CC ligaments (conoid and trapezoid)
  - *Type II:* Displaced medial to CC ligaments
  - *Type III:* Nondisplaced occurs through AC joint
  - *Type IV:* Pediatric displaced fracture, periosteum attached to ligaments
- *Group III:* 5%; proximal third fractures
  - *Type I:* Minimally displaced ligaments intact
  - *Type II:* Displaced with ligaments ruptured
  - *Type III:* Involves articular surface of SC joint
  - *Type IV:* Epiphyseal separation may be confused with SC dislocation

Treatment: Most fractures can be treated with sling or figure-of-eight brace immobilization for 4 to 6 weeks. General surgical indications include neurovascular injury, open or severely tented skin, floating shoulder, or conditions not allowing patient to tolerate immobilization (seizure disorder).

Fracture-Specific Indications: Middle third clavicle fractures, severely angulated or shortened 2 cm or more; distal third type II fractures have a high rate of nonunion when treated closed.

Complications: Nonunion is most common with middle third fractures (75%), but the highest rate is in the type II distal clavicle. Nonunions occur due to inadequate period of immobilization, refracture, or marked initial displacement. Malunion may result in cosmetic problems. Neurovascular problems, including thoracic outlet syndrome, occur most frequently with greatly displaced fractures.

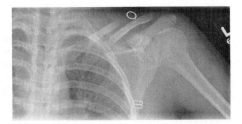

Fig. 50-1 A 13-year-old sustained a left clavicle fracture in a boating accident. Significant shortening at the fracture site ultimately warranted open reduction and internal fixation. *(From Auerbach PS: Wilderness Medicine, 5th ed. Philadelphia, Mosby, 2007.)*

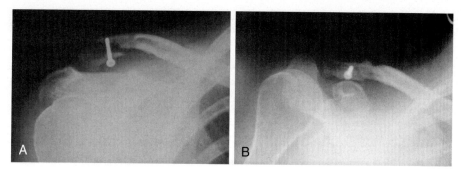

Fig. 50-2 *A,* This radiograph was obtained at presentation of a 40-year-old woman who was referred 26 months after open reduction and internal fixation of a distal clavicle fracture. The patient did not want any type of surgical intervention and therefore was treated with external electrical stimulation. *B,* A radiograph after 8 months of electrical stimulation shows solid bony union. *(From Browner BD: Skeletal Trauma: Basic Science, Management, and Reconstruction, 3rd ed. Philadelphia, Saunders, 2003.)*

Definition: Congenital clubfoot, talipes equinovarus, is a musculoskeletal deformity of the foot. Clubfeet are considered flexible if they are correctable without surgery and resistant if surgical release is required for correction.

Incidence: Clubfoot is present in approximately 1 in 1000 live births in the United States. The percentage of clubfoot varies greatly with ethnicity.

Age: Clubfoot is congenital. It is observable at birth and ultrasound may be used to diagnose it prenatally.

Gender: Clubfoot is more common in males with the male-to-female ratio at approximately 2.5:1.

Etiology and Pathophysiology: The exact cause of clubfoot is unproved; however, it has a genetic component. There are several theories including defective talus cartilaginous anlage, fetal developmental disturbances in the fibular stage, abnormal tendon insertions, neurogenic causes, and retracting fibrosis.

Clinical Presentation: Clubfoot may be bilateral or unilateral. The midfoot is adducted and supinated while the internally rotated heel is in varus and the ankle is in equinus. The foot is unable to reach dorsiflexion greater than 90 degrees. Clubfeet are usually shorter and wider than normal feet and may have creases at the midfoot and ankle. Clubfoot results in atrophy of the calf. Palpation reveals a small and soft heel and a talar neck that is laterally uncovered.

Pathology: Clubfoot consists of bone deformity and soft tissue contracture. It has several tissue abnormalities, including muscle and cartilage anomalies, bone primary germ plasm defects, and vascular abnormalities such as hypoplasia/absence of the anterior tibial artery.

Diagnostic Procedures: Radiographs can be used to determine the extent of deformities. For optimal radiographs, the foot should be weight bearing and placed in the best possible correction. However, incomplete ossification of bones in young patients as well as positioning problems of the foot may lead to radiographic difficulties.

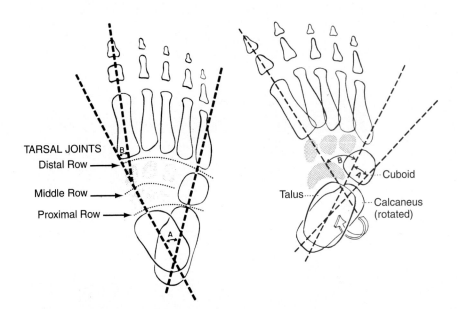

Fig. 51-1 Radiographic evaluation of clubfeet. Note the "parallelism" of the talus and calcaneus with a talocalcaneal angle (*A*) of <20 degrees and negative talus-first metatarsal angle (*B*) on the clubfoot side. (*From Simons GW: Analytical radiology of club feet. J Bone Joint Surg. 59-B:485-489, 1977.*)

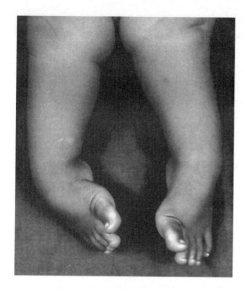

Fig. 51-2 Clinical picture demonstrating clubfoot deformity. *(From Kliegman RH: Nelson Textbook of Pediatrics, 18th ed. Philadelphia, Saunders, 2007.)*

Treatment: Clubfoot is initially treated by nonoperative means. Flexible clubfeet may be treated with serial manipulation, casting, and splinting in order to lengthen ligaments and tendons. If nonoperative treatment fails, surgery may be necessary. Surgical correction includes medial plantar release and posterior release. The subtalar joint should be internally rotated. Lateral release is often required to allow for the calcaneus to rotate outwardly.

Definition: Carpometacarpal (CMC) arthritis, or basal joint arthritis, is a form of osteoarthritis that affects the basilar joint at the base of the thumb where the metacarpal bone and the trapezium meet.
Incidence: Far more common in women than men. Usually occurs after age 40 years.
Etiology and Pathophysiology: Several small ligaments are responsible for the stability of the basilar joint. If these ligaments stretch or loosen, there is too much friction among the bones, resulting in arthritis.
Associations: Caused by chronic or acute trauma to the base of the thumb.
Signs and Symptoms: First, patients experience difficulty with pinching and grasping, such as opening car doors and turning keys. As the disease progresses, patients may avoid activities that cause the thumb pain, resulting in muscle weakening. This may lead to a tendency to lose grip or drop objects.
Diagnostic Studies: Edema and tenderness are indications of CMC arthritis. The physician may also perform a "grind test" in which the first metacarpal is grasped, pushed down, and rotated. Pain and a crunching sound indicate a positive test. Finally, x-rays are the best way to observe the status of the joint.
Micropathology: Stretching of ligaments and wearing of cartilage in the basilar joint.
Macropathology: Localized edema and tenderness. In some cases, bony spurs may develop around the joint. In severe cases, an inward collapse of the metacarpal may occur.
Treatment: Nonsteroidal anti-inflammatory drugs, cortisone injections, and/or splinting of the thumb joint may be helpful in early stages. In advanced stages, surgical options include ligament reconstruction and tendon interposition (LRTI), trapezium excision, CMC fusion, or prosthetic replacement.

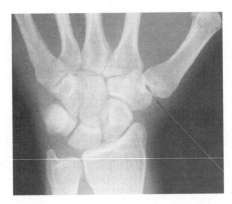

Fig. 52-1 Anteroposterior radiograph of the hand demonstrating needle placement into the first carpometacarpal joint. *(Reprinted with permission from Lennard TA. Pain Procedures in Clinical Practice, 2nd ed. Philadelphia, Hanley & Belfus, 2000.)*

History: Collagen means "glue producer" (*kolla* is Greek for "glue"), derived from the early process of boiling the skin and sinews of horses and other animals to obtain glue. The oldest glue in the world, carbon-dated as being more than 8000 years old, was found to be collagen, which was used as a protective lining on rope baskets and embroidered fabrics, and to hold utensils together.

Definition and Characteristics: Collagen is the main protein of connective tissue in animals and is the most abundant protein in mammals, making up about 25% of the total protein content. It is one of the long, fibrous structural proteins whose functions are different from those of globular proteins, such as enzymes. Tough bundles of collagen, called *collagen fibers,* are a major component of the extracellular matrix that supports most tissues and gives cells structure from the outside, but collagen is also found inside certain cells. Collagen has great tensile strength, and is the main component of cartilage, ligaments, tendons, bone, and teeth. Along with soft keratin, it is responsible for skin strength and elasticity, and its degradation leads to wrinkles that accompany aging. It strengthens blood vessels and plays a role in tissue development. It is also used in cosmetic surgery and burns surgery.

Composition and Structure: The tropocollagen, or "collagen molecule" subunit, is a rod about 300 nm long and 1.5 nm in diameter, made up of three polypeptide strands, each of which is a left-handed helix. These three left-handed helices are twisted together into a right-handed coiled coil, a triple helix, a cooperative quaternary structure stabilized by numerous hydrogen bonds. Tropocollagen subunits spontaneously self-assemble, with regularly staggered ends, into even larger arrays in the extracellular spaces of tissues. There is some covalent cross-linking within the triple helices, and there is a variable amount of covalent cross-linking between tropocollagen helices, forming the different types of collagen found in different mature tissues— similar to the situation found with the α-keratins in hair.

A distinctive feature of collagen is the regular arrangement of amino acids in each of the three chains of these collagen subunits. The sequence often follows the pattern Gly-X-Pro or Gly-X-Hyp,

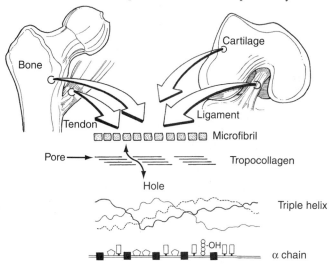

Fig. 53-1 Microstructure of collagen. Collagen is composed of microfibrils that are packed in a quarter-staggered fashion (tropocollagen). Note hole and pore regions for mineral deposition (for calcification). Tropocollagen, in turn, is made up of a triple helix of α chains of polypeptides. *(From Brinker MR, Miller MD: Fundamentals of Orthopaedics. Philadelphia, WB Saunders, 1999, with permission.)*

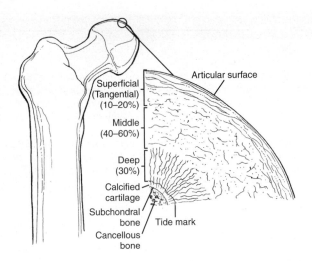

Fig. 53-2 Articular cartilage layers. *(From Brinker MR, Miller MD: Fundamentals of Orthopaedics. Philadelphia, WB Saunders, 1999, with permission.)*

where X is any of various other amino acid residues. Gly-Pro-Hyp occurs frequently. The triple helix tightens under tension, resisting stretching, making collagen inextensible.

Because glycine is the smallest amino acid, it plays a unique role in fibrous structural proteins. In collagen, glycine is required at every third position, because the assembly of the triple helix puts this residue at the interior (axis) of the helix, where there is no space for a larger side group than glycine's single hydrogen atom. For the same reason, the rings of the Pro and Hyp must point outward. These two amino acids thermally stabilize the triple helix—Hyp even more so than Pro.

In bone, entire collagen triple helices lie in a parallel, staggered array. Gaps measuring 40 nm between the ends of the tropocollagen subunits probably serve as nucleation sites for the deposition of long, hard, fine crystals of the mineral component, which is (approximately) hydroxyapatite, $Ca_5(PO_4)_3(OH)$, with some phosphate. It is in this way that certain kinds of cartilage turn into bone. Collagen gives bone its elasticity and contributes to fracture resistance.

In addition, major interest has been focused on endostatin, a fragment released from type XVIII collagen, which potently inhibits angiogenesis and tumor growth.

Types of Collagen: Collagen occurs in many places throughout the body and occurs in different forms known as types. There are more than 20 types of collagen; 13 are described in Table 53-1.

Histology: In staining, collagen is brightly eosinophilic (pink) in standard hematoxylin and eosin slides. The dyes methyl violet and methyl blue are used to stain the collagen in tissue samples, and immunohistochemical stains are available if required. The best stain for use in differentiating collagen from other fibers is Masson's trichrome stain.

Diseases: Collagen diseases commonly arise from genetic defects that affect the biosynthesis, assembly, post-translational modification, secretion, or other processes in the normal production of collagen. The most common genetic disease associated with collagen defects is osteogenesis imperfecta or "brittle bone disease." This results from decreased quantity or quality of type I collagen in the bone. Connective tissue diseases that are due to genetic inheritance include Marfan's syndrome and Ehlers-Danlos syndrome.

Other diseases of connective tissue not defined by gene abnormalities are characterized as a group by the presence of spontaneous overactivity of the immune system, resulting in the production of extra antibodies into the circulation. These include rheumatoid arthritis, polyarteritis nodosa, systemic lupus erythematosus, systemic sclerosis, and dermatomyositis.

Table 53-1. COLLAGEN TYPES

	Notes
I	Most abundant collagen of the human body; present in scar tissue, the end product when tissue heals by repair; found in tendons, the endomysium of myofibrils, and the organic part of bone
II	Articular cartilage and hyaline cartilage
III	Collagen of granulation tissue; produced quickly by young fibroblasts before the tougher type I collagen is synthesized; reticular fiber
IV	Basal lamina; eye lens
V	Most interstitial tissue; associated with type I; associated with placenta
VI	Most interstitial tissue; associated with type I
VII	Forms anchoring fibrils in dermal epidermal junctions
VIII	Some endothelial cells
IX	FACIT collagen, cartilage; associated with type II and XI fibrils
X	Hypertrophic and mineralizing cartilage
XI	Cartilage
XII	FACIT collagen, interacts with type I–containing fibrils, decorin, and glucosaminoglycans
XIII	Transmembrane collagen; interacts with integrin a1b1, fibronectin, and components of basement membranes, such as nidogen and perlecan

Deficiencies in other collagen types have been linked to other diseases, including the congenital muscular dystrophies. For example, Ulrich myopathy and Bethlam myopathy are caused by mutations in collagen VI. Mutations to genes coding for collagen type IV lead to Alport's syndrome. Also notable are cartilage pathologies, known as chondrodysplasia, and collagen type VII disease, which causes certain subtypes of epidermolysis bullosa. There are also cases of osteoporosis, arterial aneurysms, osteoarthrosis, and intervertebral disk disease.

Further characterization of mutations in additional collagen genes will add more diseases to this list. Mice with genetically engineered collagen mutations have proved valuable for defining the functions of various collagens and for studying many aspects of the related diseases.

Medical Uses: Collagen has been widely used in cosmetic surgery and certain skin substitutes for burn patients. The cosmetic use of collagens is declining because (1) there is a fairly high rate of allergic reactions, causing prolonged redness and requiring inconspicuous patch testing before cosmetic use; (2) most medical collagen is derived from cows, posing the risk of transmitting prion diseases such as bovine spongiform encephalopathy; and, (3) alternatives using the patient's own fat or hyaluronic acid are readily available. Collagens are employed in the construction of artificial skin substitutes used in the management of severe burns. These collagens may be bovine or porcine, used in combination with silicones, glycosaminoglycans, fibroblasts, growth factors, and other substances. Collagen is sold commercially as a joint mobility supplement (glucosamine, glucosamine and chondroitin).

Spina Bifida (Myelodysplasia):
- Disorder of incomplete spinal cord closure or secondary rupture.
  - *Spina Bifida Occulta:* Defect in the vertebral arch with confined cord and meninges
  - *Meningocele:* Sac without neural elements protruding through defect
  - *Myelomeningocele:* Protrusion of sac with neural elements
  - *Rachischisis:* Neural elements exposed with no covering
- Diagnosed in utero with increased alpha-fetoprotein; related to folate deficiency in utero.
- Level based on lowest functional level; the L4 level is key because it innervates the quadriceps, allowing independent ambulation.
- Sudden changes in function (scoliosis curvature, spasticity, new deficit, increase in urinary tract infections) can be related to tethered cord, hydrocephalus, or hydromyelia.
- Maintain a latex-free environment during surgery (there is a high incidence of sensitivity).
- Hip dislocation (most common at L3-4 level) common; fractures are common.

Torticollis:
- Congenital deformity resulting in contracture of the sternocleidomastoid muscle.
- Associated with other "packaging" disorders, such as hip dysplasia and metatarsus adductus.
- Cause remains uncertain; may be the result of an intrauterine compartment syndrome involving the sternocleidomastoid muscle compartment.
- *Treatment:* Most cases respond to passive stretching within the first month of life; surgery or Z-plasty may be required if torticollis persists beyond 1 year of life.

Syndactyly:
- Most common congenital hand anomaly.
- Classified as *simple* (absence of bony connections) or *complex* (bony connections) and *complete* (joining extends to tip of finger) or *incomplete* (joining stops short of tip of finger).
- Remember 5-15-50-30: Thumb-index (5%), index-middle (15%), middle-ring (50%), and ring-small (30%).
- Syndactylized digits are typically released at 1 year of age; both sides of the digit are never separated at the same time to protect circulation; full thickness skin grafts are always required.

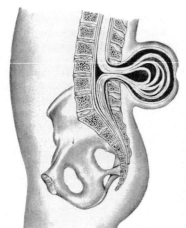
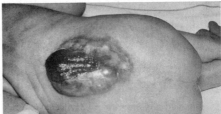

Fig. 54-1   Meningomyelocele. *(From Wong DL: Whaley's and Wong's Nursing Care of Infants and Children 5th ed, St Louis, 1995, Mosby.)*

- *Poland's Syndrome:* Rare, nongenetic; characterized by unilateral short fingers, simple complete syndactyly, hand hypoplasia, and ipsilateral absence of sternocostal head of pectoralis major.
- *Apert's Syndrome:* Acrocephaly, hypertelorism, bilateral complex syndactyly with symphalangism.

Clubfoot (Congenital Talipes Equinovarus):
- Forefoot adductus/supination; hindfoot equinus/varus.
- Talar neck deformity (medial and plantar deviation), medial rotation of calcaneus, medial displacement of navicular and cuboid.
- More common in males; one half of cases are bilateral.
- Associated with shortened and contracted muscles, joint capsules, ligaments, and fascia.
- Can be associated with hand anomalies (Streeter's dysplasia), diastrophic dwarfism, arthrogryposis, prune belly, tibial hemimelia, and myelomeningocele.
- *Radiographs:*
  - *Dorsiflexion Lateral View (Turco's):* Talocalcaneal angle is smaller than 35 degrees with a flat talar head
  - *Anteroposterior View:* Talocalcaneal angle is less than 20 degrees; a negative talus-first metatarsal angle also seen with clubfeet
  - *Parallelism of Talus and Calcaneus:* Both views
- *Treatment:* Ponsetti's method of serial casting is preferred.

Developmental Dysplasia of the Hip (DDH):
- Abnormal development or dislocation of the hip.
- *Capsular Laxity/Mechanical-Intrauterine Positioning:* Breech, females, first born, family history (risk factors)
- *Potential Obstructions to Obtaining a Concentric Reduction:* Iliopsoas tendon, pulvinar, contracted inferomedial hip capsule, and transverse acetabular ligament.
- Diagnosed with Ortolani's test and Barlow's test; limited hip abduction (later); positive Galeazzi sign (foreshortening of femur); asymmetrical gluteal folds; Trendelenburg stance (older).
- *Radiographs:* Acetabular index (normal < 25 degrees), Perkins' line, Shenton's line.
- *Dynamic Ultrasound:* Especially in young children before ossification of femoral head.
- *Treatment:*
  - Younger than 6 months, Pavlick harness
  - 12 to 18 months with failed closed reduction, open reduction
  - 18 months and older, open reduction
  - Older than 2 years, osteotomies are indicated to achieve and maintain early concentric reduction

Congenital Scoliosis:
- Most common congenital spinal disorder; progression risk depends on vertebral morphology.
- Fully segmented hemivertebra (normal disk spaces on both sides) results in higher risk of progression.
- Unsegmented hemivertebra (fused above and below) results in lower risk.
- Incarcerated hemivertebra (within lateral margins of vertebrae) results in better prognosis than an unincarcerated hemivertebra.
- Block vertebra (bilateral failure of segmentation) results in best prognosis.
- *Worst Prognosis:* Unilateral unsegmented bar with a contralateral, fully segmented hemivertebra; indication for surgery at presentation.
- *Treatment:* Posterior fusion in situ is gold standard of treatment for most progressive curves; bracing is largely ineffective. Avoid crankshaft phenomenon (continued anterior spinal growth).

Definition: Compartment syndrome (CS) is a condition in which the perfusion pressure falls below the tissue pressure in a closed anatomic space, with subsequent compromise of circulation and function of the tissues. Each muscle and muscle group is enclosed in a compartment bound by rigid walls of bone and fascia. The compartments of the lower extremity are prone to developing elevated compartment pressures. Exercise-induced CS is the result of elevated compartment pressure that leads to ischemia of the muscles or nerves.

Etiology: In 45% of cases, CS is caused by tibial fractures. Other causes include long bone fractures, vascular injuries, bleeding in enclosed spaces, intramuscular injections, drug overdose, or a tight cast dressing.

Incidence: Acute CS varies depending on the inciting event. In 1981, DeLee and Stiehl found that 6% of patients with open tibia fractures developed CS, whereas only 1.2% of patients with closed tibia fractures developed CS.

Age-Gender: Young adult males are especially at risk due to their muscle bulk and noncompliant fascia.

Race: There is no evidence of differences between the races.

Clinical Presentation: On a physical evaluation, the evidence of trauma and gross deformity should alert the physician to the possible development of CS. Compartment pressures greater than 40 mm Hg or a differential of less than 30 mm Hg with the diastolic is indicative of possible CS.

Pathophysiology: CS develops after elevated compartment pressure causes muscle and nerve ischemia. When fluid is introduced into the compartment, the tissue pressure increases and raises the venous pressure.

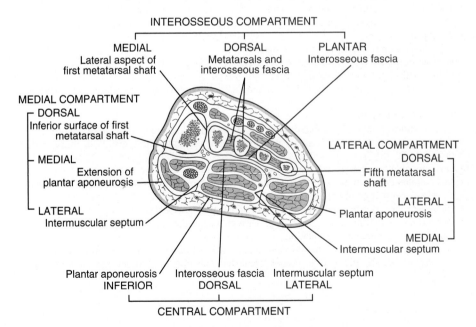

Fig. 55-1 Compartments of the foot. Similar detail can be seen with magnetic resonance imaging. *(Redrawn with permission from AAOS. Orthopaedic Knowledge Update: Foot and Ankle. Rosemont, IL, American Academy of Orthopaedic Surgeons, 1994, p. 263; from Browner BD: Skeletal Trauma: Basic Science, Management, and Reconstruction, 3rd ed. Philadelphia, Saunders, 2003.)*

Signs and Symptoms: Patients with CS often have pain, a sensation of tightness, and weakness of the muscles involved. Pain on passive stretch is the most sensitive sign. Loss of pulses, sensation, or motor function occurs late.

Treatment: Surgical treatment consists of an emergent fasciotomy (compartment release) with subsequent orthopedic reduction or fracture stabilization and vascular repair, if needed. The goal of decompression is restoration of muscle perfusion within 6 hours. Although several surgical techniques have been described, the double incision fasciotomy of the lower leg is the most common approach. To minimize soft tissue injury, especially in the setting of fracture/CS, some surgeons prefer a single incision approach. Regardless of the approach used, adequate decompression of all compartments is paramount.

Definition: A rare affliction resulting from trauma to an extremity with pain that is disproportionate in intensity and duration.
- Type I: Formerly known as Reflex Sympathetic Dystrophy (RSD). Diagnosed when pain is present but no identifiable nerve injury can be found. However, this does not mean that no nerve injury has occurred.
- Type II: Formerly known as Causalgia. Diagnosed when a nerve injury can be identified that leads to the pain symptoms. The symptoms are the same as in Type 1.

Incidence: Current studies indicate an incidence rate of 26.2 per 100,000 patients annually, with a higher prevalence in postmenopausal women (50 to 70 years of age), and more commonly found in the hand than the foot. Twenty percent of cases are the result of surgical trauma; of these, most are orthopedic procedures.

Etiology: The most common cause is a sprain or fracture, although it may also follow other trauma such as surgery, myocardial infarction, cerebrovascular accident, electric shock, or even phlebotomy. The trauma is thought to result in an elevated adrenergic sensitivity by the nociceptors in the affected extremity. The circulating or locally secreted sympathetic neurotransmitters in turn trigger the excessive radiating pain. A recent study has shown that depression is not a precursor to CRPS but a potential result.

Symptoms and Course: Symptoms of CRPS are not limited locally to the point of trauma; instead they radiate distally from this point. The following is a list of symptoms organized by the phases over which they progress. The first phase is marked by burning or aching pain, and hypersensitivity to thermal or mechanical stimulation. Other symptoms include edema, hyperhidrosis, mild to moderate osteopenia, and a red or slightly cyanotic appearance. The second phase occurs at approximately 3 months following the precipitating event and is primarily characterized by constant pain; intolerance to cold temperatures, clothing, and even wind; thin, dry, and glossy skin; changes in nail and hair production; indurated tissue; joint motion limitation; localized vasomotor instability; moderate to severe osteopenia; and a decrease in temperature in comparison with the contralateral extremity. The

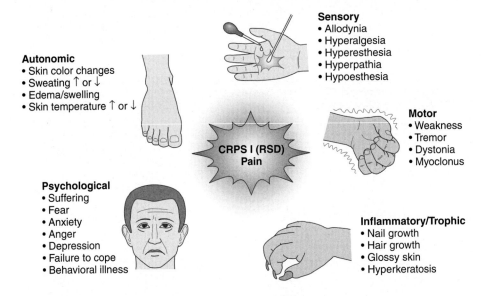

Fig. 56-1   Clinical features of complex regional pain syndrome type I (reflex sympathetic dystrophy) (CRPS I [RSD]). *(From Rutherford RB: Vascular Surgery, 6th ed. Philadelphia, Saunders, 2005.)*

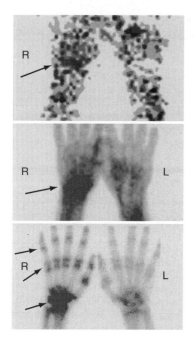

Fig. 56-2 Reflex sympathetic dystrophy in a patient with a history of right wrist fracture. Three-phase bone scintigraphy shows increased tracer delivery to the right distal upper extremity diffusely (*arrow*) on flow (*top*) and blood pool (*middle*) images. Delayed images (*bottom*) reveal diffuse abnormal uptake in the wrist (*arrow*) and increased activity in a juxta-articular distribution (*arrowheads*). (*From DeLee D, Drez D: DeLee and Drez's Orthopaedic Sports Medicine, 2nd ed. Philadelphia, Saunders, 2003.*)

third and final stage of CRPS generally begins at approximately 6 months following the initial trauma. Symptoms in this stage include thinning of the skin; atrophy; constant diffuse pain; extreme nocturnal pain; decreased temperature in affected area; hyperhidrosis; continued intolerance of cold temperatures, clothing, and wind; significant decrease in joint mobility; and severe osteopenia.

Diagnostic Studies: Diagnostic studies are limited primarily to thermal imaging, radiographs, and electromyography/nerve conduction of the affected and contralateral extremities for comparison, and are not sufficient for diagnosis. Proper diagnosis is complicated and generally lengthy in duration due first to the many other possible origins of the symptoms, second to the frequent misconception that the pain is psychophysiologic in origin, and third to the frequency with which these patients are referred to other specialists before being seen by a pain specialist who is most likely to make the accurate diagnosis. Proper diagnosis depends on the observation of symptoms from three of the four following categories: positive sensory abnormalities, vascular abnormalities, edema and sweating abnormalities, and motor and trophic changes.

Treatment: If diagnosed during the first phase, the treatment is fairly conservative, including physical therapy consisting of active and passive exercises combined with a mild anxiolytic. Or opioids, in conjunction with corticosteroids, have demonstrated varying degrees of success. In more resilient cases, sympathetic blocks combined with rigorous physical therapy have been shown to have varying degrees of effectiveness. In cases in which relief is only temporary, permanent results may be achieved with a sympathectomy. Prognosis for advanced CRPS is quite poor.

Definition: Syndactyly, also known as webbed fingers, occurs when fingers fail to separate, resulting in joined fingers. Polydactyly occurs when an extra separation occurs, leading to development of extra fingers.

Mechanism: Both of these disorders are a result of differentiation errors during development of the embryo. This differentiation usually occurs around the seventh week of development.

Incidence: Both syndactyly and polydactyly are the most common types of congenital abnormalities of the hand. Syndactyly occurs at a rate of 1 per 2000 to 2500 births. The actual incidence of polydactyly is not known, because birth defect registries do not keep track.

Gender: Syndactyly occurs in males twice as often as in females.

Race: Polydactyly is 10 times more likely to occur in African American children than in white children.

Etiology/Pathophysiology: Both disorders are believed to be familial with variable penetrance.

Associations: Syndactyly is particularly associated with craniofacial syndromes such as Apert's syndrome or acrocephalosyndactyly; Poland's syndrome and constriction band syndromes are also associated. Polydactyly is associated with several dozen syndromes, some of which are Mohr's syndrome, Pallister-Hall syndrome, and basal cell nevus syndrome.

Classification: Syndactyly is classified according to the severity of the union. Simple syndactyly occurs when the fingers are joined by only soft tissue. This can take the form of incomplete (union does not extend to fingertips) or complete (union extends to end of fingertips). Complex syndactyly occurs when the bones of the fingers are joined at the distal end. Complicated syndactyly occurs when the union is proximal to the hand. Polydactyly is classified into preaxial, central, and postaxial types. Preaxial involves the duplication of the first finger. Central involves the duplication of the second through fourth fingers. Postaxial involves the duplication of the fifth finger.

Diagnostic Studies: X-ray imaging is often necessary to determine extent of union in syndactyly.

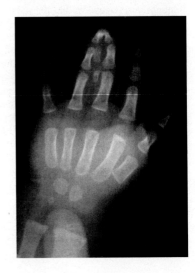

Fig. 57-1 Simple syndactyly. Fingers are bridged only by skin and other soft tissues. Radiograph. Note angular deformity of ring finger. *(From Canale ST, Beaty JH: Campbell's Operative Orthopaedics, 11th ed. Philadelphia, Mosby, 2007.)*

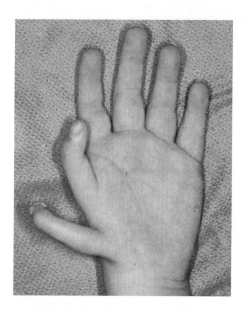

Fig. 57-2 A congenital hand anomaly: Wassel type VI polydactyly. *(From Townsend CM Jr: Sabiston Textbook of Surgery, 18th ed. Philadelphia, Saunders, 2007.)*

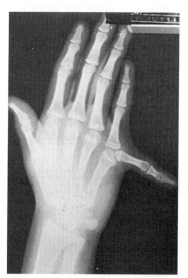

Fig. 57-3 Type 2 postaxial polydactyly: partial duplication of digit, including osseous structures. *(From Canale ST, Beaty JH: Campbell's Operative Orthopaedics, 11th ed. Philadelphia, Mosby, 2007.)*

Treatment: In both cases, surgery is the only option; however, in the case of polydactyly, often surgery is chosen for cosmetic and psychological reasons. In syndactyly, the earlier the release occurs, the better the outcome. The surgeries must also be timed according to growth rates of fingers. In simple syndactyly and complex syndactyly, the incisions are made in a zigzag pattern to minimize the chance of scars interfering with growth. Skin grafts are then used to cover any areas that lack skin following separation. Surgery in a patient with complicated syndactyly is challenging, depending on the location of neurovascular structures and tendons.

Definition: To agree, to give approval, assent, or permission. The process by which a fully informed patient can participate in choices about his or her health care. "Consent" originates from the legal and ethical rights of the patient to direct what happens to his or her body and from the ethical duty of the physician to involve the patient in his or her health care decisions.

In order for an informed consent to be valid, every adult must be considered completely (of sound mind) able to make their own decisions regarding what is to be done with their own body. With this understanding, the informed consent process should be seen as inviting the patient to participate in his or her own health care participation. The physician is obligated to have a discussion with the patient about what will take place during the rest of the process with the surgery or procedure.

Most health care institutions have policies that state which health interventions require a signed consent form. For example, surgery, anesthesia, and other invasive procedures are usually in this category. These signed consent forms are really a culmination of a dialogue required to foster the patient's informed participation in the clinical decision to have surgery.

In most cases, it is clear whether or not patients are competent to make their own decisions. Occasionally, it is not so clear. Patients are under a huge amount of stress during their illness and can experience anxiety, depression, and fear. The stress associated with illness should not necessarily preclude one from participating in one's own care. However, precautions should be taken to ensure that the patient does have the capacity to make a good decision. There are several standards to making good decisions. Generally, the health care worker should assess the patient's ability to understand his or her own situation and to understand the risks associated with the surgery or procedure. When it is unclear, a psychiatric consultation may be helpful.

If the patient is incapacitated or incompetent to make decisions, a surrogate decision maker must speak for the patient. There must be a specific hierarchy of appropriate decision makers defined by law to make the patient's decisions; this is called *power of attorney*.

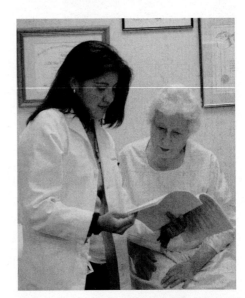

Fig. 58-1 Consent between a patient and doctor.

In an emergency situation, there is such a thing as *presumed consent*. In this case, the patient must be unconscious or incompetent and have no surrogate decision maker to make decisions at that particular time. In general, the patient's presence in the hospital ward or the intensive care unit does not represent implied consent to all treatments and procedures. The patient's wishes and values may be quite different from the physician's. Although the principle of respect for the person obligates health care workers to do their best to include the patient in the health care decisions that affect his or her life and body, the principle of beneficence may require one to act on the patient's behalf when the patient's life is at stake.

Corticosteroids have an extraordinary ability to prevent or suppress inflammation, whether the insulting agent is infectious, immunologic, or mechanical. Corticosteroids include the primary endogenous glucocorticoid, cortisol, and exogenous therapeutic agents such as prednisone and methylprednisolone.

The peak effects are seen within 4 to 6 hours. The durability of effect is related to the solubility of the compound. It is believed that corticosteroids induce their effects on the cell through a glucocorticoid receptor in the cytoplasm. The steroid-receptor complex translocates into the nucleus of the cell, where it attaches to DNA and causes transcription of specific messenger RNA, which sythesizes proteins that mediate glucocorticoid activity. Mediators result in neutrophilia, through accelerated release from the bone marrow into the circulation and inhibition of leukocyte endothelial transit. Corticosteroids inhibit the ability of neutrophils to adhere to vessel walls, which is an essential step in the migration of cells from the circulation into the tissue. It is believed that this process is mediated by the inhibition of the transcription of mRNA encoding endothelial-leukocyte adhesion molecule 1 (ELAM-1) and intercellular adhesion molecule 1 (ICAM-1).

Corticosteroids cause monocytopenia by blocking responses to chemotactic factors and MAF. This results in decreased phagocytosis, pyrogen production, and secretion of collagenase, elastase, and plasminogen activator, resulting in an overall decrease in tissue destruction. Lymphocytopenia occurs mostly due to redistribution of T and B cells to lymphoid compartments. Interestingly, corticosteroids also inhibit interleukin (IL)-2 and IL-1. IL-2 is produced by T cells to promote proliferation. IL-1 is related to prostaglandin production, which is also stunted by reducing the availability of fatty acid precursors (arachidonic acid).

Intra-articular and Extra-articular Injections in Orthopedics

Literature and double-blind trials have shown that repeated intra-articular corticosteroid injections into the knee for relief of osteoarthritis and rheumatoid arthritis symptoms are safe and effective for up to 2 years. Whereas no differences were shown in joint space narrowing, corticosteroids do improve range of motion and reduce pain. Injections have also been shown to improve symptoms of overuse syndromes (tendinitis, bursitis, ligament sprain, tenosynovitis), acute athletic injuries, and nerve compression. The generally accepted recommendation for frequency of intra-articular injections is no more than once every 3 months into the same joint.

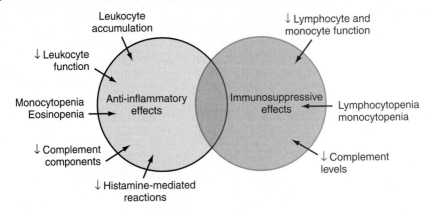

Fig. 59-1 Corticosteroid effects.

In rat models of rheumatoid arthritis, corticosteroids were shown to decrease cartilage oligomeric matrix protein (COMP), a candidate biomarker for the monitoring of cartilage destruction. The picture for osteoarthritis is less clear because inflammation is only a component of the underlying disease; however, evidence from animal models shows modifying effects (reduction in osteophyte size and cartilage proteolytic activity). Many believe wear macromolecules and calcium crystals initiate a process that activates the synovium to release inflammatory factors. IL-1 has been implicated due to its association with degradative enzymes (collagenases and stromelysin), prostaglandins, and plasminogen activators. It is also important to recognize that relief of symptoms of osteoarthritis may also stem from the reduced production of inflammation related to pain. Bradykinin and histamine directly stimulate afferent nociceptive nerve fibers.

COX-1 and COX-2: The body produces several different forms of cyclooxygenase (COX), including COX-1 and COX-2. COX-1 is primarily a constitutively expressed enzyme with important roles in gastrointestinal mucosa protection, platelet aggregation, renal function, pain, clotting, and protecting the stomach, whereas COX-2 is an enzyme that is primarily upregulated in response to tissue damage during inflammation. The inhibition of COX-1 is therefore undesirable, whereas the inhibition of COX-2 has a desirable effect. Drugs such as celecoxib (Celebrex) are now commercially available for the treatment of rheumatoid arthritis, osteoarthritis, and postoperative pain.

COX-1 is now known to be present in most tissues as the "housekeeper" enzyme. COX-2 is inducible by inflammation. It is not present at baseline but increases in response to inflammation, including arthritis. It has 60% homology with COX-1. Both have the same affinity to convert arachidonic acid to prostaglandin.

COX-2 to COX-1 Ratio: This concept provides a mechanism to assess the balance of inhibition of the inducible COX-2. Analyses of these ratios and side effects of the older, conventional nonsteroidal anti-inflammatory drugs (NSAIDs) show that the lower the ratio, the lower the COX-1 inhibition and the lower the overall side-effect profile. Celecoxib, for example, is 375-fold more selective for COX-2 compared with COX-1.
NSAIDs vs. COX: Conventional NSAIDs inhibit both isoforms of COX; hence, the inflammatory process is limited and the previously mentioned side effects arise. Celecoxib, as a selective COX-2-inhibitor, primarily interferes with inflammation and has limited influence on the gastrointestinal mucosa, platelet aggregation, and renal function.

In addition, the newer COX-2 inhibitor drugs, such as rofecoxib (Vioxx) and celecoxib, are much more active against COX-2 than COX-1.

COX-2 inhibitors are effective against inflammation and seem to avoid damage to the gastrointestinal tract. Unfortunately, they increase the risk of blood clots, which can cause heart attacks and strokes because they do not block the synthesis of thromboxane A2 by platelets (which contain only COX-1). This means that people depending on NSAIDs for their heart-protective effects must monitor any use of COX-2 inhibitors carefully. In fact, because of the apparent increased risk of heart attacks and strokes, the manufacturer of Vioxx removed it from the market in 2004.

"Preferential" COX-2 Inhibitors: Such drugs are not COX specific. Problems in classifying drugs as selective agents resulted in the standardization of the science of COX-2. Discussion as to what constituted true COX selectivity has resulted in a classification of the drugs into specific versus preferential COX-2 inhibitors.
Corticosteroids: A class of steroid hormones that are closely related to cortisol and that are produced in the adrenal cortex. Corticosteroids are involved in a wide range of physiologic systems such as stress and immune response, regulation of inflammation, carbohydrate metabolism, protein catabolism, blood electrolyte levels, and behavior.
Role of Cortisol: Plays an important part in controlling salt and water balance in the body and regulating carbohydrate, fat, and protein metabolism. When the body becomes stressed, the pituitary gland at the base of the brain releases adrenocorticotropic hormone, which stimulates the adrenals to produce cortisol. The extra cortisol allows the body to cope with stress, such as that produced by infection, trauma, surgery, or emotional problems.
How They Work: Corticosteroids act on the immune system by blocking the production of substances that trigger allergic and inflammatory actions, such as prostaglandins. However, they also impede the function of white blood cells, which destroy foreign bodies and help keep the immune system functioning properly. The interference with white blood cell function yields a side effect of increased susceptibility to infection.

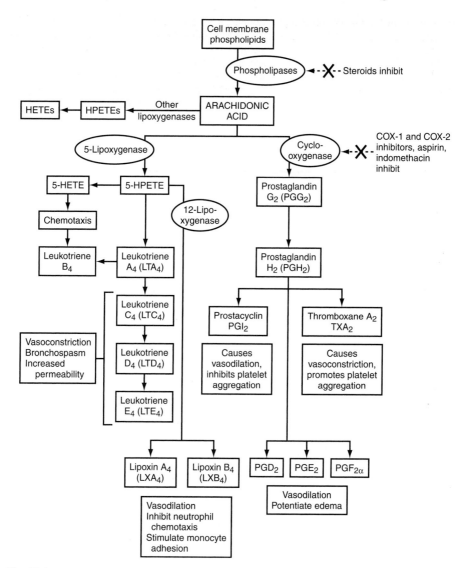

Fig. 60-1 Generation of arachidonic acid metabolites and their roles in inflammation. The molecular targets of action of some anti-inflammatory drugs are indicated by an X. COX, cyclooxygenase; HETE, hydroxyeicosatetraenoic acid; HPETE, hydroperoxyeicosatetraenoic acid. *(From Kumar V, et al: Robbins and Cotran Pathologic Basis of Disease, 7th ed. Philadelphia, Saunders, 2005.)*

Conditions They Treat: Corticosteroids are widely used for many conditions. They are also used to control inflammation of the joints and organs in diseases such as rheumatoid arthritis, systemic lupus erythematosus, ankylosing spondylitis, juvenile arthritis, inflammatory bowel disease, dermatomyositis, polymyositis, mixed connective tissue disease, Behçet's disease, polymyalgia rheumatica, scleroderma systemic sclerosis, giant cell arteritis, and vasculitis. Corticosteroids are not used systemically for osteoarthritis, although they are sometimes used as a local injection into an affected joint.

Side Effects and Adverse Reactions: The potent effect of corticosteroids can result in serious side effects that mimic Cushing's disease, a malfunction of the adrenal glands resulting in an overproduction of cortisol. The list of potential side effects includes increased appetite and weight gain, deposits of fat in the chest, face, upper back, and stomach, water and salt retention leading to swelling and edema, high blood pressure, diabetes, slowed healing of wounds, osteoporosis, cataracts, muscle weakness, thinning of the skin, increased susceptibility to infection, stomach ulcers, increased sweating, and psychological problems.

Definition: Coxa vara exists when the femoral neck shaft angle is less than 120 to 135 degrees.
Incidence: Congenital coxa vara is present in 1 per 13,000 to 25,000 births. Unilateral coxa vara occurs more commonly than bilateral coxa vara.
Age: Coxa vara may be congenital, developmental, or acquired.
Etiology/Pathophysiology: The cause of congenital coxa vara is unknown. However, it is commonly believed to be caused by a primary ossification defect resulting in varus deformity. Coxa vara may also be caused by trauma, infection, metabolic abnormalities, and as a sequela of Legg-Perthes disease.
Clinical Presentation: The main symptom of coxa vara is an abnormal but painless gait. A Trendelenburg limp is sometimes associated with unilateral coxa vara, whereas a waddling gait is often associated with bilateral coxa vara. Patients with coxa vara often have limb length discrepancy, a prominent greater trochanter, and weak abductors. Patients may also have femoral retroversion or decreased anteversion.
Pathology: Congenital coxa vara has decreased metaphyseal bone due to abnormal proximal femoral chondrocyte maturation and ossification. In congenital coxa vara, the inferior medial area of the femoral neck may be fragmented. There is progressive varus deformity, overgrowth of the trochanter, and shortening of the femoral neck.
Diagnostic Procedure: Coxa vara is evident through radiography, magnetic resonance imaging (MRI), and computed tomography (CT) scans. Symptoms of coxa vara visible through radiography are as follows: a reduced femoral shaft angle, a small and flat femoral head in retroversion or decreased anteversion, a shallow and oval acetabulum, coxa brevis, and a physeal plate with an overly vertical orientation. Radiographs of congenital coxa vara have a lucency shaped like the letter Y, representing the abnormal ossification. Radiographs can be used to determine the Hilgenreiner epiphyseal angle (HEA), which is made by the oblique line through the proximal femoral capital physes and the horizontal Hilgenreiner line through the triradiate cartilages. CT scans may be used to determine the degree of femoral anteversion or retroversion. Through MRI, it is possible to visualize the growth plate, which may be widened in coxa vara.
Treatment: Nonoperative treatment is usually insufficient for coxa vara; consequently, surgery is often needed. Surgery is recommended for patients who limp and have an HEA of more than 60 degrees as well as for patients with an HEA of 45 to 60 degrees with progression of deformity. Surgery attempts to correct the neck shaft angle to at least 140 degrees, as well as correct the abductor and ossify the femoral neck. Both intertrochanteric and subtrochanteric osteotomies often provide satisfactory results. It is recommended that an adductor tenotomy be performed along with the osteotomy.

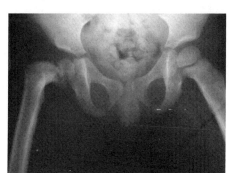

Fig. 61-1 Femoral dysplasia. Right coxa vara deformity. *(From Adam A, et al: Grainger & Allison's Diagnostic Radiology, 5th ed. Philadelphia, Churchill Livingstone, 2008.)*

Definition: Gout and pseudogout are the two most common crystalline-induced arthropathies. Lowenhook described this disorder in 1600.

Calcium Pyrophosphate Crystal Deposition Disease: A general term for a disorder characterized by the deposition of calcium pyrophosphate dihydrate (CPPD) crystals in or around joints.

Pseudogout: A term applied to one of the clinical patterns that may be associated with CPPD crystal deposition disease. This pattern, characterized by intermittent acute attacks of arthritis, simulates the findings of gout.

Chondrocalcinosis: A term reserved for pathologically or radiologically evident calcification of hyaline articular cartilage or fibrocartilage. In some cases, this calcification may not indicate deposits of CPPD crystals but accumulations of other crystals.

Pyrophosphate Arthropathy: A term used to describe a peculiar pattern of structural joint damage occurring in CPPD crystal deposition disease simulating, in many ways, degenerative joint disease but characterized by distinctive features.

Etiology: Gout is a disease of abnormal purine metabolism, resulting in precipitation and deposition of monosodium urate crystals. Pseudogout is an inflammatory response to deposition of CPPD crystals in joints.

Association: Some medications that increase serum uric acid, purine-rich foods, trauma, and alcohol, may be associated with gouty arthropathy. Pseudogout has been associated with metabolic disorders as well as with aging and trauma.

Incidence: Gout affects 2.7 out of every 1000 adults in the United States (20% in patients with a family history of gout). The annual incidence of acute attacks of pseudogout arthritic pain and swelling is about 1.3 per 1000 adults.

Age: The typical age at onset for crystalline-induced arthropathies is in the third and fourth decades.

Gender: For gout, the male-to-female ratio is 9:1. For pseudogout, the male-to-female ratio is 1.5:1.

Symptoms:
Gout: A sudden painful attack, usually in the metatarsophalangeal joint of the great toe, is the most common presentation (podagra). Other common sites of gouty arthritis are the ankle, wrist, and knee.

Pseudogout: Most commonly affects knee joint, although it may also affect other joints such as the wrist, ankle, and shoulder.

Signs: Signs of inflammation, such as redness, swelling, and tenderness are seen in the involved joint. It is usually monarticular. Extra-articular deposits of monosodium urate crystals, known as tophi, may be seen along tendons or on the ear helix and bursae.

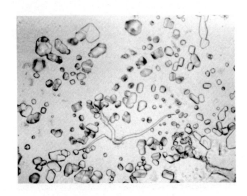

Fig. 62-1 Smear preparation of synovial fluid containing calcium pyrophosphate crystals. *(From Kumar V, et al: Robbins and Cotran Pathologic Basis of Disease, 7th ed. Philadelphia, Saunders, 2005.)*

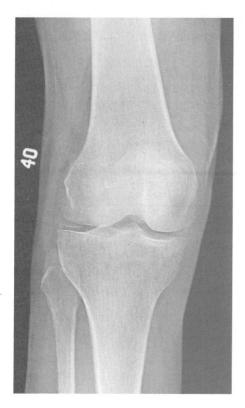

Fig. 62-2 Calcium pyrophosphate dihydrate crystal deposition disease producing chondrocalcinosis. Linear calcification is present within the lateral meniscus. *(From Firestein GS: Kelley's Textbook of Rheumatology, 8th ed. Philadelphia, Saunders, 2008.)*

Radiology:
Gout: Soft tissue enlargement, bony erosions, extensive articular destruction.
Pseudogout: Intra-articular calcification; rarely, joint destruction over a long period.

Micropathology:
Gout: Deposition of needle-shaped, negative birefringent monosodium urate crystals in the joint.
Pseudogout: Deposition of often rhomboidal shaped, weakly positive birefringent CPPD crystals in joints.

Treatment:
Gout: Acute attacks are treated with hydration, rest, indomethacin, and colchicine. Prevention of recurrent attacks includes allopurinol. Surgical intervention is warranted in severely destroyed joints with large amounts of debris and tophi.
Pseudogout: Treatment is with rest, hydration, and oral nonsteroidal anti-inflammatory drugs.

Sequelae: Severe joint destruction over a long period of time may necessitate surgical care. Pseudogout usually does not result in joint destruction.

Definition: Damage control orthopedics is the provisional management of orthopedic injuries in the multiple-injured patient that allows for stabilization of the patient's overall physiology. The goal is to avoid the "second hit" of major surgery during the acute systemic inflammatory response to trauma. This usually involves external fixation with conversion to definitive fixation (usually IM or plate fixation) at a later date.

Pathophysiology: The inflammatory response can be stimulated by the "first hit," or it may be primed, allowing a lesser proinflammatory event (the "second hit") to activate a pathologic systemic inflammatory response. Activation of polymorphonuclear leukocytes (PMNs) via endothelial release of cytokines has been related to ARDS and multiorgan failure, and HLA-DR antigen expression is related to resistance to serious infection after blunt trauma. Reamed IM nailing of femur fractures has been shown to increase the systemic inflammatory response, and reamed nailing has been shown to suppress HLA-DR antigen expression compared with unreamed nailing, presumably increasing the risk of systemic infection.

Resuscitation Measures

- Occult hypoperfusion is defined as hemodynamically normal, with a serum lactate level greater than 2.5 mmol/L.
- Preoperative hypoperfusion has been related to increased postoperative complications and infections and increased intensive care unit costs in patients treated with "early surgical stabilization" of femur fractures.

Table 63-1. GLASGOW COMA SCALE

A. Eye Opening	
Spontaneous	4
To voice	3
To pain	2
None	1
B. Verbal Response	
Oriented	5
Confused	4
Inappropriate words	3
Incomprehensible sounds	2
None	1
C. Motor Response	
Obeys commands	6
Localized pain	5
Withdraw to pain	4
Flexion to pain	3
Extension to pain	2
None	1
Total GCS Points (A + B + C)	3–15

From Browner BD: Skeletal Trauma: Basic Science, Management, and Reconstruction, 3rd ed. Philadelphia, Saunders, 2003.

Table 63-2. ABBREVIATED INJURY SCORE

Abbreviated Injury Score Examples	Score
Head	
Crush of head or brain	6
Brain stem contusion	5
Epidural hematoma (small)	4
Face	
Optic nerve laceration	2
External carotid laceration (major)	3
Le Fort III fracture	3
Neck	
Crushed larynx	5
Pharynx hematoma	3
Thyroid gland contusion	1
Thorax	
Open chest wound	4
Aorta, intimal tear	4
Esophageal contusion	2
Myocardial contusion	3
Pulmonary contusion (bilateral)	4
Two or three rib fractures	2
Abdomen and Pelvic Contents	
Bladder perforation	4
Colon transection	4
Liver laceration >20% blood loss	3
Retroperitoneal hematoma	3
Splenic laceration—major	4
Spine	
Incomplete brachial plexus	2
Complete spinal cord C4 or below	5
Herniated disc with radiculopathy	3
Vertebral body compress >20%	3
Upper Extremity	
Amputation	3
Elbow crush	3
Shoulder dislocation	2
Open forearm fracture	3

Abbreviated Injury Score Examples	Score
Lower Extremity	
Amputation	
Below knee	3
Above knee	4
Hip dislocation	2
Knee dislocation	2
Femoral shaft fracture	3
Open pelvic fracture	3
External	
Hypothermia 31°C–30°C	3
Electrical injury with myonecrosis	3
Second-degree to third-degree burns—	
20%–29% body surface area	3

Table 63-2. ABBREVIATED INJURY SCORE—cont'd

Trauma Scoring Systems

- Glasgow Coma Score
  - Sum of three scores (eye opening, verbal response, motor response)
  - Score from 3 to 15 (<8 = severe injury, 9 to 12 = moderate, 13 to 15 = minor)
- Injury Severity Score (ISS)
  - Sum of squares of three highest AIS regional scores
  - Score from 1 to 75; score greater than 60 usually fatal
- Abbreviated Injury Score
  - From 0 to 6 in six body regions
  - Score of 6 in any one region is automatic ISS of 75
  - More than one injury to one body region does not increase the ISS
  - Body regions: head and neck, face, chest, abdominal or pelvic contents, extremities or pelvic girdle, external

Criteria That Suggest Damage Control Orthopedics

1. Polytrauma and ISS greater than 20, and thoracic trauma (injury score > 2)
2. Polytrauma with abdominal/pelvic trauma and hemorrhagic shock (initial systolic blood pressure [SBP] less than 90)
3. ISS > 40
4. Bilateral lung contusions on x-ray study
5. Initial pulmonary arterial pressure greater than 24 mm Hg
6. Increase of more than 6 mm Hg in pulmonary arterial pressure during IM nailing

Soft Criteria

1. Clinically unstable/difficult resuscitation
2. Coagulopathy (platelets less than 90 K)
3. Hypothermia (<32° C)
4. Shock and >25 units of blood needed
5. Presumed operation time > 6 hours
6. Arterial injury and hemodynamic instability (SBP < 90)
7. Exaggerated inflammatory response

Definition: DDH affects the proximal femur and acetabulum, which includes distortion of the anatomy with inadequate covering and uncentered hips. Hips can also be subluxated and unstable, allowing dislocation. Early diagnosis and treatment are imperative, because failure to diagnose DDH in neonates and young infants can result in significant morbidity.

Incidence: In cases of significant DDH, 2 per 1000 live births; in cases of instability, 5 to 20 per 1000. Risk factors include first pregnancy breech presentation, multiple gestation, high birth weight, oligohydramnios, clubfoot and congenital torticollis, and familial history. Subsequent siblings of a child with DDH incur a 6% risk, and children of a parent who had DDH are at a 12% risk. Because left occiput anterior position is the most frequent presentation, it has been theorized that this may limit abduction of the left hip because it lies against the mother's spine, so the left hip is affected 3 times more often than the right hip.

Gender: The ratio of female-to-male occurrence is 7:1, attributed to increased levels of circulating estrogens and relaxin that cause a generalized ligamentous laxity.

Race: DDH is more common in Caucasian neonates than in African American or Asian neonates. Some indigenous North American groups have a higher incidence.

Signs and Symptoms: Legs of different lengths. The Barlow maneuver is used to determine whether a hip is dislocatable. The femur is flexed and adducted while posteriorly directed pressure is applied. This maneuver displaces out an unstable hip from the acetabulum. The Ortolani maneuver is used to reduce a dislocated hip. This is performed by flexing and abducting the femur; a palpable low-frequency clunk is noted as the femoral head slides back and reduces into the acetabulum. The Allis, or Galeazzi, sign is an apparent shortening of the compromised thigh.

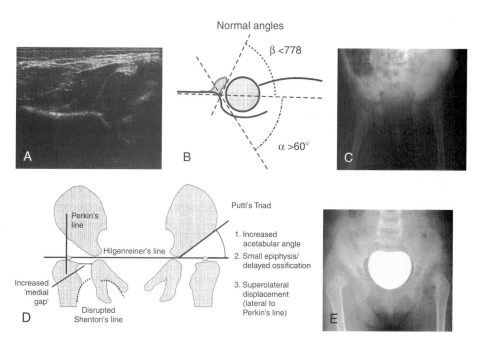

Fig. 64-1 Developmental dysplasia of the hip (DDH). **A,** Ultrasound of a dislocated hip. **B,** Normal Graf angles. **C,** AP radiograph of the pelvis with left DDH. **D,** Measurements in DDH. **E,** AP radiograph of the pelvis showing bilateral DDH. Note the early formation of pseudoacetabulae. *(From Adam A, et al: Grainger & Allison's Diagnostic Radiology, 5th ed. Philadelphia, Churchill Livingstone, 2008.)*

Diagnostic Studies: Ultrasonography (US) is the preferred method for evaluating the hip in children 6 months or younger. US enables imaging of the cartilaginous portions of the hip. X-rays are done in older infants. Measurements are acetabular angle ($\pm$ 28 degrees at birth), the "H" line or horizontal or Hilgenreiner's line, the "P" line or perpendicular or Perkins line, and the Shenton's arc line. Computed tomography scan with three-dimensional reconstruction shows spatial orientation and defects of the hip. Magnetic resonance imaging shows soft tissue related to the hip.

Treatment: The goal is to restore the joint. Treatment varies with the patient's age and the degree of instability. Most unstable hips in neonates return to normal spontaneously within the first 2 to 4 weeks after birth, so observation and reexamination in subluxating hips in the immediate neonatal period are recommended. The initial treatment for DDH is the use of a brace that keeps the hip in flexion and abduction, it is worn until the clinical and radiologic examination findings are normal. In children older than 6 months, the treatment is closed reduction under general anesthesia and application of a spica cast for several months. If this treatment fails, open reduction can be performed. In children older than 2 years, femoral or pelvic osteotomy and open reduction may be performed.

Complications: Persistent dysplasia, recurrent dislocation, and most significantly, avascular necrosis of the femoral head.

Sequelae: The failure to diagnose and treat DDH in the immediate neonatal period can result in significant morbidity, including closed treatment failure, the need for open reduction, and the eventual development of osteoarthritis.

Definition: Infection of the deep periprosthetic tissues surrounding the artificial joint replacement, resulting in sepsis, bacteremia, pain, and loss of function, with or without loosening of the prosthesis.

Etiology: The organism most frequently found in infected total knee replacements is *Staphylococcus aureus.*

Incidence: The incidence of infection after total knee arthroplasty ranges from 1.1% to 12.4%, depending on various factors and comorbidities listed below. The incidence of infection following total hip arthroplasty in patients with primary osteoarthritis is around 0.5%, with the incidence increasing depending on multiple factors.

Associations: Risk of sepsis is increased in patients with severe rheumatoid arthritis who are on steroids, have poorly controlled diabetes, prior hip surgery, a prior history of infection in or about the hip, skin ulceration, obesity, recurrent urinary tract infections, taking oral corticosteroids or other immunosuppressants, undergoing tooth extractions and other procedures causing bacteremia, chronic renal insufficiency, and with neoplasms requiring chemotherapy.

Age and Gender: Men of advanced age seem to have a higher incidence of sepsis.

Classification: Segawa and colleagues proposed the following classification system:
- *Type 1* is characterized by positive cultures after a revision procedure.
- *Type 2* is characterized by an acute infection diagnosed within 30 days after an arthroplasty.
- *Type 3* is characterized by an acute hematogenous infection in a patient with an otherwise well-functioning prosthesis.
- *Type 4* is characterized by a chronic or late indolent infection.

A simpler version of classifying these infections is "early" versus "late." Early infections are defined as within 3 months following surgery, whereas a late infection is more than 3 months after surgery. Late infections are much more common than early infections.

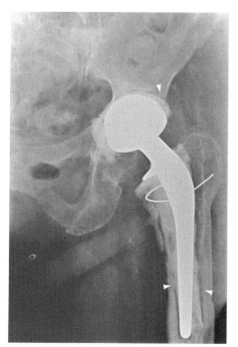

Fig. 65-1 A plain radiograph of an infected total hip prosthesis demonstrates lucencies at the bone-cement interface of both femoral and acetabular components *(arrowheads) (From Mandell GL, Bennett JE, and Dolin R [eds]: Principles and Practice of Infectious Diseases, 6th ed. Philadelphia, Churchill Livingstone, 2005.)*

Signs and Symptoms: Deep periprosthetic infection may be associated with clear signs and symptoms of sepsis, including wound drainage, erythema, swelling, pain, fevers, chills, and loss of motion and function. Late subclinical infection may not have any of the above signs.

Investigations: The white blood cell count, C-reactive protein levels, and the erythrocyte sedimentation rate remain elevated. The diagnosis of an infection after total knee or total hip arthroplasty rests solely on the results of examination of joint fluid aspirated under strict aseptic conditions. Radiographic analysis or radioisotope scans are also of limited value.

Treatment: The six basic treatment options are:
- Antibiotic suppression (type 1)
- Open débridement (types 2 and 3)
- Resection arthroplasty (types 3 and 4)
- Arthrodesis
- Amputation
- Implantation of another prosthesis

Complications: Complications of a septic joint include loss of the joint, limb, or life due to septicemia.

Upper Extremity:

Dermatomes:
- C5: Anterior elbow halfway between biceps tendon and lateral epicondyle
- C6 Median Nerve: Palmar distal thumb
- C6 Radial Nerve: Dorsal MP joint of thumb
- C7 Median Nerve: Palmar, distal long finger

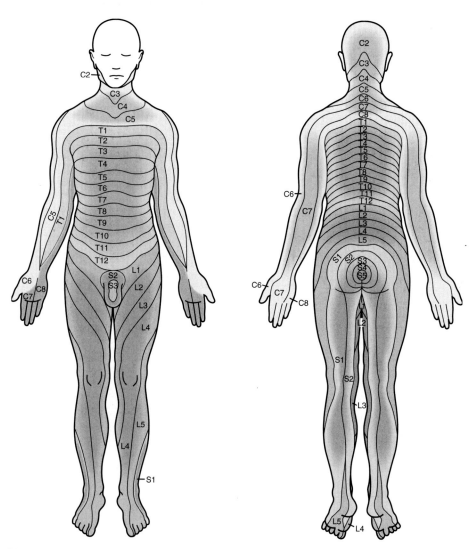

Fig. 66-1 Sensory dermatomes. *(From Marx J: Rosen's Emergency Medicine: Concepts and Clinical Practice, 6th ed. Philadelphia, Mosby, 2006.)*

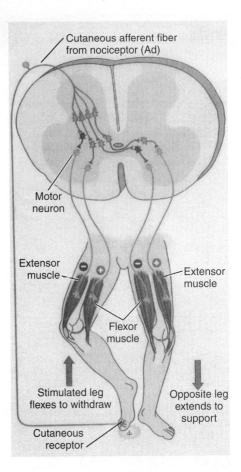

Fig. 66-2 The crossed extensor reflex. When a painful stimulus activates the flexor reflex and withdrawal of the leg, a reflex extension of the opposite leg maintains support of the body. *(From Purves D, Augustine GJ, Fitzpatrick D, et al: Neuroscience, 2nd ed. Sunderland, MA, Sinauer, 2001.)*

- C7 Radial Nerve: Dorsal MP joint of long finger
- C8 Ulnar Nerve: Palmar, distal little finger
- C8 Medial Antebrachial Cutaneous Nerve: Approximately 3 inches proximal to ulnar side of wrist
- T1: Medial epicondyle of elbow

Reflexes:
- C5: Biceps
- C6: Extensor carpi radialis longus
- C7: Triceps
- C8: Finger flexors

Lower Extremity:

Dermatomes:
- L2: Midline of thigh halfway between inguinal ligament and patella
- L3: Medial condyle
- L4: Medial malleolus
- L5: Base of second toe
- S1: Little toe

Peripheral Cutaneous Branches of Lower Leg:
- Saphenous Nerve: Medial half, lower leg from knee to medial malleolus
- Superficial Peroneal Nerve: Lateral half, lower leg and dorsum of foot excluding first web space and lateral malleolus
- Deep Peroneal Nerve: First web space of foot

Reflexes:
- L4: Quadriceps
- L5: Medial hamstring
- S1: Achilles

Definition: A desmoid tumor, also known as *aggressive fibromatosis*, is a histologically benign yet infiltrative fibrous tumor in skeletal muscle. These tumors are believed to be caused by myofibroblast cells.

Incidence: Desmoid tumors are rare. The incidence of these tumors is approximately 0.03% of neoplasms; however, they have been suggested to occur in 10% to 15% of patients with familial adenomatous polyposis.

Age: All ages are susceptible to desmoid tumors; however, young adults are most commonly affected ages (younger than 40 years).

Gender: Desmoid tumors are more common in women than in men (2:1). This may be due to the tendency of these tumors to arise in women during or after pregnancy.

Etiology: The exact cause of desmoid tumors is uncertain. It may be due to trauma, hormones, or genetic factors. Desmoid tumors may be associated with colonic polyposis, which is also known as *Gardner's syndrome*.

Clinical Presentation: This tumor occurs most often in the shoulder girdle, abdominal wall, and the thigh. The skin above the tumor appears normal and the tumor feels smooth when palpated. The tumor is mobile, although it may adhere to surrounding tissues.

Associations: This tumor can cause deformity, morbidity, and mortality resulting from the effects of pressure and the potential obstruction of vital structures and organs.

Pathology: This tumor consists of overgrowths of fibrous tissue that is locally aggressive. The tissue tends to surround muscle bundles, which may lead to deterioration of the bundles. Electron microscopy of the tumor reveals dense collagen, bundles of spindle-shaped fibroblasts, and peripherally located lymphocytes and macrophages. These tumors do not normally metastasize.

Diagnostic Procedures: Desmoid tumors are diagnosable through biopsy. Immunostaining may also be useful in diagnosing these tumors. The size and limits of the tumor may be visualized by magnetic resonance imaging and computed tomography.

Treatment: Desmoid tumors are normally treated by complete surgical resection. Radiation therapy, chemotherapy, and/or estrogen blockade may be used in conjunction with surgery, when the tumor is recurrent, or when surgery is not possible. Despite treatment, this type of tumor is often recurring.

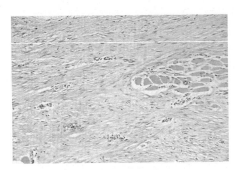

Fig. 67-1   Fibromatosis infiltrating between skeletal muscle cells. *(From Kumar V, et al: Robbins and Cotran Pathologic Basis of Disease, 7th ed. Philadelphia, Saunders, 2005.)*

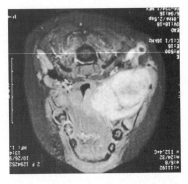

Fig. 67-2   Axial magnetic resonance image showing juvenile aggressive fibromatosis of the parapharyngeal space in a patient who presented with new onset of symptoms of OSAS. *(From Cummings CW: Otolaryngology: Head & Neck Surgery, 4th ed. Philadelphia, Mosby, 2005.)*

Definition: A chronic disease in which an abnormally high amount of glucose is present in the blood. Type 1 diabetes occurs when the pancreas is unable to produce insulin due to destruction of the beta cells in the pancreas due to an autoimmune process. Type 2 diabetes arises because the pancreas is either unable to secrete enough insulin to metabolize glucose in the blood or the cells in the body are not receptive to insulin.

Incidence: Diabetes mellitus is a common disease, afflicting about 15 million people in the United States alone. About 10% of those living with this disease have type 1 diabetes while the other 90% are categorized as having type 2 diabetes.

Age: Type 1 diabetes is usually diagnosed in childhood, adolescence, or early adulthood. In rarer instances, this type of diabetes may also develop in older individuals. Type 2 diabetes usually arises in adults 40 years of age and older and, to a lesser extent, in adolescents and young adults. Obese children may also develop this type of diabetes.

Gender: Type 1 diabetes occurs equally in males and females, whereas type 2 diabetes mellitus manifests somewhat more in older women than men.

Symptoms: People with type 1 diabetes commonly are the ones who present with symptoms, such as polyuria, polydipsia, polyphagia, blurred vision, and lower extremity paresthesias. Type 2 diabetics typically may not develop symptoms for many years.

Signs: Polyuria, weight loss, polydipsia, and polyphagia are common signs accompanied by either hyperglycemia or hypoglycemia.

Pathology: Commonly, diabetic patients' random blood glucose measurement will be greater than 200 mg/dL. Additionally, diabetic patients' urinalysis will be positive for greater than 30 mg/g of microalbumin on at least two of three consecutive sampling dates. Type 2 diabetics who have had diabetes mellitus for more than 2 years will usually have a fasting C-peptide level greater than 1.0 ng/dL. Patients with type 1 diabetes will have islet cell and anti-insulin autoantibodies present in their blood within 6 months of diagnosis. These antibodies, though, usually fade after 6 months.

Sequelae: Diabetes can lead to microvascular, macrovascular, neurosensory, and renal damage. Microvascular injuries can lead to retinal damage, which can result in blindness, kidney failure, and hypertension. Macrovascular problems can produce serious complications, such as myocardial infarction, cerebrovascular accident, and peripheral vascular disease, which can eventually lead to amputation of extremities. Diabetes can also lead to an increased incidence of infection and poor wound healing.

Prognosis: Regular monitoring of blood glucose and control of glucose levels with either insulin or oral antidiabetic agents, along with lifestyle modifications, such as smoking cessation, exercise, and dieting can lessen the severity of complications related to this disease.

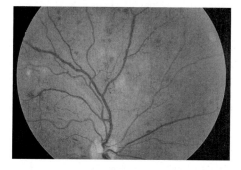

Fig. 68-1   Severe proliferative diabetic retinopathy with cotton-wool spots, intraretinal microvascular abnormalities, and venous bleeding. *(From Duker JS: Ophthalmology. London, CV Mosby, 1999.)*

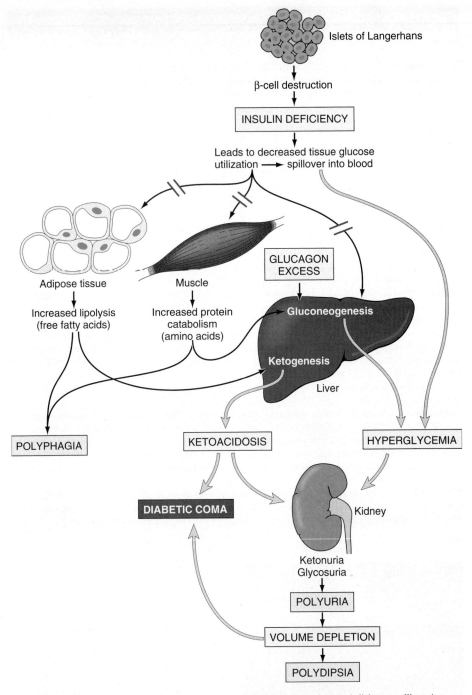

Fig. 68-2 Sequence of metabolic derangements leading to diabetic coma in type 1 diabetes mellitus. An absolute insulin deficiency leads to a catabolic state, eventuating in ketoacidosis and severe volume depletion. These cause sufficient central nervous system compromise to lead to coma and eventual death if left untreated. *(From Kumar V, et al: Robbins and Cotran Pathologic Basis of Disease, 7th ed. Philadelphia, Saunders, 2005.)*

Definition: Diabetic foot is a condition in which foot ulcers form on patients with diabetes. People with diabetic foot ulcers (DFUs) have a decreased quality of life and an 8% higher incidence of needing a lower extremity amputation (LEA) in the future.

Incidence: 3% to 4% of people with diabetes have foot ulcers and 15% will develop them within their lifetime. There is no age, gender, or racial preference.

Etiology and Pathophysiology: Peripheral neuropathy in diabetes causes the foot ulcers by affecting the sensory, motor, and autonomic pathways. Motor peripheral neuropathy or Charcot osteoarthropathy produces bony deformities. The deformities create severe pressure on the skin, which is increased by the edema caused by autonomic neuropathy. The patient does not feel this pressure or pain due to the dysfunction of the sensory system. This results in tissue failure and skin ulceration.

Associations: History of foot infection or ulceration and previous partial or whole foot amputation.

Signs and Symptoms: Ulcers of the foot.

Diagnostic Studies: Visible detection. Classified by depth from 0 to 3, with 0 meaning no ulceration and 3 meaning extensive ulceration or abscesses. Also classified by ischemia from A to D, with A being not ischemic through D being complete foot gangrene.

Micropathology: Bone destruction, tissue degeneration, and ulcer formation occur.

Macropathology: Open sores, visible edema, and sometimes infection are visible.

Treatment: Rest, relief of pressure, and elevation of the affected foot are the initial necessary treatments. Antibiotics are prescribed to treat polymicrobial infection. Vascular débridement or resection are surgical procedures that may be needed in severe cases. Untreated ulcers may lead to full or partial amputation.

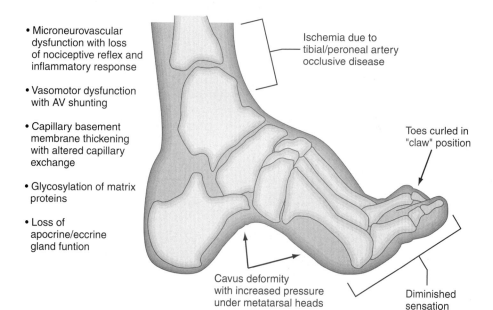

Fig. 69-1   Some of the pathophysiologic mechanisms contributing to ulceration in the diabetic foot. AV, arteriovenous. (*Modified from LoGerfo FW: Bypass grafts to the dorsalis pedis artery. Adv Vasc Surg 10:173–181, 2002; from Rutherford R: Vascular Surgery, 6th ed. Philadelphia, Saunders, 2005.*)

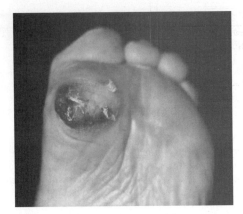

Fig. 69-2   Patient with diabetes mellitus and neuropathy had severe claw toes, and shear forces across plantar surface of first metatarsal head caused recurrent ulceration. *(From Canale ST, Beaty JH [eds]: Campbell's Operative Orthopaedics, 11th ed. Philadelphia, Mosby, 2007.)*

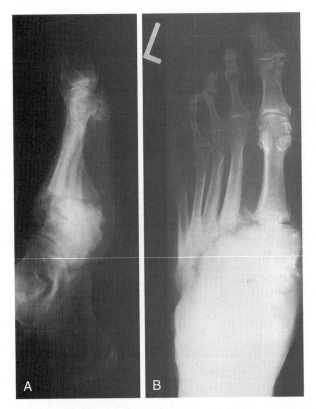

Fig. 69-3   Diabetes mellitus and neuropathic arthritis. Note lateral displacement of metatarsals (**A**) and fragmentation and osseous debris (**B**). *(From Goldman L, Ausiello D [eds]: Cecil Textbook of Medicine, 22nd ed. Philadelphia, Saunders, 2004.)*

Definition: Frequent source of back pain, spasms, and lower extremity discomfort and weakness. Disk degeneration starts in the third decade with loss of water content and height, and with onset of bulging. Annular tears can cause pain with or without herniation. Direct compression and production of inflammatory factors (e.g., interleukins, substance P) cause radiculopathy in the lumbar spine and either radiculopathy or myelopathy in the cervical or thoracic spine.

Etiology: Progressive dysfunction is associated with age, activity (especially torsion), smoking (40% increased incidence in back pain due to disk degeneration), obesity, vibration, sedentary lifestyle, and psychosocial factors.

Incidence: Disk degeneration is a normal process associated with aging. Incidence of back pain occurrence over a lifetime: 80%. Prevalence of back pain in the population at any given day: 10% to 25%. Sciatica incidence: 1% to 10% in the U.S. population.

Age: The group most commonly affected is adults age 25 to 45 years.

Gender: The male-to-female ratio is approximately 1:1.

Signs and Symptoms:

Cervicothoracic Spine: Upper back or neck pain with *radiculopathy*—shoulder/arm weakness/pain or numbness/paresthesias. Upper back or neck pain with *myelopathy*—long tract findings, balance/bowel/bladder dysfunction, hyperreflexia in the legs and difficulty with fine motor skills in the hands (opening jars, buttoning shirts, manipulating small objects). Bandlike pain around the chest for a thoracic disk herniation.

Lumbar Spine: Radiculopathy with dermatomal pain/numbness and isolated muscle weakness according to the anatomic motor unit.

Clinical Findings: Weakness/numbness as explained above. Provocative Spurling's testing for cervical radiculopathy and (reverse) straight leg raise test positive for lumbar spine radiculopathy. Back pain worse after sitting indicates diskogenic back pain; worse after walking indicates neurogenic back pain.

Staging: No clear stages for clinical symptoms. Magnetic resonance imaging staging of disk degeneration.

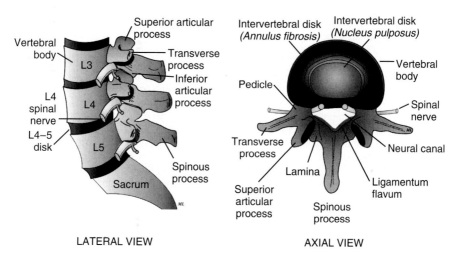

Fig. 70-1 Lateral and axial views of lumbar vertebral anatomy. *(From Marx J: Rosen's Emergency Medicine: Concepts and Clinical Practice, 6th ed. Philadelphia, Mosby, 2006.)*

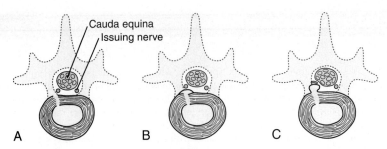

Fig. 70-2 Stages in prolapse of an intervertebral disk. **A,** The annulus fibrosus is torn, but there has been no extrusion of the nucleus pulposus. **B,** Extrusion of nuclear material through the rent. The posterior longitudinal ligament is stretched, but the protrusion has not reached the nerve. **C,** The protraction is larger, and the nerve is stretched over it. Sometimes, a fragment of the torn annulus itself protrudes backward. *(Redrawn from Adam JC, Hamblen DL: Outline of Orthopedics, 13th ed. New York, Churchill Livingstone, 2001; from Rakel R: Textbook of Family Medicine, 7th ed. Philadelphia, Saunders, 2007.)*

Micropathology: Microtearing caused by repetitive microtrauma eventually results in loss of circumferential annular fibers and herniation. Lack of nutrient inflow from the vertebral and disk endplate interface (due to smoking, diabetes, and vascular disease, for example) accelerates the degenerative cascade.

Medical Treatment: Successful outcome is achieved with symptomatic treatment, such as with physical therapy (e.g., hamstring stretching, dynamic lumbar stabilization exercises, electrical stimulation) and over-the-counter medications (e.g., nonsteroidal anti-inflammatory drugs and acetaminophen). Stronger pain therapy (narcotics) is only advised for short-term use. Acute flare may require muscle relaxants (Valium), oral steroids, or steroid injection (epidural vs. select nerve root block). Using these kinds of treatment, 95% of people will recover and return to normal activities.

Surgical Treatment: Microdiskectomy is the standard treatment after failing nonoperative management for radiculopathy in the lumbar spine. Anterior diskectomy is required for cervical or thoracic spine, usually followed by one-level fusion. Lumbar fusion surgery for diskogenic back pain is frequently performed when intervertebral segments are unstable, or after positive provocative diskography testing. One-level fusion does not significantly change the mechanics of the spine. Adjacent segment degeneration in the cervical spine after fusion of one level is 25% after 10 years and lower after more fusion levels.

Studies: Radiographs are used to show degenerative disease, bone spur formation, instability (flexion-extension), and disk height loss; magnetic resonance imaging (MRI) is used to visualize reduced water content, annular tears, and nerve or spinal cord compression (myelomalacia = signal change of the cord). Computed tomography (CT) myelogram is used for neurogenic compression if MRI is impossible (e.g., in patients with pacemakers), provocative diskogram for disk pathology and evidence of annular tearing (on post-diskogram CT), and electromyography/ nerve conduction testing for paraspinal muscle involvement in cervical radiculopathy and general peripheral root/nerve compression.

Sequelae: Although chronic pain can occur, diskogenic back pain typically burns out after 3 to 5 years. Persistent radiculopathy can lead to irreversible nerve damage; myelopathy progresses predictably in a stepwise pattern of degeneration. Decompression needs to be recommended strongly.

Complications: Can result in chronic back or neck pain, or permanent spinal cord injury if myelopathy is left untreated. Loss of sensation and strength in arms or legs and potential loss of bowel and bladder function can result from irreversible nerve damage.

Epidemiology: Most common upper extremity fracture. Older patients sustaining a fall on outstretched hand with a history of osteopenia. Female-to-male ratio of 4:1.

Anatomy: Articular surface is divided into two hyaline cartilage–covered facets for articulation with the carpal scaphoid and lunate. A well-defined ridge traversing from the dorsal to the palmar surface separates the two facets.

Weight-bearing distribution of the wrist is 80% radius and 20% ulna and triangular fibrocartilage complex (TFCC). The articular end of the radius slopes in an ulnar and palmar direction. A reversal of palmar tilt will result in excessive load transfer to the ulna and TFCC, resulting in ulnar-sided pain, also known as *ulnar abutment syndrome.*

Numerous ligaments attach the radius to the proximal carpal, thus reduction is achieved with *ligamentotaxis.* Dorsal stronger than volar.

Dorsal comminution is a result of dorsal cortical failure in compression with tension failure of the volar cortex.

Radiographic Parameters: Radial height is 11 to 13 mm. Radial inclination is 22 degrees. Palmar tilt is 11 degrees.

Distal Radius Fracture: For Frykman classification, see Table 71-1.

Table 71-1. FRYKMAN CLASSIFICATION OF DISTAL RADIUS FRACTURES

Distal Ulna Fracture:	No	Yes
Extra-articular	I	II
Intra-articular into radiocarpal joint	III	IV
Intra-articular into radioulnar joint	V	VI
Intra-articular into RC + RU joints	VII	VIII

Eponyms:

Extra-articular Fractures: (90% of Distal Radius Fractures)
• Colles fracture (dorsal angulation, apex volar). Fall on extended wrist with pronation.
• Smith fracture (volar angulation, apex dorsal). Fall on flexed wrist with supination.

Intra-articular Fractures:
• Die Punch Fracture: Lunate impaction injury into distal radius.
• Barton's Fracture: High energy shear forces result in intra-articular fracture; carpal bones move with sheared radial rim fragment.
    • Volar Barton's: Wrist in flexion
    • Dorsal Barton's: Wrist in extension
• Chauffeur Fractures/Backfire Fractures/Hutchinson Fractures: Fractures of the radial styloid.

Treatment:

Nonoperative: Closed Reduction and Casting
• Reduction and splinting in the emergency department followed by casting 3 to 4 days after injury. Repeat radiographs are obtained to ensure accurate reduction.

Operative Treatment:
• External fixator
• Volar plating/dorsal plating
• Fix distal radioulnar joint (DRUJ) with pinning in supination

145

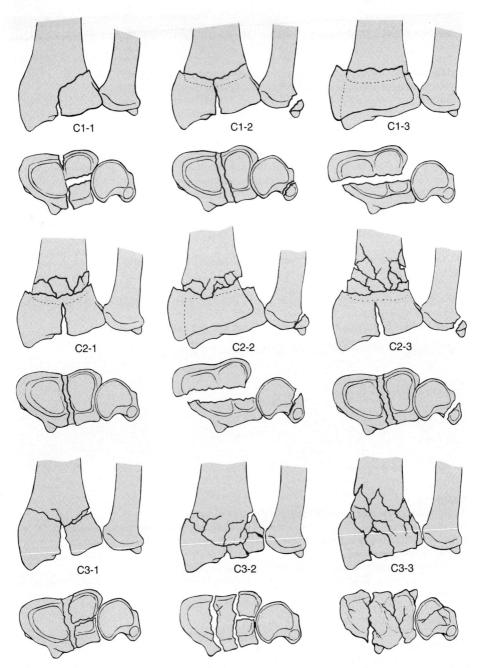

Fig. 71-1 The AO classification of complete articular distal radius fractures. *(From Browner BD: Skeletal Trauma: Basic Science, Management, and Reconstruction, 3rd ed. Philadelphia, Saunders, 2003.)*

Complications:
- Median nerve dysfunction (15% to 25%); usually from hematoma pressure or lidocaine effect from hematoma block
- Reflex sympathetic dystrophy
- Loss of active range of motion
- Tendon rupture: Extensor pollicis longus secondary to mechanical irritation over fracture callus
- DRUJ injuries
- Scaphoid lunate instability; widening greater than 2 mm

Anatomy: Five structures maintain the distal radioulnar joint (DRUJ), which all function to stabilize the joint in supination and pronation.
- Triangular fibrocartilage (TFC)
- Ulnocarpal ligament complex
- Infratendinous extensor retinaculum
- Pronator quadratus muscle
- Interosseous membrane

Injuries:
Fractures:
- Galeazzi (radial fracture with distal ulnar dislocation)
- Both-bone
- Intra-articular distal radius
- Lunate
- Ulnocarpal impaction

Others:
- Radial shortening— congenital versus post-fracture
- Radioulnar subluxation
- Ligamentous tear (triangular fibrocartilage complex)

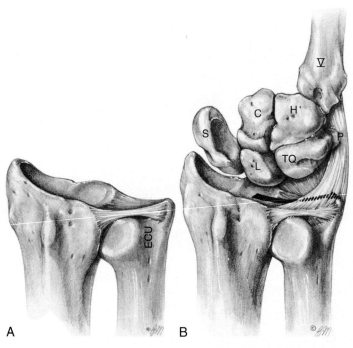

Fig. 72-1 The triangular fibrocartilage complex. **A,** The combined triangular fibrocartilage and ulnocarpal V ligament. **B,** Meniscal reflection that extends from the radius, over the triangular fibrocartilage, and distally to the base of the fifth metatarsal. The *arrow* shows access to the prestyloid recess. C, capitellum; ECU, extensor carpi ulnaris; H, hamate; L, lunate; S, scaphoid; TQ, triquetrum; V, 5th metacarpal. *(A, B,From Bowers WH: In Green DP [ed]. Operative Hand Surgery, 2nd ed, Vol 2. New York, Churchill Livingstone, 1982.)*

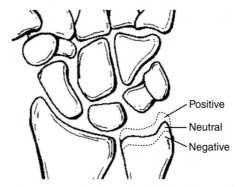

Fig. 72-2 Ulnar variance. Ulnar-minus variant is associated with an increased incidence of avascular necrosis of the lunate. *(From DeLee D, Drez D: DeLee and Drez's Orthopaedic Sports Medicine, 2nd ed. Philadelphia, Saunders, 2003.)*

Clinical Signs and Symptoms:

Piano Key Sign: DRUJ instability—Subluxation of ulna on radius when both hands are pressed forcefully downward on a table or depression of the ulnar head with support of forearm while pronated. When released, ulnar head comes back like piano key.

Other Signs: Pain on palpation, swelling, erythema, prominence of the distal ulna with dorsal dislocation. Palmar dislocation harder to recognize with swelling. Marked dysfunction of wrist.

Diagnostic Tests: Lateral x-ray shows displacement in relation to radius. Posteroanterior view shows gap between the ulnar head and distal radius (increased in dorsal dislocation, decreased, even superimposed if palmarly displaced). Computed tomography increases sensitivity. Magnetic resonance imaging is used for ligamentous injury; arthroscopy is the gold standard.

Treatment:

Isolated DRUJ Dislocation: Closed reduction with casting.

Fractures with DRUJ Instability: Treatment of choice is open reduction and internal fixation; without surgery, there is poor outcome.

Table 72-1.	BOWERS CLASSIFICATION
I	Acute fracture
II	Acute joint injury
III	Chronic joint disruption
IV	Chronic joint disorder
V	ECU tendon avulsion
VI	Fixed rotational deformity

Table 72-2.

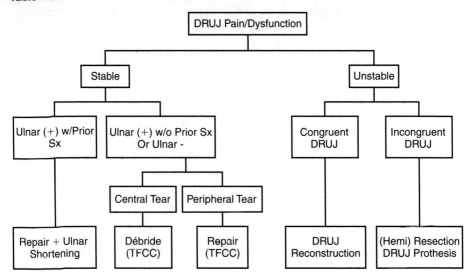

Historical Background: Developed in the 1950s by Gavriil A. Ilizarov in Kugan, Siberia, as an outgrowth of traditional fracture care with Kirschner wires, threaded rods, and frames, the technique of distraction osteogenesis arose serendipitously when a patient accidentally distracted his frame at a nonunion site, regenerating bone.

Principles:
- Stable external fixation that rigidly opposes shear but allows a small degree of micromotion at the fracture/osteotomy site to stimulate bone formation
- Percutaneous correction in any plane
- Preservation of marrow blood supply
- Latency
- Physiologic use of limb

Indications: Extensive bone/soft tissue defects, one-stage treatment for congenital or traumatic pseudarthrosis, limb length inequality, osteotomy, malunion, osteomyelitis–bone transport.

Mechanics: A combination of external fixators with pins and rings with tensioned wires can be used. Biomechanical principles of external fixators apply; that is, (1) Bending stiffness of pins is proportional to the fourth power of the pin radius and the third power of the bone rod distance, (2) Strength of construct is proportional to the number of pins through the bone, and (3) Near-near, far-far orientation provides strength. Circular frames are used in combination with a 1.8-mm diameter wire fixed in tension (between 90 and 130 kg). Strength of the construct is enhanced by decreased ring diameter, increased wire tension, orientation of wires or half pins at 90 degrees to one another, highest possible tension, decreased spacing of rings, and use of olive wires and additional rings or wires.

Technique for Distraction Osteogenesis: (1) A percutaneous osteotomy at the level of the apex of correction or point of distraction. (2) Constructs are placed in the operating room. (3) Construct is locked statically for latency period of 1 week to 10 days. (4) Regenerate is distracted at 1 mm per day (in 0.25-mm increments) until correction is achieved. (5) Once length/correction is achieved, construct is locked statically for approximately twice the duration of the lengthening-consolidation.

Biology: Bone forms in three distinct stages. (1) The latency period corresponds to an inflammatory period of cell migration to the osteotomy site. (2) The distraction period accounts for the lengthening of bone through intramembranous osteosynthesis; soft tissues are lengthened through tension in the process. (3) Mineralization and ossification of matrix occur during consolidation.

Advantages: Percutaneous, regenerate from host tissue, versatile.

Disadvantages: Cumbersome, lengthy treatment, risk of infection.

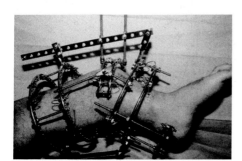

Fig. 73-1 Ilizarov technique; external fracture care.

151

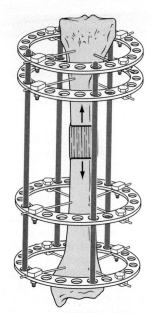

Fig. 73-2 Ilizarov ring fixator with four rings and four connecting rods. A stable, adaptable, component-based fixator used for bone transport is shown. Potentially complex to apply, cumbersome, and ill-suited for soft tissue care, these devices are valuable for reconstructive applications. *(From Browner BD: Skeletal Trauma: Basic Science, Management, and Reconstruction, 3rd ed. Philadelphia, Saunders, 2003.)*

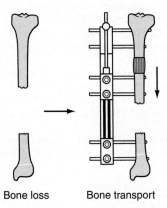

Bone loss   Bone transport

Fig. 73-3 Distraction-compression transport (i.e., bone transport) can be used to treat bone defects. *(From Browner BD: Skeletal Trauma: Basic Science, Management, and Reconstruction, 3rd ed. Philadelphia, Saunders, 2003.)*

Definition: A benign, progressive fibroproliferative disease of the palmar fascia (characterized by thickening and contracture of the fibrous bands on the palmar surfaces of the hand and fingers) that has no clear etiology or pathogenesis. First described in 1614 (Platter), Dupuytren later presented a detailed anatomic study in 1831 establishing the palmar fascia as the site of origin.

Etiology: Etiology is unclear. A total of 27% to 68% of patients relate a positive family history.

Two Theories:
• *Intrinsic Theory:* Metaplasia of the existing fascia
• *Extrinsic Theory:* Arises in the fibrofatty subdermal tissue and attaches to the underlying fascia

Incidence: Approximately 5% to 15% of males older than 50 years of age are affected in the United States. In Europe, up to 25% of males older than 65 years are affected.

Associations: Increased incidence in people of Anglo-Saxon origin; family history—autosomal dominant; 68% prevalence in first-degree relatives, epileptics (42%), alcohol-induced liver disease, diabetes mellitus, chronic obstructive pulmonary disease (COPD), hypertension, and IHD.

Age and Gender: More common in males older than 65 years. Male-to-female ratio 2-5:1.

Symptoms: Fingers get in the way of activities of daily living, such as washing face, combing hair, putting hand in the pocket, and putting hand in glove. Men may also present with deformity associated with pits and nodules in the palm of the hand.

Signs: Firm nodules that may be tender to palpation, atrophic grooves or pits in the skin, denoting adherence to the underlying fascia, tender knuckle pads (*Garrod's knuckle pad*) over the dorsal aspect of the proximal interphalangeal (PIP) joints, PIP joint flexion contractures.

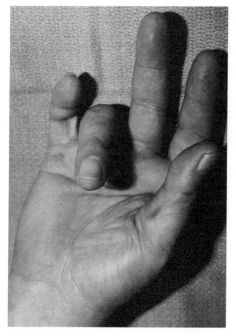

Fig. 74-1 Dupuytren's contracture, anteroposterior. *(From Noble J, et al: Textbook of Primary Care Medicine, 3rd ed. St. Louis, Mosby, 2001.)*

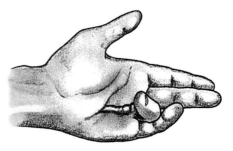

Fig. 74-2 Dupuytren's contracture. A flexion deformity of the finger is present, with nodular thickening of the fascia to the ring finger. *(From Ferri F: Ferri's Clinical Advisor 2009. Philadelphia, Mosby, 2009.)*

Clinical Findings: *Tabletop Test of Hueston:* Place the hand and fingers prone on a table. Positive = hand won't go flat. If negative, surgery is not indicated (Table 74-1).

Micropathology: Early disease shows nodules with a predominance of fibroblasts and type III collagen. In the active contractile phase, fibroblasts are replaced by myofibroblasts, and collagen types III and V predominate.

Treatment: Depends on the stage of disease and wishes of the patient (see Table 74-1).

Medical Care: No medical treatment (collagenase) has long-term value in halting or reversing the progression of contracture.

Surgical Care:

- *Closed Fasciotomy:* Risk of nerve or tendon damage and increased incidence of recurrence.
- *Limited Fasciotomy:* Only a short portion of fascia is removed through multiple short curved incisions.
- *Regional Fasciotomy:* The most common operation performed. Only the diseased fascia is removed, leaving the normal-appearing fascia.
- *Extensive Fasciectomy:* Reserved for those who have extensive involvement or have an increased diathesis to the disease. The diseased and normal looking fascia is removed.
- *Dermofasciectomy:* Skin as well as fascia are excised and replaced by a full-thickness skin graft. Amputation may be indicated for severe deformity with fixed contractures.

If PIP contracture is not corrected following excision of fascia, then soft tissue release of PIP is done as follows: Incision of the fibrous flexor sheath, release of check rein ligaments, excision of junction of accessory collateral ligament and volar plate.

Complications: The overall incidence of complications following surgery is 20%; recurrent disease is approximately 50%. Other complications include ischemic digit, digital nerve division, skin loss/necrosis, infection, and scar contracture.

Table 74-1. STAGING-WOODRUFF, 1998

Stage	Description	Management
1	Early palmar disease with no contracture	Leave alone
2	One finger involved, with only metacarpophalangeal joint contracture	Surgery
3	One finger—metacarpophalangeal joint + proximal interphalangeal joint	Surgery difficult
4	Stage 3 + more than one finger involved	Surgery prolonged and only partly successful
5	Finger-in-palm deformity	Consider amputation

Definition: The presence of thrombus, which is composed primarily of platelets and fibrin, within the deep venous system and the associated inflammatory response of vessel walls.

Incidence: One in nine patients diagnosed with DVT when younger than age 80 years. The true incidence in the general population is likely underestimated because it relies on clinical recognition of the condition. It occurs less frequently in upper extremities than in lower extremities.

Etiology: Unknown, but factors that predispose to increased risk include stasis, vascular injury, and hypercoagulability (Virchow's triad). Any clinical situation that contributes to Virchow's triad increases the risk of developing DVT (e.g., trauma, immobilization, pregnancy).

Associations: Patients who undergo orthopedic or abdominal/thoracic surgery and those with cancer or any underlying disease that results in systemic hypercoagulability tend to have a disproportionately higher risk of developing DVT. End-stage renal disease and congestive heart failure may also predispose patients to DVT.

Signs and Symptoms: Pain/tenderness along involved veins. Unilateral leg swelling, warmth, and erythema with possible palpable cord over involved veins. In some patients, there may be a cyanotic hue (*phlegmasia cerulean dolens*) or pallor (*phlegmasia alba dolens*).

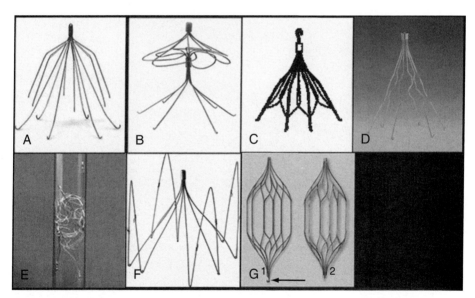

Fig. 75-1   The six types of inferior vena cava (IVC) filters available in the United States are: **(A)** G2 (C.R. Bard, Murray Hill, NJ); **(B)** Simon Nitinol (C.R. Bard); **(C)** Günther-Tulip (Cook Medical, Bloomington, IN); **(D)** Greenfield (Boston Scientific, Natick, MA); **(E)** Bird's Nest (Cook Medical, Bloomington, IN); **(F)** VenaTech (B. Braun Medical, Bethlehem, PA); **(G)** OptEase (Cordis J&J, Roden, The Netherlands), **(1)** (retrieval hook, *arrow*); and TrapEase (Cordis, Miami Lakes, FL). There is no prospective, randomized study that compares the safety and efficacy of these filters. Therefore, the choice is made simply on the basis of operator preference, technical feasibility (diameter of IVC), and the need for retrievability. The Günther-Tulip **(C)** and OptEase **(G1)** have Food and Drug Administration indication for retrievability. Studies have shown this to be feasible up to 3 to 4 weeks postplacement. Beyond that, epithelial overgrowth may increase the risk of IVC injury if removal is attempted. The G2 filter **(A)**, although not approved for retrievability, can technically be removed because it is the same design as its G1 predecessor, which had approval for indefinite retrieval. *(From Cameron JL: Current Surgical Therapy, 9th ed. Philadelphia, Mosby, 2008.)*

Diagnostic Studies: Elevation of D-dimer is sensitive, but not specific. Detection of thrombus using duplex venous ultrasonography via direct visualization or inference when vein does not collapse on compressive maneuvers is commonly used. Magnetic resonance imaging is useful for suspected superior and inferior venae cavae or pelvic vein thrombosis. Invasive procedures such as venography are also available but less frequently used.

Treatment: Anticoagulation with unfractionated heparin (intravenous administration of initial bolus of 5000 IU, followed by continuous infusion of 1000 to 1500 IU/hr) or low-molecular-weight heparin (subcutaneous administration of enoxaparin 1 mg/kg twice daily). Unfractionated heparin requires monitoring of activated partial thromboplastin time (aPTT) and switching to an oral anticoagulant for extended treatment. A direct thrombin inhibitor, such as lepirudin or argatroban can be used if heparin is contraindicated. Anticoagulation should be continued for at least 3 to 6 months to decrease likelihood of recurrence. Warfarin 2 to 5 mg PO/IV to maintain an INR of 2.5 can also be used as a treatment option. If anticoagulation is contraindicated, a permanent or temporary inferior venous cava filter can be inserted, or a catheter-directed thrombolysis, mechanical thrombectomy, and stenting of venous obstructions may be considered.

Sequelae: Post-thrombotic syndrome, pulmonary embolism, and paradoxical embolism can result from DVT. Other sequelae can be due to the treatment of DVT.

Definition: A genetic disorder that is composed of at least 10 distinct types that result in aberrant functioning of the connective tissue matrix.

Etiology: Ehlers-Danlos syndrome (EDS) is associated with autosomal dominant inheritance of defective genes that control the development of connective tissue.

Incidence: The incidence in the United States is estimated to be 1 in 400,000.

Age and Gender: EDS affects both genders equally. Type V EDS is an X-linked syndrome, which is found more in males. Some of the symptoms of the syndrome (e.g., hypermobile joints) are present at birth; however, some patients develop symptoms later in life.

Symptoms and Signs:

Classic Type (Formerly Types I and II): Joint hypermobility, skin laxity, easy bruising, joint dislocations, and scoliosis.

Hypermobility Type (Formerly Type III): Joint hypermobility is the major sign.

Vascular Type (Formerly Type IV, the arterial form): Spontaneous rupture of arteries and bowel and clubfoot are manifestations of this type.

Kyphoscoliosis Type (Formerly Type VI): Significant skin and joint laxity, and severe scoliosis and fragile globes of the eyes are typical features.

Arthrochalsia Type (Formerly Type VIIB, Arthrochalasis Multiplex Congenita): Shortness in height, severe joint laxity and dislocations, and variable skin involvement.

Dermatosparaxis Type (Formerly Type VIIC): Severe fragile skin that is soft with sagging and folding.

Tenascin—X-Deficient Type: Joint hypermobility, hyperelastic skin, and fragile tissue, lacking multiple shrinking (atrophied) scars in the skin.

Pathology: In the skin samples, irregularities of the diameters of the fibrils, irregular collagen shapes, and decreased or absence of some types of collagen are some of the findings.

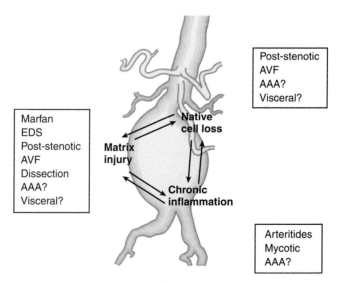

Fig. 76-1 The interrelationship of pathophysiologic features of aneurysmal degeneration. Boxed diseases represent potential entry points into the cycle. EDS, Ehlers-Danlos syndrome; AAA, abdominal aortic aneurysm; AVF, arteriovenous fistula. *(From Rutherford R: Vascular Surgery, 6th ed. Philadelphia, Saunders, 2005.)*

157

Treatment: A medical alert bracelet can be helpful. Skin care, avoiding contact sports, extreme caution during surgical maneuvering, and using a brace to maintain joint stability if necessary are some of the measures taken to treat these patients. Some studies have shown that high-dose (1 to 4 g/day) vitamin C has a potential effect in the treatment of scars and bleeding in type VI EDS.

Definition: A method of examining and treating pathology of the elbow joint with a minimally invasive technique, avoiding complications associated with open surgery.

Indications: Diagnostic arthroscopy, osteophyte excision, synovectomy, capsular release, loose body removal, osteochondritis dissecans, septic arthritis, lateral epicondylitis, and some fractures.

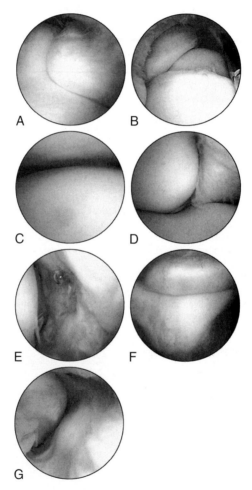

Fig. 77-1 View of medial side of elbow with coronoid process on right and trochlea on left. **B,** Anterior aspect of elbow viewed from medial portal with coronoid and trochlea in foreground and radiocapitellar joint. Annular ligament is clearly seen. **C,** Radiocapitellar joint with varus stress applied to expose undersurface of radial head. **D,** With elbow flexed 90 degrees, patient supine, and 2.7-mm arthroscope in direct lateral portal, articulation of three bones is seen. Radial head is superior left, ulna is superior right, and capitellum is inferior. **E,** Bare area of olecranon is right inside with trochlea on left. Scope is in direct lateral portal. **F,** Posterior compartment viewed through posterolateral portal. Tip of olecranon is superior, trochlea is inferior, and olecranon fossa is in foreground. **G,** Medial gutter viewed through posterolateral portal with posterior aspect of ulnar collateral ligament on right and distal humerus on left. *(From Canale ST, Beaty JH: Campbell's Operative Orthopaedics, 11th ed. Philadelphia, Mosby, 2007.)*

159

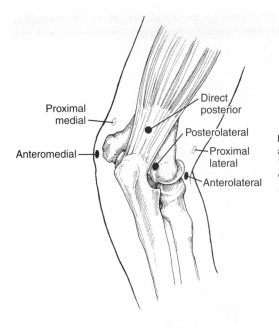

Proximal medial

Anteromedial

Direct posterior

Posterolateral

Proximal lateral

Anterolateral

Fig. 77-2 Arthroscopic portals for elbow arthroscopy. *(From Miller MD, Osborne JR, Warner JJP, Fu FH [eds]: MRI-Arthroscopy Correlative Atlas. Philadelphia, Saunders, 1997.)*

Contraindications: Severe arthrofibrosis or ankylosis, previous ulnar nerve transposition, subluxating ulnar nerve (relative contraindication), and skin infection overlying the elbow.

Complications: Compartment syndrome, septic arthritis, cellulitis, synovial-cutaneous fistula, vascular injury, and transient or permanent nerve injury. Transient ulnar neuritis is the most common complication following an elbow arthroscopy.

Positioning and Setup: The patient can be positioned supine, lateral decubitus, or prone. Either a 4-mm or 2.7-mm 30-degree arthroscope may be used. Anatomic landmarks should be drawn on the skin: radial head, medial and lateral epicondyles, olecranon, and ulnar nerve.

Portals: (Table 77-1)

Table 77-1. ARTHROSCOPIC PORTALS

Name	Location	Visualization/Use	Danger
Proximal anteromedial	2 cm superior to medial epicondyle; 1 to 2 cm anterior to intermuscular septum	Full access to anterior elbow	Ulnar nerve, medial antebrachial cutaneous nerve
Standard anteromedial	2 cm anterior and 2 cm distal to medial epicondyle	Full access to anterior elbow	Medial antebrachial cutaneous nerve, median nerve, ulnar nerve, brachial artery
Standard anterolateral	1 cm distal and 3 cm anterior to lateral epicondyle		Radial nerve, lateral antebrachial cutaneous nerve, posterior interosseous nerve

Table 77-1.   ARTHROSCOPIC PORTALS — cont'd

Name	Location	Visualization/Use	Danger
Mid-anterolateral	2 cm directly anterior to lateral epicondyle	Anterior radial head débridement	Radial nerve, lateral antebrachial cutaneous nerve
Proximal anterolateral	1 cm proximal and 1 cm anterior to lateral epicondyle	Anterior compartment, lateral epicondylectomy	Radial nerve, lateral antebrachial cutaneous nerve
Straight lateral	Soft spot between lateral humeral condyle, olecranon process, and radial head	Anterior	
Straight posterior (posterocentral)	3 cm proximal to olecranon tip	Medial/lateral compartments, olecranon fossa	
Superior posterolateral	Within 3 cm proximal to olecranon tip, just lateral to triceps tendon	Olecranon fossa, lateral gutter	
Inferior posterolateral	Posterolateral gutter at level of radiocapitellar joint	Posterolateral gutter, osteochondritis dissecans capitellum, radial head excision	

Osteology

Ulnohumeral Joint:
- One of the most congruous joints
- Olecranon locks into olecranon fossa in extension, as do the radial head and the coronoid into their respective fossa in full flexion
- Coronoid process is essential in preventing posterior subluxation; no soft tissue attachments can lead to small flake fractures, which represent shear injuries and can lead to instability
- Radial head is an important secondary stabilizer

Radiohumeral Joint:
- Anterolateral aspect of radial head lacks strong subchondral bone, which can predispose to fractures
- Central radial head is stiffer than capitellum; shear forces with valgus forces can lead to osteochondritis dissecans

Capsule and Ligaments

- Maximum capsular volume—15 to 30 mL at 80 degrees flexion; illustrated by position of elbow with hemarthrosis
- Medial collateral ligament (MCL) and lateral collateral ligament (LCL)—capsular thickenings important for elbow stability
- *MCL:*
  - Anterior bundle is the main constraint to valgus instability
  - Nonisometry creates cam-like effect between the anterior and posterior bundles; tension throughout flexion and extension
- *LCL:*
  - Ulnar–lateral ulnar collateral ligament (LUCL), radial and annular portions
  - Interdependent fibers that are intimately associated with extensor tendons superficially and the underlying joint capsule
- *LUCL:* Primary constraint against PLRI (posterolateral rotatory instability); homologous with anterior bundle of MCL

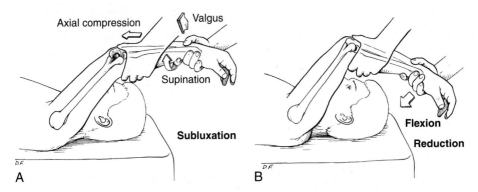

Fig. 78-1   Pivot shift test of the elbow. **A,** With extension valgus and supination, the elbow subluxes. **B,** Flexion and pronation reduce the subluxation. *(Reproduced by permission of the Mayo Foundation. From DeLee D, Drez D [eds]: DeLee and Drez's Orthopaedic Sports Medicine, 2nd ed. Philadelphia, Saunders, 2003.)*

Muscles—Key Points

Brachialis: Inserts average 11 mm distal to coronoid; accessory capsular insertion predisposes to heterotopic ossifications (HO) and post-traumatic flexion contracture
Triceps: Athletes with olecranon fractures or distal triceps ruptures may maintain some active elbow extension due to wide aponeurotic insertion via anconeus
Flexor-Pronator Group: Provides dynamic stability against valgus stresses
Supinator-Extensor Group: Augments the LCL

Elbow Biomechanics—Stability

The two most common injury mechanisms that cause elbow instability in athletes:
Chronic Valgus Extension Overload
- Commonly seen in overhead athletes—wind-up, cocking, acceleration, deceleration, follow-through phases
- Valgus torque peaks are seen during the late cocking and acceleration phases; internal rotation of the shoulder initiates humeral internal rotation, which approximates MCL failure load
- In the pitching motion, during the deceleration phase, a combination of torques and compressive forces "wedge" the olecranon into its fossa during extension → articular shear injuries initiating pathologic changes
- Pathway of degenerative changes—olecranon impingement → cartilage erosion on articular surface → osteophyte formation with osteoarthritic changes → shape of trochlear fossa changes from an O to a U, blocking extension and flexion

Acute Posterolateral Rotatory Instability (PLRI)
- Most common acute instability
- A three-dimensional injury pattern—the ulna supinates/external rotation beyond its normal limit → radiohumeral joint subluxes posterolaterally → ulna swings into valgus and clears the coronoid under the trochlea
- LUCL is the primary ligamentous restraint; disruption produces the posterolateral pivot shift phenomenon
- Typically occurs as a fall on an outstretched arm; the humerus internally rotates on the elbow, which experiences external rotation and valgus moment as it flexes; coronoid passes beneath the trochlea → dictates the posterolateral direction
- A "circle" concept of soft tissue injury from lateral to medial—LUCL → LCL → anterior and posterior capsule → posterior MCL → anterior MCL → flexor pronator origin

Medial Elbow

Medial elbow pain can have multiple causes, but one of the most common is medial epicondylitis, an overuse injury of the wrist flexors and forearm pronator muscles. This manifests itself with tenderness at or around the medial condyle. This injury is commonly known as "golfer's elbow." The pain can be reproduced by having the patient pronate and flex the wrist against resistance.

The most common ligamentous injury of the medial elbow is damage to the ulnar collateral ligament. While this is an unusual injury in an adult, it can commonly be found on the Little League baseball diamond. Young pitchers who throw with a sidearm motion (and young tennis players) are more likely to present with a strain of the ulnar collateral ligament. This can be elicited with a valgus stress of the elbow, with the pain localized to the medial joint line.

Another less common reason for medial elbow pain is the presence of an epitrochlear node. This can be found immediately proximal to the medial epicondyle of the elbow. An enlarged node is associated with infection (usually of the hand), sarcoid, or lymphoma.

The elbow should also be looked at grossly for the presence of bruising, fracture, or any other indication of direct trauma to the area that may be causing the pain.

Posterior Elbow

Posterior elbow pain has a much more narrow differential diagnosis due to the lack of many posterior structures. The most common cause of posterior elbow pain is olecranon bursitis. This can manifest as a swelling over the olecranon process. Inflammation can either be serous, which is usually nontender, or infectious, which presents as a hot, red, "angry" joint.

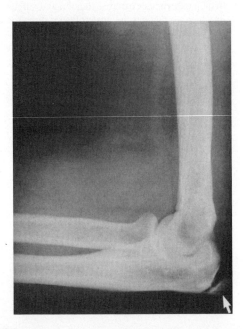

Fig. 79-1   Radiograph showing an olecranon spur (*arrow*). (*From DeLee D, Drez D [eds]: DeLee and Drez's Orthopaedic Sports Medicine, 2nd ed. Philadelphia, Saunders, 2003.*)

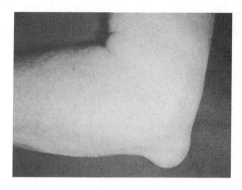

Fig. 79-2 Photograph of an enlarged olecranon bursa. *(From DeLee D, Drez D [eds]: DeLee and Drez's Orthopaedic Sports Medicine, 2nd ed. Philadelphia, Saunders, 2003.)*

Next on the differential is a triceps strain or tear. In this type of injury, the patient has a tender posterior arm, pain and weakness with elbow extension, and possibly a palpable defect accompanied by bruising over the triceps insertion if the tear is substantial.

Also of note causing pain over the posterior elbow is dislocation. This manifests itself with pain over range of motion, or possible inability to move the joint. The joint should be relocated as soon as possible to prevent compromise of the neurovascular structures.

Lateral Elbow

As with the medial side, lateral epicondylitis is the most common cause of pain on the lateral side of the elbow. This is the infamous "tennis elbow," and is associated with pain and tenderness over the area of the lateral epicondyle. This pain can be reproduced by having the patient supinate the forearm and extend at the wrist, because the muscles that produce these actions originate at the lateral epicondyle.

Trauma, as always, should be a consideration. The elbow again should be grossly examined for any evidence of trauma.

Definition: Electrolytes are substances that contain free ions, which behave as electrically conductive mediums. They commonly exist as acids, bases, and salts. The main electrolytes in humans are Na^+, K^+, Ca^{2+}, Mg^{2+}, Cl^-, PO_4^{3-}, and HCO_3^-. The levels of these ions must be strictly regulated in the intracellular space as well as the extracellular space in order to maintain homeostasis. This chapter focuses primarily on the imbalances of Na^+ and Ca^{2+}.

Incidence: Hypercalcemia develops in 20% to 30% of cancer patients. There are approximately 50,000 new cases of hypercalcemia each year. Hypernatremia is a rare occurrence, because sodium levels are strictly controlled by different systems. However, when it does occur, it has a very high mortality rate. Hypocalcemia occurs more frequently than hypercalcemia and occurs in 15% to 50% of intensive care unit (ICU) patients. Hyponatremia is the most common electrolyte disorder, with an overall incidence of 1% to 2.5%. Furthermore, 4.4% of surgical patients develop hyponatremia 1 week postoperatively and 30% of ICU patients are treated for it.

Pathophysiology: Serum calcium levels in the body are controlled by the hormones parathyroid hormone (PTH), calcitonin, and calcitriol. These hormones have receptors in bone, kidney, and gastrointestinal tissue. PTH works to raise the $[Ca^{2+}]$ in blood through bone erosion and Ca^{2+} reabsorption in the kidneys. Calcitriol, also known as vitamin D, increases the absorption of Ca^{2+} in the gastrointestinal tract. Calcitonin increases the excretion of Ca^{2+} in the kidneys and the trapping of Ca^{2+} in bone. Serum sodium level is controlled through thirst, antidiuretic hormone (ADH), the renin-angiotensin-aldosterone system, and the renal system. ADH works by increasing H_2O reabsorption in the kidney. Aldosterone causes Na^+ to be absorbed in the distal convoluted tubules. The absorption causes H_2O to diffuse back into the body to dilute the increased osmolarity.

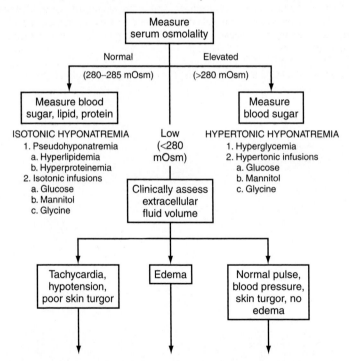

Fig. 80-1 Diagnostic approach to hyponatremia. *(Modified from Narins RG, Jones ER, Stom MC, et al: Diagnostic strategies in disorders of fluid, electrolyte, and acid-base homeostasis. Am J Med 72:496, 1982; from Ferri F: Practical Guide to the Care of the Medical Patient, 7th ed. Philadelphia, Mosby, 2007.)*

Associations: Hypercalcemia often is due to malignancy or hyperparathyroidism. Hypocalcemia is an indicator of chronic renal failure. Hypernatremia often is caused by excessive fluid loss or dehydration.

Diagnostic Studies: The first step is to take a comprehensive history and physical examination including a neurologic assessment. Important information to obtain in history taking includes use of medications (particularly thiazide diuretics), recent vomiting, diarrhea or excessive sweating with hypotonic fluid ingestion, recent surgery, and a history of psychiatric illness, congestive heart failure (CHF), cirrhosis, or nephrotic syndrome with renal failure. Physical examination should focus on assessment of volume status and include orthostatic vital signs, skin turgor, mucous membrane appearance, jugular venous distention, findings of edema, and wedge pressure and central venous pressure if available. Next, laboratory tests of serum levels need to be obtained. In cases when a calcium imbalance is suspected, albumin levels should be monitored as well. Hypercalcemia is defined as plasma Ca^{2+} greater than 10.6 mg/dL. Hypocalcemia is defined as plasma Ca^{2+} concentration less than 8.5 mg/dL. Hypernatremia is defined as plasma Na^+ concentration greater than 145 mmol/L. Hyponatremia is defined as plasma Na^+ concentration less than 135 mmol/L.

Treatment:

Hypercalcemia: The first step is to replace the extracellular fluid with saline. Once it has begun to normalize it will promote calcium excretion through saline diuresis. Throughout treatment, levels of other electrolytes must be closely monitored. In severe chronic cases caused by primary hyperparathyroidism, the only effective treatment is a parathyroidectomy.

Hypocalcemia: In the acute setting, as this is an emergency, calcium gluconate must be immediately given (this is the most effective way to obtain absorption of Ca^{2+}). On a long-term basis, calcium and vitamin D supplements can be used.

Hypernatremia: Correcting the imbalance too quickly is dangerous because it will cause a rapid shift of H_2O in brain cells, leading to seizures and/or other neurologic problems. Correction should be done slowly over 2 to 3 days. $[Na^+]$ should be lowered 0.5 mmol/L/hr.

Hyponatremia: Again, rapid correction of imbalance can cause neurologic problems to develop. The type of treatment depends on what the underlying cause is. If it is due to volume contraction, Na^+ repletion using isotonic saline is needed. If it is due to volume overload, water and Na^+ intake should be restricted while their excretion is promoted using diuretics.

Table 80-1. SIGNS AND SYMPTOMS

	Eyes	Thirst	Heart	Liver/Pancreas	Bowel
Hypercalcemia	Corneal calcification — **Bones:** Painful, fragile; Radiolucency, erosion	Increased — **Muscles:** Weakness	Cardiac Calcification; Cardiac arrhythmias — **Brain:** Mental confusion; Headache; Convulsion, coma	Ectopic calcification — **Kidneys:** Renal calculi; Polyuria; Renal failure	Emesis; Peptic ulceration; Abdominal pain; Constipation — **Bones:** Painful, fragile; Radiolucency, erosion
Hypocalcemia	**Eyes:** Papilledema; Cataract formation — **Brain:** Mood changes; Convulsion	**Chvostek's Sign:** Tapping over parotid causes facial muscles to twitch (neuromuscular excitability) — **Heart:** Cardiac arrhythmia		**Trousseau's Sign:** Blood pressure cuff causes carpopedal spasm (tetany in hand) — **Muscles:** Spasms; Cramps	**Hands/Feet:** Numbness; Paresthesia
Hypernatremia	**Thirst:** Excessive	**Kidney:** Polyuria; Nocturia	**Brain:** Irritability; Hyperreflexia; Seizures; Coma; Dizziness	**Muscle:** Lethargy; Weakness	**Skin:** Diaphoresis
Hyponatremia	**Brain:** Cerebral edema; Obtundation; Depressed reflexes; Agitation; Focal neurologic defects; Seizures; Coma		**Lungs:** Cheyne-Stokes respiration	**Muscles:** Cramps; Lethargy	**Gastrointestinal:** Nausea

Definition: A highly malignant, red bone marrow–derived tumor; first described by James Ewing in 1921. It belongs to the Ewing sarcoma family of tumors (ESFT) along with peripheral primitive neuroectodermal tumor, neuroepithelioma, atypical Ewing sarcoma, and Askin's tumor.

Incidence: More common in African Americans and Asians, it is the second most common malignant bone tumor in young patients and the most lethal bone tumor.

Age: Most commonly occurs in children and young adolescence age 4 to 15 years.

Gender: It is more common in male patients (male-to-female ratio 1.5:1).

Signs and Symptoms: The earliest symptom is worsening pain. Pathologic fracture, neurologic signs in the case of nerve compression, and weight loss are other signs found in these patients. Occasionally, this tumor manifests with a clinical picture like osteomyelitis with remittent fever, mild anemia, leukocytosis, and elevated erythrocyte sedimentation rate.

Diagnostic Studies: On x-ray study, a lytic lesion is usually found in the diaphysis or metaphysis of the bone with periosteal reaction and sometimes a soft tissue mass extending from the bone. The periosteal reaction, which often has an onion-skin or sunburst pattern, indicates an aggressive process. Magnetic resonance imaging is essential in diagnosis of soft tissue involvement.

Pathology: The t(11;22) and (q24-12) or one of a series of related translocations has been found in more than 95% of patients. CD99 expression is identified in nearly all ESFT and constitutes a useful positive marker when used as part of a panel of immunostains that can help rule out other differential diagnostic considerations. Microscopically, there are sheets and large nests of uniform, small, polygonal cells with scanty cytoplasm and indistinct cell borders with dispersed chromatin with hyperchromasia and variable mitotic figures. Rosettes are present in 10% of cases.

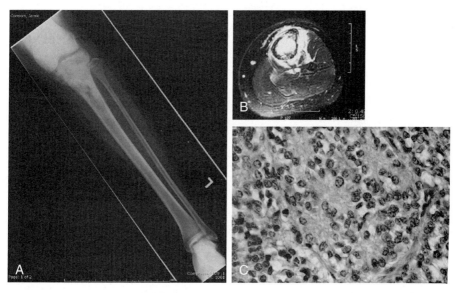

Fig. 81-1 **A,** Ewing sarcoma of the proximal tibia showing a permeative pattern of bone destruction of the metaphysis. Because the soft-tissue mass is unmineralized, it is not apparent on the plain radiograph. **B,** The axial MRI shows the extent of the soft-tissue mass. **C,** Photomicrograph of a Ewing sarcoma showing a round cell tumor. This alone would not establish the diagnosis. Immunohistochemistry and at times cytogenetics are necessary to distinguish this from other round cell tumors. *(From Abeloff M: Abeloff's Clinical Oncology, 4th ed. Philadelphia, Churchill Livingstone, 2008.)*

Prognosis: The following factors are usually associated with poor prognosis: male gender, age older than 12, pelvic tumor, anemia, elevated erythrocyte sedimentation rate and lactate dehydrogenase levels, and more than 10% viable tumor cells after chemotherapy.

Treatment: Neoadjuvant chemotherapy is the standard treatment. Chemotherapy increases survival to 65% to 70% for patients with localized tumor and 25% to 30% for patients with metastatic disease. Radiation therapy, either alone or in addition to surgery, remains useful.

Background: External fixation is a process for fracture fixation by which pins or wires are inserted into bone percutaneously and held together via an external scaffold. Initially described by Malgaigne in 1853, external fixation was proposed as an alternative to immobilization in plaster cast, traction, or internal fixation. Circular external fixation with thin wire fixation was popularized by the Ilizarov technique in the 1970s and 1980s, further evolving into hybrid fixation systems using both thin wires and standard half-pins for periarticular fractures.

Clinical Applications: Predominantly used for fracture fixation in adult and pediatric patients who have open fractures with severe soft tissue and/or wound contamination. External fixators may be used as a temporizing treatment, providing provisional alignment and stability, or as definitive treatment in select pelvic fractures, open long bone fractures, and periarticular fractures.

Frame Components:

Pins: Including half-pins, centrally threaded transfixation pins, and thin wire.

Pin Clamps: Serve to connect pins/wires to a rod or ring.

Rings: For use with Ilizarov and hybrid fixators.

Connecting Rods: Most are carbon fiber, 15% stiffer than stainless steel tubes with less deformation at 50% maximum loads.

Actions: The design of the fixator can be varied to provide compressive or distractive forces and to neutralize bending and rotational moments.

Biomechanics: Maximizing pin size, pin number, pin separation, pin proximity to the fracture, bone to clamp/bar proximity, and the diameter of the pins/connecting rod optimizes frame stability. The ideal position for pin placement is a near-far construct with a pin placed close to the fracture site on both sides and a pin placed as far away as possible on each side of the fracture. Stiffness is also increased by double stacking the connecting rods.

Pin Care: Up to 10% of external fixation pins develop signs of infection or osteolysis. No consensus on pin care treatment exists. A randomized controlled trial found fewer pin site infections in untreated patients. Loose pins should be removed and replaced, if necessary, to maintain fixator stability.

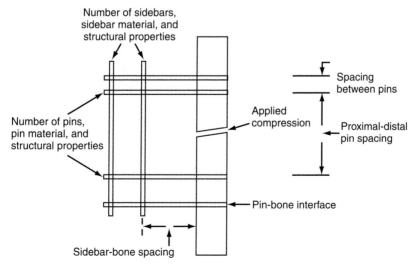

Fig. 82-1 Factors affecting the stability of an externally fixed fracture. *(From Browner BD: Skeletal Trauma: Basic Science, Management, and Reconstruction, 3rd ed. Philadelphia, Saunders, 2003.)*

Complications: Loosening and infection are the two most common complications. Thermal injury may result from pins placed under power. Chronic osteomyelitis has been reported in up to 4% of patients. Nerve and vessel injury is possible; understanding cross-sectional anatomy decreases risk of injury to vital structures.

Definition: A syndrome, first described by Zenker in 1862, whose signature findings include hypoxemia, central nervous system depression, and petechiae.

Etiology: Currently two theories exist. The *mechanical* theory states that large fat droplets are released into the venous system that eventually deposit in pulmonary capillary beds and the brain via arteriovenous shunts. Local ischemia and inflammation then persist in the areas of fat deposit. The second model, a *biochemical* theory, states that trauma and sepsis induce systemic release of free fatty acids as chylomicrons from hormonal changes. Acute-phase reactants cause the released chylomicrons to coalesce and create the reactions clinically seen.

Incidence: Frequency is unknown. Typically seen in younger adults. Diagnosis in made clinically, and patients are often missed secondary to confounding injury or illness. Fatal in 10% to 15% of cases.

Signs and Symptoms: Syndrome typically seen 24 to 72 hours after trauma. Early persistent tachycardia is often first noticed. Patients often become tachypneic and hypoxic, presenting with ventilation-perfusion deficits. High spiking temperatures are common during the syndrome. Reddish-brown nonpalpable petechiae develop over the upper body, often found in the axillae within 24 to 36 hours after injury. Additional petechiae can be found in subconjunctival and oral mucosa. Central nervous system dysfunction is often manifested by delirium, stupor, seizures, and coma. Additionally, retinal hemorrhages are visible on funduscopic examination.

Causes: Blunt trauma is associated with 90% of all cases. Long bone fractures are associated with 3% to 4% of cases. Additional recognized causes include acute pancreatitis, diabetes mellitus, burns, joint reconstruction, liposuction, cardiopulmonary bypass, decompression sickness, parenteral lipid infusion, and sickle cell crisis.

Laboratory Studies: Arterial blood gas demonstrates an alveolar-to-arterial oxygen tension difference, which, when drawn within 24 to 48 hours of a sentinel event, can be suggestive of fat embolism. Thrombocytopenia, anemia, and hypofibrinogenemia are nonspecific findings. Urinary fat stains are not thought to be sensitive or specific.

Imaging Studies: Plain chest radiography often reveals diffuse bilateral pulmonary infiltrates within 24 to 48 hours of clinical findings. Noncontrast head computed tomography may be normal or demonstrate petechial hemorrhages consistent with microvascular injury. Ventilation

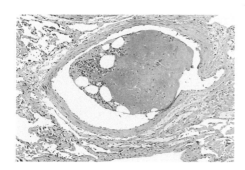

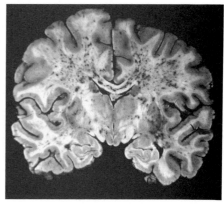

Fig. 83-1 Bone marrow embolus in the pulmonary circulation. The cleared vacuoles represent marrow fat that is now impacted in a distal vessel along with the cellular hematopoietic precursors. *(From Kumar V: Robbins and Cotran Pathologic Basis of Disease, 7th ed. Philadelphia, Saunders, 2005.)*

Fig. 83-2 Widespread white matter hemorrhages are characteristic of bone marrow embolization. *(From Kumar V: Robbins and Cotran Pathologic Basis of Disease, 7th ed. Philadelphia, Saunders, 2005.)*

perfusion scans may be normal or have subsegmental perfusion defects. Helical chest computed tomography can be normal or demonstrate lung contusion or acute respiratory distress syndrome (ARDS).

Medical Treatment: Supportive care is often needed, including adequate oxygenation and ventilation, hydration, stabilization of hemodynamics, blood products if necessary, and nutrition. Continuous pulse oximetry monitoring may help detect desaturations. Steroids do not appear to have a prophylactic role in treatment.

Surgical Treatment: Early stabilization of fractures is recommended to minimize potential fat embolism.

Sequelae: Residual diffusion capacity deficits may exist. Neurologic deficits range from nonexistent to memory impairment and cognitive dysfunction.

Physiologic Differences: Women are, on average, smaller and lighter than men, with approximately 10% more body fat and a 10% lower basal metabolic rate. Women tend to have lower cardiac output, hemoglobin levels, and muscle mass.

Female Athlete Triad: Amenorrhea, osteoporosis, disordered eating. Amenorrhea is seen due to changes in the hypothalamic-pituitary axis, increased vigorousness of training, and decreased body fat. This triad is found in both elite athletes and in a smaller percentage of normal, active females. Prevention and risk screening should be geared toward all active females.

Anterior Cruciate Ligament Injuries: A higher incidence of anterior cruciate ligament injuries has been found in females, especially soccer and basketball players. No definitive etiology has been found, but it is thought to be related to gender-specific differences in joint laxity, limb alignment, and intercondylar notch anatomy.

Patellofemoral Pain: Associated with genu valgum, ligamentous laxity, excessive pronation, and increased Q angle. Results in lateralization of patellar tracking. Pain aggravated by squatting and sitting. Treatment aimed primarily at quadriceps strengthening. Few indications for surgical intervention.

Stress Fractures: Due to overuse. Associated with amenorrhea, osteopenia. Most commonly seen in lower extremity (femoral neck, pubic rami). If suspected, patient should use crutches and limit weight bearing until fracture is ruled out by imaging (x-ray, bone scan, magnetic resonance imaging). Women with stress fractures or evidence of female athlete triad should have a DEXA scan.

Spondylolysis: Gymnasts and dancers (activities requiring hyperlordosis of the lumbar spine) are at increased risk of developing spondylolysis. Treated by rest and bracing.

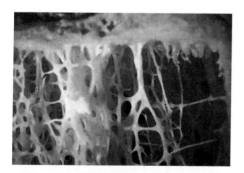

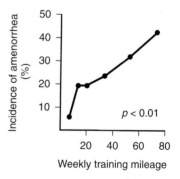

Fig. 84-1 Osteoporosis of lumbar vertebra. There is generalized loss of bone. The vertical plates have become more perforated and the number of horizontal cross-braces are decreased markedly in proportion to the vertical plates. *(From McPherson & Pincus: Henry's Clinical Diagnosis and Management by Laboratory Methods, 21st ed. Philadelphia, Saunders, 2006.)*

Fig. 84-2 Correlation between training mileage and amenorrhea. Each point represents average of 21 respondents. Statistical significance of relationship was obtained from point-biserial correlation (1 mile [1.6 km]). *(From Feicht CB, Johnson TS, Martin BJ: Secondary amenorrhoea in athletes. Lancet 2:1145, 1978; Katz VL, et al: Comprehensive Gynecology, 5th ed. Philadelphia, Mosby, 2007.)*

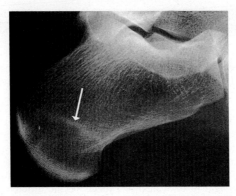

Fig. 84-3 Calcaneal stress fracture. Lateral radiograph of the foot shows a linear band of sclerosis *(arrow)* that is oriented perpendicular to the trabeculae of the posterior calcaneus. *(From DeLee D, Drez D: DeLee and Drez's Orthopaedic Sports Medicine, 2nd ed. Philadelphia, Saunders, 2002.)*

Anatomy: The femoral nerve is the largest branch of the lumbar plexus. It arises from lumbar plexus roots L2-4. The nerve descends through the fibers of the psoas muscle, and then passes anterior to the iliopsoas under the inguinal ligament before surfacing in the anterior thigh. The nerve lies deep to the fascia lata and fascia iliacus. The fascia iliacus separates it from the vascular bundle containing the femoral artery and vein. It divides into numerous branches early in the proximal anterior thigh.

Anesthesia Distribution/Considerations: Femoral nerve blockade provides sensory anesthesia for surgery on the anterior thigh, hip, femur, knee joint, quadriceps tendon, and medial aspect of the calf, ankle, and foot. When combined with a block of the sciatic nerve, anesthesia of the lower extremity from the mid-thigh level is achieved. Profound analgesia is obtained without the adverse effects associated with opioids or ketamine, such as respiratory depression or depression of consciousness. More rapid recovery and lower incidence of urinary retention may result compared with spinal anesthesia when short-acting local anesthetics are used for outpatient procedures.

Continuous Femoral Nerve Block Indications: Postoperative analgesia can be continued for days with a local anesthetic infusion when a catheter is placed within the connective tissue "sheath" of the femoral nerve. This technique significantly reduces systemic opioid requirements with a minimum of complications following knee procedures, total hip and knee arthroplasty, and femoropopliteal bypass surgery.

Specific Contraindications: The presence of a prosthetic femoral artery graft is a relative contraindication to femoral nerve block. The procedure, when combined with sciatic block, is contraindicated in situations where a dense sensory block could mask the onset of lower extremity compartment syndrome (e.g., fresh, traumatic or extensive fractures of the tibia and fibula). This contraindication is not specific for the femoral nerve block but applies to regional anesthesia of the lower extremity in general.

Sciatic Nerve Block

Anatomy: The sciatic nerve is the largest single nerve trunk of the body, with a diameter of 16 to 20 mm. It arises from the L4, L5, S1, S2, and S3 spinal roots and exits the pelvis posteriorly through the greater sciatic foramen, running laterally along the posterior surface of the ischium anterior to the piriformis muscle. The posterior cutaneous nerve of the thigh escorts the sciatic nerve as it exits the greater sciatic foramen. The sciatic nerve has medial and lateral components, which separate into the tibial and common peroneal nerves in the superior aspect of the popliteal fossa.

Anesthesia Distribution/Considerations: The posterior approach to sciatic nerve blockade results in anesthesia of the thigh, hamstrings, part of the hip and knee joint, and the entire leg below the knee, with the exception of the skin of the medial aspect of the lower leg, which is innervated by the saphenous nerve. When combined with a femoral nerve or lumbar plexus block, anesthesia of almost the entire leg is achieved.

Approach: There are four approaches to blocking the sciatic nerve: the classic posterior approach of Labat, and the anterior, lateral, and supine lithotomy approaches. The latter three approaches have the advantage of keeping the patient supine. A higher failure rate characterizes the anterior approach. The classic approach requires placing the patient in a lateral (Sims') position, which may be painful in the multiple-injured patient and contraindicated in the presence of a potential spine injury.

Complications: As in other peripheral nerve blocks, local anesthetic toxicity from intravascular injection is a risk, but is minimized by the use of epinephrine test doses and incremental injections. Nerve injury from intraneural injection is avoided by use of a nerve stimulator and avoidance of paresthesias in the awake patient. Strong motor evoked responses to low stimulation currents may indicate intraneural placement. Local anesthetic should flow easily into the perineural space on injection; resistance suggests intraneural needle placement.

Neuromuscular-Blocking Agents

Neuromuscular-blocking drugs block neuromuscular transmission at the neuromuscular junction, causing paralysis of the affected skeletal muscles. This is accomplished either by acting presynaptically via the inhibition of acetylcholine synthesis or release, or by acting postsynaptically at the acetylcholine receptor. Clinically, neuromuscular block is used as an adjunct to anesthesia to induce paralysis so that there are fewer complications at surgery. These drugs fall into two groups.

Nondepolarizing Blocking Agents: These act as competitive antagonists against acetylcholine. They compete by blocking the binding sites, or interrupting inotropic activity, of nicotinic cholinergic receptors. This prevents depolarization of the motor end plate (end-plate potentials do not reach the threshold potential needed for activation of muscle fiber contraction), resulting in paralysis of varying onset and duration. Side effects include increased cardiovascular activity and myopathy.

Depolarizing Blocking Agents: These agents act by noncompetitive inhibition of acetylcholine at nicotinic receptors on the neuromuscular junction, causing depolarization of the neuron. These agents are resistant to degradation by acetylcholinesterase and can persistently depolarize the muscle fibers as opposed to the transient depolarization by acetylcholine, which is rapidly degraded. Prolonged depolarization causes all receptors to remain inactive and no further action potentials are conducted. This results in a rapid onset of paralysis and fasciculations. Duration is short, due to metabolism by plasma cholinesterase. Side effects include myalgia, malignant hyperthermia, hyperkalemia, and phase II block—postsynaptic plasma membrane is no longer sensitive to further stimulation even though repolarized.

Reversal: Nondepolarizing blockers are reversed by anticholinesterase inhibitor drugs. Because they are competitive antagonists at the acetylcholine receptor, they can be reversed by increases in acetylcholine. The depolarizing blockers already have acetylcholine-like actions, so these agents have a prolonged effect under the influence of anticholinesterase inhibitors.

Definition: Femoroacetabular impingement (FAI) can be described as the abutment between the proximal femur and the acetabular rim. This leads to labral and chondral injury, which if not corrected, may progress to early onset of osteoarthritis of the hip.

Types of Femoroacetabular Impingement: Two distinct types of FAI have been described, the cam and the pincer. Cam type affects young males with morphologic abnormalities involving the femoral head. Impingement occurs during hip flexion in a nonspherical femoral head with increased radius, producing an abrasion in the anterosuperior area of the acetabulum cartilage, labrum, and subchondral bone. Pincer-type impingement is more common in middle-aged women and is the result of abnormal contact between the acetabular rim and the femoral neck. The abutment is a result of overcoverage of the femoral head in conditions such as coxa profunda or acetabular retroversion.

Clinical Presentation: FAI manifests as groin pain of slow onset, usually noticed after an episode of minor trauma. The pain is intermittent and may be exacerbated by excessive demand on the hip such as athletic activities or prolonged walking. The pain may also manifest after sitting for a prolonged period. Examination of the hip often reveals limitation of motion, particularly the internal rotation and adduction in flexion. The impingement test is done with the patient supine; the hip is internally rotated as it is passively flexed to approximately 90 degrees and adducted. The provocative test to elicit posteroinferior impingement is performed with external rotation in extension, giving rise to severe deep groin pain, and is indicative of posteroinferior impingement.

Radiography: An anteroposterior pelvis and a lateral film of the hip are the initial tests used in the diagnostic approach of FAI. The radiographic findings are subtle and include a bony prominence in the anterolateral head and neck junction, which can be objectively measured using the alpha angle. Acetabular abnormalities that lead to overcoverage are also identified in anteroposterior pelvis views.

Magnetic Resonance Imaging (MRI): Direct MRI arthrography is the best diagnostic test in the evaluation of FAI. It is capable of detecting bony abnormalities such as nonsphericity of the femoral head, low offset of the neck, and fibrocystic lesions, and most importantly allows visualization of the labrum and acetabular cartilage. Most patients present with a triad of MRI findings consisting of abnormal head-neck morphology (increased alpha angle), osteochondral lesions, and labral tears.

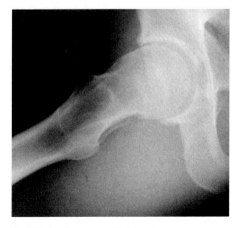

Fig. 86-1   Damage to the hip joint.

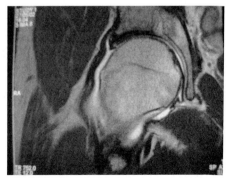

Fig. 86-2   Damage to the hip cartilage.

Treatment: Open femoroacetabular osteotomy is performed after dislocation of the hip. The acetabulum is inspected to identify labral and chondral lesions. The torn labrum is débrided and osteotomy of the acetabular rim to remove the chondral lesion is performed, then the labrum is reattached using nonabsorbable anchor sutures. Analysis of the outcome of femoroacetabular osteotomy is ongoing, but preliminary results indicate that improvement of the head and neck offset is successful in addressing the symptoms arising from the underlying impingement.

Definition: Fibrous dysplasia is a benign intramedullary fibroosseous lesion.

Incidence: Accounts for 7% of all benign bone tumors.

Age: The polyostotic form usually manifests before the age of 10 and the monostotic form between 5 and 20 years.

Gender: Distribution between genders is equal.

Etiology/Pathophysiology: Mutation in the $\gamma_s\alpha$ subunit located at chromosome 20q13.2-13.3 that leads to sustained activation of adenylate cyclase and elevated cyclic adenosine monophosphate (cAMP) levels and interleukin (IL)-6. The high cAMP stimulates osteoblastic expression of c-fos, which leads to altered cellular differentiation and osteoblastic proliferation. IL-6 may be responsible for increased osteoclast numbers and bone resorption.

Associations: Endocrine disorders, such as hyperthyroidism, hypophosphatemia, acromegaly, hyperprolactinemia, and Cushing's disease, have been associated with fibrous dysplasia, especially the polyostotic form. Fibrous dysplasia is characteristic of McCune-Albright syndrome (polyostotic fibrous dysplasia, café-au-lait spots, and endocrine dysfunction) and Mazabraud's syndrome (polyostotic fibrous dysplasia and soft tissue myxomas). Malignant transformation is rare and ranges from 0.5% to 4%, transforming most commonly to osteosarcoma, fibrosarcoma, and chondrosarcoma.

Signs and Symptoms: The majority of monostotic lesions are asymptomatic, while localized pain may be the presenting symptom in those with fatigue fractures. Diffuse polyostotic lesions in large weight-bearing bones are prone to bowing deformities that increase with age and skeletal growth.

Diagnostic Studies: Plain radiographs show a lesion that is more radiolucent than normal bone, with a grayish "ground glass" pattern without any trabecular pattern. In the proximal femur,

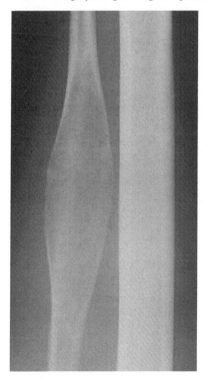

Fig. 87-1 Fibrous dysplasia. A characteristic expansile lesion with a ground-glass appearance has caused thinning of the cortex in the mid-diaphysis of the fibula. *(From Whyte MP: Fibrous dysplasia. In Favus MJ [ed]: Primer on the Metabolic Bone Diseases and Disorders of Mineral Metabolism, 3rd ed. Philadelphia, Lippincott-Raven, 1996.)*

microfractures and remodeling over a long time lead to varus deformity (shepherd's crook). Bone scans reveal increased uptake but are most useful for identifying the distribution of lesions in polyostotic disease. Computed tomography scanning is the best technique to delineate the extent of the lesion and its cortical boundary. The major benefit of magnetic resonance imaging is that it allows for coronal and sagittal evaluation of the extent of bony involvement.

Macropathology: Fibrous dysplasia rises most commonly in the ribs, craniofacial bones, and pelvis, and within the medullary canal of the metaphysic or diaphysis of the femur and tibia. The more extensive and aggressive lesions are found in polyostotic disease that can involve as few as two bones to 75% of the skeleton.

Micropathology: Fibrous dysplasia is composed of avascular fibrous stroma of dysplastic spindle-shaped cells that lack atypia and mitotic figures. The trabeculae have abnormally thick osteoid and lack osteoblast rimming.

Treatment: Asymptomatic lesions can be observed for progression. Surgery is indicated when the patient has progressive deformity, large symptomatic lesions, or malignancy. Curettage and bone grafting with internal fixation work in smaller monostotic lesions but are limited in younger patients with polyostotic disease. Medial displacement osteotomy can be used for shepherd's crook deformity, whereas valgus osteotomy is adequate for coxa vara. Large or extensive lesions that are not surgical candidates are treated with intravenous or oral bisphosphonates.

Definition: Flatfoot is a condition in which the longitudinal arch of the foot is lost. It also involves abduction of the forefoot and valgus deformity of the hind foot. In flexible flatfoot, the arch is present during non–weight bearing but is lost during weight bearing. In rigid flatfoot, the arch is absent in weight-bearing and non–weight-bearing positions.

Incidence: Flexible flatfoot is common in young children and may or may not resolve without treatment. Adult-acquired flatfoot is also common; however, the exact incidence is unknown because it is often misdiagnosed.

Age: This disorder may be congenital or acquired.

Etiology and Pathophysiology: Flexible flatfoot is caused by laxity of the ligaments. Adult-acquired flatfoot, or fallen arches, is commonly believed to be caused by posterior tibial tendon insufficiency. Obesity, neuropathy, soft tissue trauma, and bone trauma are possible causes of tibial tendon insufficiency. Rigid flatfoot is caused by bone anomalies such as tarsal coalition, congenial vertical talus, or arthritis.

Clinical Presentation: Loss of the foot's longitudinal arch, valgus hindfoot, and an abducted forefoot may be evident during examination (Table 88-1).

Diagnostic Procedures: The foot should be weight bearing for radiographs. Radiographs should be obtained in the lateral and anteroposterior views. Magnetic resonance imaging (MRI) may be used for cases that are difficult to diagnose. Computed tomography scans aid in indicating the presence of bone loss or damage due to flatfoot.

Treatment: The goal for flatfoot treatment is to establish optimal soft tissue support and bone alignment. Flexible flatfoot often does not need to be treated. However, if it is painful or if equinus contracture exists, then treatment may be necessary. Conservative treatment for flexible flatfoot may include stretching, corrective shoe wear, and/or casting. Operative treatment for flexible flatfoot may include soft tissue correction, fusion, and/or osteotomy. Conservative treatment for rigid flatfoot includes nonsteroidal anti-inflammatory drugs, corrective shoe wear, and/or casting. Surgical correction of rigid flatfoot may include excision of a cuneonavicular or a talocalcaneal coalition, osteotomy, or lateral column lengthening.

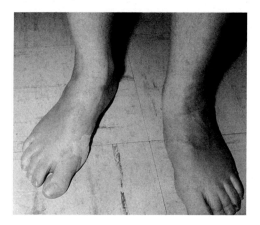

Fig. 88-1 Unilateral acquired adult flatfoot caused by posterior tibial tendon rupture of left foot. *(From Noble J, et al: Textbook of Primary Care Medicine, 3rd ed. St. Louis, Mosby, 2001.)*

183

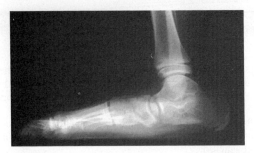

Fig. 88-2 Lateral weight-bearing radiograph demonstrating features of flatfoot. *(From Kliegman RM, et al: Nelson Textbook of Pediatrics, 18th ed. Philadelphia, Saunders, 2007.)*

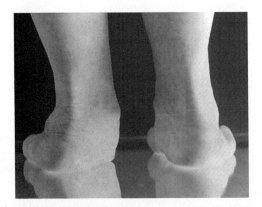

Fig. 88-3 A standing view from behind shows a patient with long-standing flatfeet and mild heel valgus. A couple of years earlier, he experienced proximal medial arch pain on the left side and progressive flattening of the arch with severe heel valgus. Examination of that side revealed a very tight gastrocnemius, inability to do a single-leg heel rise, and inability to plantar flex and invert the foot. The first metatarsal is hypermobile and elevated. These symptoms are classic indications of rupture of the posterior tibial tendon. *(From Browner BD: Skeletal Trauma: Basic Science, Management, and Reconstruction, 3rd ed. Philadelphia, Saunders, 2003.)*

Table 88-1. STAGES OF ADULT-ACQUIRED FLATFOOT

I	Mild tenderness of the posterior tibial tendon with slight or no loss of tendon strength
II	Forefoot abduction and hindfoot valgus with a loss of corrective heel inversion during heel rise
III	Hindfoot fixed in a valgus deformity and forefoot fixed in supination often with lateral pain

From Johnson KA, Strom DE: Tibialis posterior tendon dysfunction. Clin Orthop Relat Res 239:196-206, 1989.

Definition: Congenital or acquired anomaly with variable levels of union between two tarsal bones. Most commonly occurs at the calcaneonavicular joint and middle facet of the talocalcaneal joint. Calcaneocuboid, talonavicular, and cubonavicular tarsal fusions also occur, but are less common.

Incidence: One percent prevalence in the United States with a 50% incidence of bilateral coalition.

Etiology: Genetic studies indicate that tarsal coalitions are probably inherited as an autosomal dominant trait with almost complete penetrance. A failure of primitive mesenchymal differentiation and a possible link to weight-bearing biomechanical activity have been implicated.

Age: Calcaneonavicular coalition typically manifests in 8- to 12-year-olds. Talocalcaneal typically manifests in 12- to 15-year-olds.

Gender: No predilection, although some research suggest a slightly higher association with males.

Race: No predilection.

Signs and Symptoms: Coalition typically manifests with pain in a flat-footed child. Hindfoot may stay in valgus when rising to toes rather than swinging to normal varus. Terminology for completeness of ossification: *synostosis*—completely ossified bar; *synchondrosis*—partially cartilaginous bar; *syndesmosis*—spanned by fibrous tissue.

Associations: Fibular hemimelia, symphalangism, carpal coalition, Apert and Nievergelt-Pearlman syndrome.

Imaging: A solid bony bar forms a bridge if an osseous coalition is present. Anteroposterior, lateral, oblique, and axial views are indicated with the calcaneonavicular best seen on a 45-degree oblique view and the talocalcaneal best viewed in an axial plane. However, a follow-up computed tomography scan is indicated if such condition is suspected. Magnetic resonance imaging is the best modality for differentiating osseous from fibrous coalitions.

Treatment:

Conservative: Short leg walking cast in varus position for 2 to 4 weeks, followed by UCBL (University of California Berkeley Laboratory) orthosis. If no relief occurs, surgery is recommended.

Surgical:

- Calcaneonavicular Coalition: Typically uses the lateral approach, a 1-cm wide resection of osseous bar, interposition of the extensor digitorum brevis, and a non–weight-bearing short leg cast for 3 weeks. Eighty percent of patients achieve pain relief; however, a triple arthrodesis should be considered if no relief is experienced, in older patients, and in cases of advanced degenerative joint disease.

- Talocalcaneal Coalition: Medial approach, 1-cm wide resection of bar with fat grafting into defect, and a non–weight-bearing short leg cast for 3 weeks. Triple arthrodesis is recommended if no pain relief is experienced.

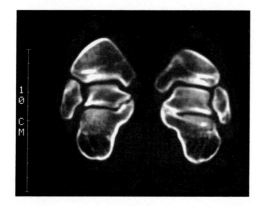

Fig. 89-1   CT scan of the talocalcaneal complex demonstrating tarsal coalition. *(From Kliegman RM, et al: Nelson Textbook of Pediatrics, 18th ed. Philadelphia, Saunders, 2007.)*

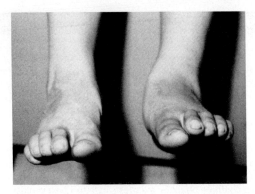

Fig. 89-2 This patient had a tarsal coalition in the left foot. Note that the foot is held in an everted position. Attempted inversion caused pain and resistance. *(From DeLee D, Drez D: DeLee and Drez's Orthopaedic Sports Medicine, 2nd ed. Philadelphia, Saunders, 2003.)*

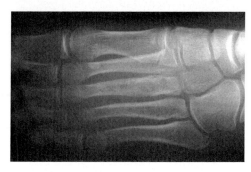

Fig. 90-1 Ewing sarcoma. Mixed lytic and sclerotic lesion of the third metatarsal bone. *(From Adam A: Grainger & Allison's Diagnostic Radiology, 5th ed. Philadelphia, Churchill Livingstone, 2008.)*

Tumor	Character	Location	Treatment
Giant cell tumor	Benign, aggressive Lytic	Distal tibial epiphysis and metaphysis	Curettage and filling with bone graft or cement
Osteochondroma	Benign Arises from bone as a cartilage-capped mass	Distal tibia, metatarsals, phalanges	Observation Marginal excision if painful, deforming, or aggressive
Enchondroma	Benign Lytic with "popcorn" chondroid calcification	Centrally in small long bones	Observation Immobilize if fracture Curettage and filling with bone graft or cement if fracture does not heal
Osteoid osteoma	Benign Lytic nidus of stroma and osteoid		NSAIDs Marginal excision or CT-guided radiofrequency ablation if no relief with NSAIDs
Osteoblastoma	Benign Resembles osteoid osteoma, but is larger and more lytic		Curettage and filling with bone graft or cement

Tumor	Character	Location	Treatment
Chondroblastoma	Benign Lytic with chicken-wire calcifications	Hindfoot, long bone epiphyses	Curettage and filling with bone graft or cement
Bizarre parosteal osteochondromatous proliferation	Benign Sclerotic	Periosteum of small long bones	Marginal excision
Osteosarcoma	Malignant Lytic	Distal tibia	Wide resection or amputation with adjuvant chemotherapy
Chondrosarcoma	Malignant Lytic		Wide resection or amputation
Lipoma	Benign	Deep to fascia	Observation Marginal resection if symptomatic
Plantar fibroma	Benign	At medial plantar fascia	Nonoperative with NSAIDs, shoe modifications
Schwannoma	Benign		Marginal resection
Neurofibroma	Benign		Marginal resection
Synovial sarcoma	Malignant Made of epithelial and spindle cells	Deep to fascia	Wide resection with adjuvant radiation
Clear cell sarcoma	Malignant Nests of cells with clear cytoplasm	Associated with tendons	Wide resection with adjuvant radiation

CT, computed tomography; NSAIDs, nonsteroidal anti-inflammatory drugs.

ANATOMY

Bones (2):
- Radius and ulna
- Derived from the somatic layer of the lateral plate mesoderm
- Forms by endochondral ossification (primary at 8 to 9 weeks of gestation, secondary at up to 10 years)
- Fusion occurs between 14 and 21 years for the radius and between 16 and 20 years for the ulna
- Ossification of the elbow is used to determine bone age in pediatric patients

Joints (3):
- Elbow, proximal/distal radioulnar

Muscles (20):
- *Flexors:* Flexor pollicis longus (FPL), flexor digitorum profundus (FDP), flexor digitorum superficialis (FDS), flexor carpi ulnaris (FCU), flexor carpi radialis (FCR), palmaris longus (PL), brachioradialis (BR)
- *Pronators:* Pronator teres (PT), pronator quadratus (PQ)
- *Extensors (six compartments, I to VI, arranged lateral to medial):*
  - I: Abductor pollicis longus (APL), extensor pollicis brevis (EPB)
  - II: Extensor carpi radialis longus (ECRL) and brevis (ECRB)
  - III: Extensor pollicis longus (EPL)

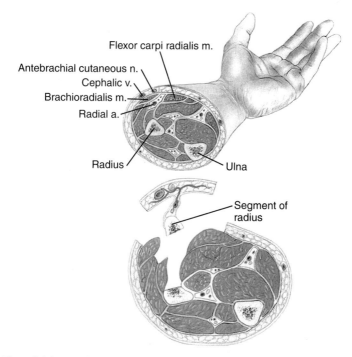

Fig. 91-1 The radial forearm free flap is harvested as a fasciocutaneous free flap based on the radial artery. *(Modified from Urken ML: Radial forearm. In Urken ML et al [eds]: Atlas of Regional and Free Flaps for Head and Neck Reconstruction. New York, Raven Press, 1995. By permission of Lippincott Williams & Wilkins.)*

189

- IV: Extensor digitorum communis (EDC), extensor indicis proprius (EIP)
- V: Extensor digiti minimi (EDM)
- VI: Extensor carpi ulnaris (ECU)
- *Supinators:* Supinator (S)
- *Miscellaneous:* Anconeus (A)
- Muscles can be classified by level (superficial/deep), or as extrinsic/intrinsic
- Forearm is divided into two or three compartments:
  - Mobile wad (considered by some as part of the dorsal compartment)
  - Dorsal
  - Volar
- Derived from the myotome portion of the somites (paraxial mesoderm)

Nerves:
- Musculocutaneous (C5-7): Only sensory over lateral aspect of forearm
- Median (C5-T1): Runs between PT heads, under FDS into the carpal tunnel
  - Anterior IO Nerve (AIN): Compression sites include PT, FDS, FCR
- Radial (C5-T1):
  - Superficial Branch (Sensory Only)—courses along the radial aspect of the forearm
  - Deep branch
- Posterior IO Nerve (PIN): Compression sites include the fibrous tissue of radial head, leash of Henry, Arcade of Frohse, distal Supinator, and ECRB
- Ulnar (C7-8, T1): Runs in the ulnar tunnel, between the ECU heads, under the FCU, and Guyon's canal

Vasculature:
- Brachial Artery
- Radial
  - Radial recurrent
- Ulnar
  - Anterior/posterior ulnar recurrent
  - Common interosseous
- IO recurrent
  - Anterior interosseous (AIA)
  - Posterior interosseous (PIA)

Miscellaneous Structures of Note:
- IO membrane of the forearm
- Annular/orbicular ligament of the ulna
- Cubital tunnel
- Ulnar tunnel
- Guyon's canal

An open fracture is defined as one in which a break in the skin and underlying soft tissues leads directly into, or communicates with, the fracture. Associated wounds are therefore at extremely high risk for environmental contamination at the time of the injury.

Gustilo and Anderson Classification System:

Type I: <1-cm wound, low-energy fracture, often from an inside to outside injury.

Type II: 1- to 10-cm wound, higher energy fracture, usually displays some comminution and has a minimal to moderate crushing component.

Type III: >10-cm wound, high-energy fracture, usually with significant comminution and a great deal of soft tissue damage. Injury results usually from high-velocity gunshots, motorcycle accidents, or injuries with contamination from outdoor sites (tornado disasters, farming accidents).

Type IIIA: Moderate periosteal stripping; wound closure not requiring soft tissue flap.

Type IIIB: Marked periosteal stripping; wound closure requires soft tissue flap.

Type IIIC: Any open fracture with a vascular injury that requires repair.

Initial Treatment:
- *Examination:* Neurologic status, head, spine, abdomen, and pelvis
- Cover wound with dry sterile dressing and splint
- Tetanus updated or immunoglobulin administered if unsure
- Antibiotics started with first generation cephalosporin (cefazolin)
  - Add aminoglycoside (gentamicin) for type III
  - Add penicillin for barnyard or heavily contaminated wounds

First Objective:
- Removal of all contamination from the wound and fracture site
- Irrigation with 9 to 12 L of normal saline
- Removal of all foreign material (gunshot wadding, clothing, etc), débridement/excision of necrotic tissue and devitalized bone

Closure:
- Types I and II open fractures undergo successful primary wound closure
- Type III fractures defy primary closure at all levels; flap coverage may be necessary
  - If no necrotic tissue or contamination is present, ideal time frame for closure is 5 to 7 days

Fracture Stabilization:
- Open fractures in children can be managed in a cast, same as closed fractures (wounds will close by secondary intention)
- In general, external fixation is used following multiple irrigation and débridements (type III) treatments
- Internal fixation with plates and screws may be used in type I open fractures and articular fractures that require anatomic reduction; primary and delayed intramedullary fixation has been used in types I, II, and III open fractures of the long bones
- The trend at the present is for greater use of intramedullary fixation, less plate fixation, less external fixation, and less cast fixation
- Keep added risks in mind:
  - Plate fixation requires additional exposure, external fixation can contribute to fracture distraction, and intramedullary fixation can spread contamination from an imperfectly cleaned fracture site

Current Controversy: Amputation versus salvage for treatment of type IIIC open fractures of the tibia.

Amputation: Might be the better option.
- Negatives: Results in the loss of a limb and requirement of a prosthesis. High-activity-requiring sports, jobs, labor could no longer be possible.
- Positives: Shorter hospital stay, fewer surgeries, rapid return to work.

Salvage:
- Negatives: Multiple surgical procedures (fracture repair, vascular, soft tissue transfers, débridement/infected bone excision, nerve repair, and reconstruction. Amputation may still be required following infection, painful limb, or non-union results. The "4 Ds" (divorce, destitution, depression, and disability) may result from attempted salvage.
- Positives: Potential to keep limb, some abilities. The advent of microvascular surgery has somewhat reduced the absolute indication for amputation resulting from limb ischemia.

Absolute Indications for Amputation:
- Warm ischemia time > 6 hours and/or disruption of the posterior tibial nerve
- If Mangled Extremity Severity Score (MESS) >7, amputation should be strongly considered

Table 92-1. MANGLED EXTREMITY SEVERITY SCORE

Score	Interpretation
0 to 6	Probably viable limb
>	Very high likelihood of amputation
Skeletal/Soft Tissue Injury	
Low-energy (stab, simple fracture, pistol gunshot wound)	1
Medium-energy (open or multiple fractures, dislocation)	2
High-energy (high-speed MVA or rifle gunshot wound)	3
Very high-energy (high-speed trauma + gross contamination)	4
Limb Ischemia	
Pulse reduced or absent but perfusion normal	1*
Pulseless, paresthesias, diminished capillary refill	2
Cool, paralyzed, insensate, numb	3*
Shock	
Systolic blood pressure always > 90 mm Hg	0
Hypotensive transiently	1
Persistent hypotension	2
Age (years)	
<30	0
30 to 50	1
>50	2

* Score doubled for ischemia > 6 hours

Stability

Absolute Stability: The compressed surfaces of the fracture fragments do not displace under applied functional load. Examples: Lag screw, plates, tension band.
Relative Stability: A fixation device that allows small amounts of motion in proportion to the load applied. The deformation or displacement is inversely proportional to the stiffness of the implant. Examples: Intramedullary rod, bridge plating, external fixation.

Screw Types:

- Cortical Screws: Designed to engage the cortex, shallower thread, smaller pitch (distance between threads) and outer diameter; designed for diaphyseal bone
- Cancellous Screws: Larger outer diameter, deeper threads and larger pitch; designed for use in metaphyseal or epiphyseal bone

Absolute Stability:

Lag Screw: Produces interfragmentary compression by driving the bone fragments together. A "lag screw" is partially threaded so that it only engages the distal bone fragment with its threads. A fully threaded screw can be put in with a *lag technique* by over-drilling the proximal bone fragment (gliding hole). Produce their best efficiency when placed perpendicular to the plane of the fracture. Application of a plate across the fracture site (neutralization plate) can enhance the stability of the construct. Self-tapping screws should not be used for lag screws because of insertion/removal/insertion and they might tend to cut a new path with each insertion.

Plates: Provide rigid internal fixation, articular fractures are best treated with plate osteosynthesis, compromise of cortical blood supply is a major drawback, and resistance to bending is proportional to the plate thickness cubed.

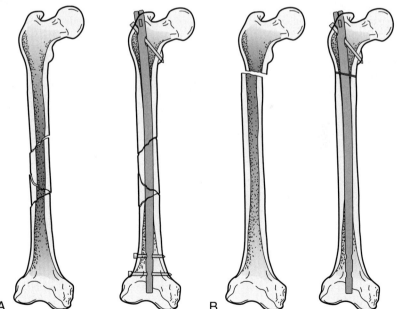

Fig. 93-1 **A,** *Static* locked intramedullary nail fixed to *both* the proximal and the distal fragments. **B,** *Dynamic* locked intramedullary nail fixed to *either* the proximal (as shown) or the distal fragment, but not to both. *(From Wolinsky PR, Johnson KD: Femoral shaft fractures. In Browner BD, Jupiter TB, Levine AM, Trafton PG [eds]: Skeletal Trauma, 2nd ed. Philadelphia, WB Saunders, 1998.)*

Tension Band: The principle is to convert a tension force into a compressive force by applying a device eccentrically or to the convex side of a curved bone.

Relative Stability:

Intramedullary Nails: Currently, nails are generally reamed and locked. Give better rotational stability (interlocking) and increased stability due to the ability to use larger nails. Nonreamed, nonlocked nails (Enders/Nancy nails, rush rods) are still used for some fracture types (pediatric femur fractures). Reaming damages the internal cortical blood supply (reversible in 8 to 12 weeks). It is a particular insult to a patient's pulmonary system in a polytrauma setting. Studies have shown solid emboli (via transesophageal echocardiography) in a reamed group vs. an unreamed group.

Bridge Plating: Combines adequate mechanical stability with natural fracture biology. Plate acts as an extramedullary splint fixed to the two main fracture fragments, while the fracture zone is left relatively untouched (bridged). Primarily used for fractures with complex fragmentation.

External Fixation: A device placed outside of the skin that stabilizes the bone fragments through wires or pins connected to longitudinal bars or tubes.

- Advantages: Less soft tissue/bone damage, useful for stabilizing open fractures, rigidity is adjustable without surgery, good in the setting of infection, quicker application
- Disadvantages: Pin/wires penetrate soft tissues, restricted joint motion, pin-track infections (including joint infections), more cumbersome/not well tolerated, limited stiffness

Stiffness: Too little or too much stiffness can delay fracture healing. Consider:

- Distance of pins from fracture line (closer is better)
- Distance between pins (farther apart is better)
- Diameter of pins (larger is better); bending rigidity is proportional to the fourth power of the diameter
- Distance of the bars to the bone (closer is better)
- Number of bars (two is better than one)
- Rods in different planes
- Configuration (unilateral, V-shaped, bilateral, triangular)

Special Considerations:

- Change over to intramedullary device considered safe if performed within first 2 weeks (provided there are no pin tract infections)
- When using external fixation around the knee, the minimum distance from the joint is 14 mm
- *Pilon Fractures (Tibial Plafond Fractures):* Can be initially treated with limited open reduction and internal fixation (ORIF) (plate the fibula to bring it out to length) and external fixation; then convert to ORIF between 10 and 21 days (provided soft tissues are adequate)

The fracture of a bone initiates healing that is broken up into three phases: inflammation, repair, and remodeling. Inflammation begins immediately after the assault and creates a callus where large volumes of new matrix are created. A hematoma accumulates in the medullary canal, damaging blood vessels, creating a necrotic nidus at the fracture site. Inflammatory cells, first polymorphonuclear leukocytes followed by macrophages and lymphocytes, release cytokines that stimulate angiogenesis.

As this phase subsides, fibroblasts and chondrocytes create the *callus,* possibly initiated by the release of transforming growth factor β (TGF-β), as necrotic tissue and exudates are resorbed. The formation of the callus represents the beginning of the reparative phase. The callus evolves from a disorganized woven bone to lamellar bone with type I collagen organized in parallel and unnecessary callus being reabsorbed over the course of the remodeling phase.

The hematoma is a critical structure in the repair of a fracture in that it provides a fibrin scaffold, facilitates the migrations of repair cells, and releases growth factors critical to fracture repair. A fracture with reduced blood flow will become necrotic and resorbed because it is denied the pluripotential mesenchymal cells that form fibrous tissue, cartilage, and eventually bone. The blood flow also provides oxygen, which stimulates bone formation at the fracture site.

In addition to adequate blood flow, the fracture repair is dependent on the correct gene expression of repair cells, which responds to mechanical stresses. For example, compression inhibits fibrous tissue, intermittent shear forces promote calcification, and hydrostatic pressure inhibits calcification. According to Wolff's Law, bone formation occurs where there is loading of the fracture site. The remodeling phase, which can go on for months to years, represents the transition from soft callus to hard callus as type I collagen arranges and orderly fibers align according to stress placed on the bone.

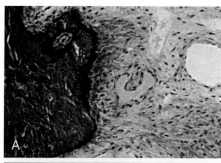
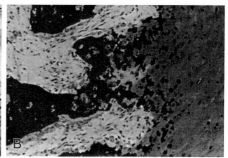
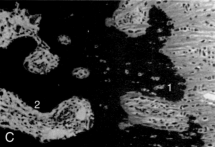

Fig. 94-1   Three types of secondary (indirect) bone formation in fracture gaps. **A,** Intramembranous bone formation. **B,** Bony substitution of fibrocartilage (von Kossa's and acid fuchsin stains, ×100). **C,** Bony substitution of dense fibrous tissue. Fibrous tissue undergoes mineralization (1) and is subsequently resorbed and substituted by bone (2) (von Kossa's and acid fuchsin stains, ×100). *(From Browner BD: Skeletal Trauma: Basic Science, Management, and Reconstruction, 3rd ed. Philadelphia, Saunders, 2003.)*

This elaborate sequence of cell and matrix changes results in mechanical stability, which can be described in four stages according to White and colleagues:
- Stage I: Torsional testing fails the original fracture site.
- Stage II: The bone still fails, but now demonstrates high stiffness and hard tissue.
- Stage III: There is failure through the fracture site and through intact bone with high stiffness.
- Stage IV: There is no failure, indicating fracture site duplicates uninjured bone.

In the absence of any stabilization, the above sequence of events will happen with the evolution of the callus as the cornerstone of healing. When a fracture is rigidly stabilized, *primary bone healing* occurs, obviating the need of the callus. The term *contact healing* refers to direct contact between cortical bone, which provides a bridge for osteons to extend from one fracture surface to the other. Despite optimal fixation, some fractures experience delayed healing due to severe injury, poor blood supply, or poor nutrition. Failure to heal or nonunion results from an arrest of the healing process with either a large-volume callus *(hypertrophic nonunion)* or little/no callus formation *(atrophic nonunion)*. Research in the last decade has discovered electrical stimulation to be efficacious in the healing of fractures. Abeed and associates determined that the distance of 80 mm or less resulted in healing in 11 of 16 nonunions.

There are numerous variables that go into the success or failure of fracture healing (Table 94-1). In addition to controlling variables that affect fracture healing, there are methods to promote healing, including bone grafting with either autograft or allograft, electrical stimulation, ultrasound, and biologicals, such as demineralized bone matrix, growth factors, and autologous bone marrow.

Table 94-1. VARIABLES IN FRACTURE HEALING

Injury Variables	Patient Variables	Tissue Variables	Treatment Variables
Open fracture	Age	Cancellous vs. cortical bone	Apposition of fracture fragments
Severity of injury	Nutrition	Bone necrosis	Loading and micromotion
Intra-articular	Systemic hormones	Bone disease	Fracture stabilization
Segmental fracture	Nicotine	Infection	
Soft tissue interposition			
Damaged blood supply			

Definition: Freiberg's disease is a painful collapse of the second metatarsal.
Incidence: This rare disease occurs most often in the second metatarsal, sometimes in the third or fourth, and rarely in the first and fifth.
Age: Frequently found in athletic adolescents, but occurs in all age groups.
Gender: About 4 to 5 times more common in females than in males.
Race: No racial preference.
Etiology and Pathophysiology: There is no agreement to the process by which this disease occurs. It often is included with a group of diseases called *osteochondroses,* diseases in which there is a loss of blood supply to the growing ends of bones in adolescent years, resulting in necrotic bone and tissue death. However, this explanation does not account for the adult cases. The metatarsal epiphysis is the joint affected and, without treatment, Freiberg's disease may develop into degenerative joint disease.
Associations: The cause is debated, but many experts believe the disease is caused by acute or chronic trauma.
Signs and Symptoms: Can be asymptomatic. Forefoot pain is the primary symptom. Other symptoms include tenderness in the area, pain when running or walking, calluses, and stiffness.
Diagnostic Studies: Detected by x-ray study. Occurs in stages. Stage I is difficult to detect and includes fissuring of the epiphysis of the metatarsal bone. In stages II and III, a central depression forms and the bones gradually degrade. In stage IV, loose bodies form and in stage V severe deformity occurs.

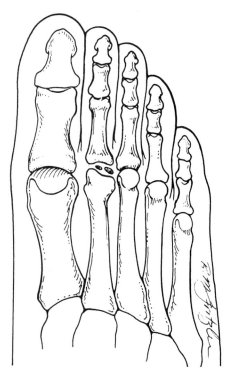

Fig. 95-1 Freiberg's infarction with loose bodies in joint. *(From DeLee D, Drez D [eds]: DeLee and Drez's Orthopaedic Sports Medicine, 2nd ed. Philadelphia, Saunders, 2003.)*

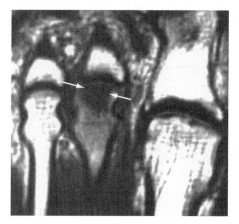

Fig. 95-2 Coronal T_1-weighted image shows crescent-shaped marrow infarction of the second metatarsal head *(between arrows)* in a patient with Freiberg's infarction. *(From DeLee D, Drez D [eds]: DeLee and Drez's Orthopaedic Sports Medicine, 2nd ed. Philadelphia, Saunders, 2003.)*

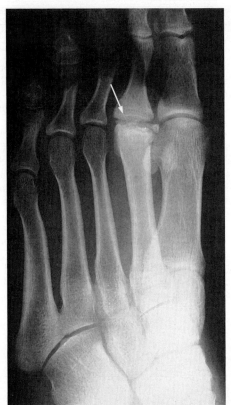

Fig. 95-3 Aseptic necrosis of the second metatarsal head. This usually occurs in teenagers and is referred to as a Freiberg osteonecrosis. Subsequent degenerative arthritis in this region is common. *(From Mettler FA, Jr: Essentials of Radiology, 2nd ed. Philadelphia, Saunders, 2005.)*

Micropathology: Bone decalcification and tissue regeneration occur.

Macropathology: Deformities may occur in the area. The pain may cause a limp, leading to added stress on other joints and therefore additional pain.

Treatment: Possible nonsurgical treatments include bed rest, a plaster cast, or metatarsal cushions. In severe cases, there are three surgical options: removing debris from on and around the metatarsal, removing part of the metatarsal, or shortening the length of the metatarsal. Sometimes nonsteroidal anti-inflammatory drugs help as an additional treatment option.

Definition: A shoulder disorder characterized by the gradual loss of motion and onset of pain within the shoulder.

Etiology: Reported etiologic agents include trauma, surgery (including but not limited to the shoulder), inflammatory disease, diabetes, regional conditions, and various shoulder maladies. An autoimmune theory has been postulated, with elevated levels of C-reactive protein and an increased incidence of HLA-B27 histocompatibility antigen reported in patients with frozen shoulder versus control subjects.

Incidence: Five percent of new patients at shoulder clinic.

Associations: Diabetes (40% of those with bilateral capsulitis have severe diabetes), hyperlipidemia. Trauma often elsewhere on the limb. Dupuytren's nodules in 50% of cases.

Age and Gender: Females affected more often than males; usually affects patients 40 to 70 years of age.

Symptoms: Gradual loss of function, onset of pain, and increasing stiffness. Patients are unable to sleep on the affected side, awaken on turning, and have pain localized to the deltoid region diffusely. Patients may describe a sequence of pain, then stiffness, then thawing.

Signs: Little if any wasting; limited elevation; external rotation (ER) normally less than 50% of the contralateral, both passive and active; differentiate from shoulder osteoarthritis, which also restricts movement. In ER, *beware* of bone tenderness that is not part of the frozen shoulder because malignancy may masquerade as frozen shoulder.

Investigations: Erythrocyte sedimentation rate, full blood count, and urea and electrolytes are normal; lipids may be raised; arthrogram shows reduced volume and loss of the axillary recess—therapeutic and diagnostic (magnetic resonance imaging not required but will show capsular thickening).

Staging: Classically, symptoms of primary frozen shoulder have been divided into three phases: (1) the painful phase, (2) the stiffening phase, and (3) the thawing phase.

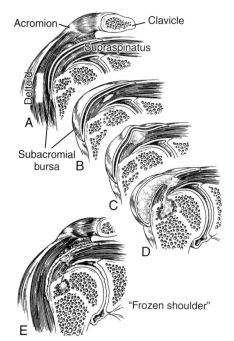

Acromion — Clavicle
Supraspinatus
Deltoid
A
Subacromial bursa B
C
D
"Frozen shoulder"
E

Fig. 96-1 Sequence of events terminating in frozen shoulder. **A,** Normal structures of the shoulder. **B,** Supraspinatus tendinitis, sometimes calcific, in the "critical zone." **C,** Spread of inflammation to the tendon sheath and a bulge into the floor of the subacromial bursa. **D,** Rupture into the subacromial bursa and extension of the inflammatory process as an osteitis into the humeral head and greater tuberosity. **E,** Frozen shoulder with involvement of tendons, bursa, capsule, synovium, and muscle with fibrous contracture and markedly diminished volume of the shoulder joint space. *(From Noble J, et al: Textbook of Primary Care Medicine, 3rd ed. St. Louis, Mosby, 2001.)*

199

Pathology: Capsule and coracohumeral ligaments are particularly affected. There is fibrous contracture of the joint capsule similar to Dupuytren's.

Treatment:

Medical Care: Physical therapy along with intra-articular injection of corticosteroids has been shown to improve function and range of motion. Oral corticosteroids provide an even stronger anti-inflammatory effect than do nonsteroidal medications.

Surgical Care: Management is controversial, but a reasonable sequence is steroid injection with physical therapy then manipulation under anesthesia (MUA). Caution must be taken when performing MUA on those with osteoporosis. If MUA is not successful, arthroscopy should be considered.

Complications: Prolonged pain and stiffness; fracture from MUA.

Definition: A fracture of the radial shaft with disruption of the distal radioulnar joint (DRUJ). The fracture is usually in the distal third of the radial shaft, just proximal to the pronator quadratus. DRUJ instability is due to disruption of the triangular fibrocartilage complex (TFCC). This injury pattern was actually first described by Cooper in 1842, 92 years before the Italian surgeon, Ricardo Galeazzi, reported his results of 18 cases.

Incidence: Trauma usually in children/adolescents. Galeazzi fractures represent 3% to 7% of all forearm fractures.

Gender: No preponderance.

Pathophysiology: Brachioradialis, pronator quadriceps, thumb extensors, and the weight of the hand are the causal forces involved with this fracture.

Etiology: Usually from fall onto outstretched hand where an axial load is placed on a hyperpronated forearm.

Symptoms: Pain with pronation/supination of forearm. Soft tissue swelling is usually present at the distal third radius fracture site and at the wrist joint.

Signs: Usually accompanied with gross deformity of the forearm and confirmed by radiographic evaluation. Anterior interosseous nerve palsy may also be present.

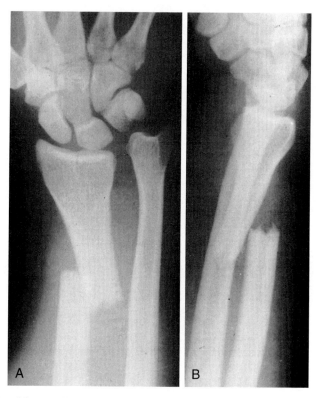

Fig. 97-1 Galeazzi fracture-dislocation of the distal forearm. AP (**A**) and lateral (**B**) views of the distal arm demonstrate a displaced fracture of the radius and diastasis of the distal radioulnar joint, with ulnar dislocation. *(From Adam A: Grainger & Allison's Diagnostic Radiology, 5th ed. Philadelphia, Churchill Livingstone, 2008.)*

Diagnostic Studies: Radiographs including the standard anteroposterior (AP) and lateral forearm views should be obtained as well as AP and lateral views of both the wrist and elbow. Additionally, contralateral views should be obtained for comparison.

Treatment: Poor results with closed reduction and cast application have shifted the standard to require compression plates and screws for the radial shaft fracture. The surgeon must evaluate the DRUJ following ORIF of the radius. If instability remains, further treatment may require percutaneous pinning or additional ORIF. Following surgical management, a long arm cast with the forearm supinated should be applied for 6 to 8 weeks.

Complications: Complication rates are approaching 40% for these fractures. Extensor carpi ulnaris injury or transposition into the DRUJ, ulnar styloid avulsion, and compartment syndrome of the forearm have been described in addition to nonunion, malunion, and infection.

Definition: A rapidly progressive infection of the muscle and soft tissue by a gas-forming organism, primarily by *Clostridium* species (estimated 80% to 95%) that is commonly found in grossly contaminated traumatic wounds.

Incidence: Ranges from 0.03% to 5.2% have been reported in the literature.

Age: No predilection.

Gender: Comorbid conditions may contribute to increased mortality, although gender is not a prognostic factor.

Race: No predilection.

Etiology: At the time of trauma or any time after the injury, the wound becomes infected by *Clostridium perfringens* or *Clostridium septicum*, both gram-positive, anaerobic, spore-forming rods that produce exotoxins. The gas formed promotes rapid spread, and the exotoxin creates local edema, fat and muscle necrosis, and thrombosis of local blood vessels.

Signs and Symptoms: Myonecrosis, gas production, and sepsis. Progressive pain and edema, high fevers, chills, tachycardia, and confusion may be present. A foul-smelling serosanguineous discharge can be found draining from the wound and there is often soft tissue crepitus over the infected region.

Micropathology: Standard tissue biopsy reveals *Clostridium* species are present, a Gram stain may demonstrate gram-positive rods. Microorganisms that colonize the skin surface often do not contribute to the underlying infection.

Macropathology: Necrotic tissue accompanied by odorous discharge.

Radiographic Findings: Widespread gas in the soft tissues surrounding the wound.

Treatment: Wide surgical débridement with fasciotomies is essential in treating this life-threatening infection. Initial antibiotic therapy should include penicillin G and clindamycin; some reports suggest the use of metronidazole, linezolid, and/or vancomycin. Analgesics are used for pain management; hyperbaric oxygenation has been reported to have varying results of success.

Complications: Early diagnosis and treatment may decrease mortality; however, the mortality associated with traumatic gas gangrene is greater than 25%, whereas nontraumatic gas gangrene mortality is estimated between 67% and 100%.

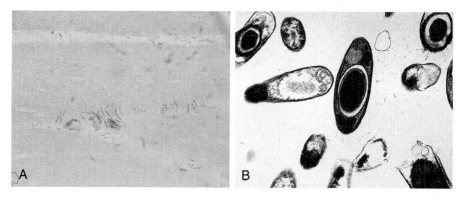

Fig. 98-1 *Clostridium perfringens* in a patient who has extensive gas gangrene. **A,** Gram stain of tissue removed from the arm of a patient. Note that the bacteria are rod shaped but gram variable. Note also that there are few if any acute inflammatory cells at the site of infection. **B,** Transmission electron micrograph of *C. perfringens*. Note the endospores. *(From Cohen J, Powderly W: Infectious Diseases, 2nd ed. Philadelphia, Mosby, 2004.)*

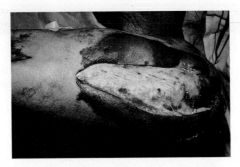

Fig. 98-2 Spontaneous necrotizing fasciitis due to *Clostridium septicum*. This patient developed the sudden onset of severe pain in the forearm. Swelling rapidly ensued and he sought medical treatment. Crepitus was present on physical examination and gas in the soft tissue was verified with routine radiographs. Immediate surgical débridement revealed necrotizing fasciitis but sparing of the muscle. *(From Cohen J, Powderly W: Infectious Diseases, 2nd ed. Philadelphia, Mosby, 2004.)*

Background

DNA:
- Composed of nucleotides (adenine, thymine, cytosine, guanine)
- Three to form codons, along with RNA, regulates protein synthesis

Proteins:
- Transcription—DNA → mRNA
- Translation—mRNA → 20 amino acids → proteins
- Proteins form enzymes = genes

Chromosomes:
- 22 pairs and 2 sex chromosomes
- Contain more than 150,000 genes encoded in DNA

Inheritance:
- Majority dictated by Mendelian modes
- Each has two alleles (form of gene), which may be dominant or recessive
- Autosomal dominant
  - Only one disease-associated allele required
  - Results in structural deficiency

Table 99-1. MODES OF INHERITANCE

Autosomal Dominant	Autosomal Recessive	X-Linked Dominant	X-Linked Recessive
Achondroplasia	Diastrophic dysplasia	Hypophosphatemic rickets	Becker's dystrophy
Charcot-Marie-Tooth	Friedreich's ataxia		Duchenne's muscular dystrophy Hunter's syndrome
Dupuytren's contracture Ehlers-Danlos Kniest's dysplasia Limb-girdle muscular dystrophy	Hereditary vitamin D–dependent rickets Hurler's syndrome Hypophosphatasia Laron's dysplasia		
Marfan syndrome	Osteogenesis imperfecta (II and III)		
Metaphyseal chondrodysplasia	Sickle cell		
Osteochondromatosis	Spinal muscular atrophy		
Osteogenesis imperfecta (I and IV) Osteopetrosis Polydactyly			

Non-Mendelian: Ewing's sarcoma, Albright's hereditary osteodystrophy, scoliosis, Osgood-Schlatter, slipped capital femoral epiphysis.

205

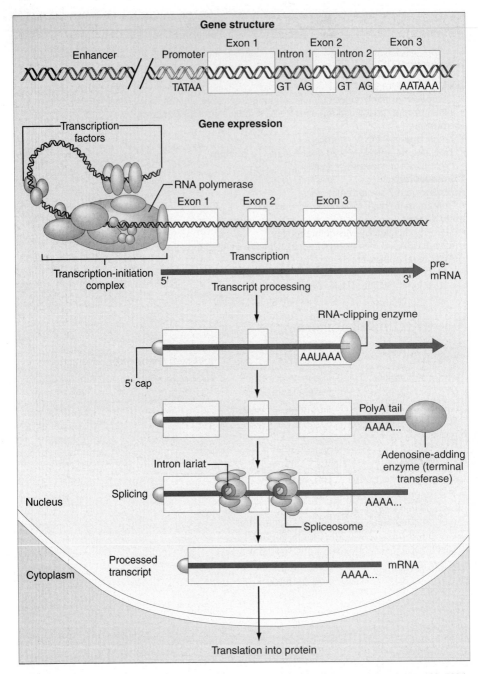

Fig. 99-1 *(Adapted from Rosenthal N: Regulation of gene expression. N Engl J Med 331:931–932, 1994; From Abeloff M: Abeloff's Clinical Oncology, 4th ed. Philadelphia, Churchill Livingstone, 2008.)*

- Autosomal recessive
  - Two disease-associated alleles required
  - Results in enzymatic deficiency
- X-Linked dominant: Only one disease-associated allele specifically on the X chromosome required
- X-Linked dominant: Requires either two disease-carrying X chromosomes in a female or more likely the mother's in a son

Definition: Giant cell tumor (GCT) of bone is a benign but locally aggressive tumor characterized by proliferation of mononuclear stromal cells interspersed with many multinucleated giant cells.

Incidence: Accounts for 20% of all benign bone tumors and 5% of all primary bone tumors. Higher incidence in the Chinese population and a slight female predominance. Most commonly occurs between 20 and 40 years of age.

Etiology and Pathophysiology: There are three types of cells found in GCT of bone. Type I cells look like fibroblasts, produce collagen, and have capacity to proliferate. This population of cells share some features of mesenchymal stem cells and is likely the tumor component of GCT. Type II cells are interstitial but resemble the monocyte/macrophage family and express surface receptors but not on the multinucleated giant cells. Type III cells are the multinucleated giant cells that share characteristics of and have morphologies similar to those of osteoclasts.

Clinical: Ninety percent of GCTs occur in the metaphyses-epiphyseal location of long bones, often extending to the articular subchondral bone; however, the joint or its capsule is rarely invaded. Fifty percent of GCTs occur about the knee at the distal femur or proximal tibia, with the proximal humerus and distal radius being the third and fourth most common sites, respectively. Spine involvement can occur. Pain is the most common presenting symptom, along with swelling, deformity of joint, joint effusion, and limited range of motion, if there is involvement about the joint, and soft tissue mass with extension outside of the bone. Pathologic fractures occur at presentation in approximately 10% to 30% of cases. Lung metastasis occurs in 3% of cases.

Macropathology: These lesions are lucent and eccentrically located within the bone. GCTs can appear aggressive, characterized by extensive local bony destruction, cortical breakthrough, and soft tissue expansion.

Micropathology: The tumor appears geographic with ill-defined borders and often without any identifiable sclerosis. Bone contour can be expanded with faint and thin periosteal new bone formation. Tumor matrix is of similar density to the surrounding soft tissue and devoid of any ossification or calcification. Computed tomography (CT) scan shows cortical involvement and soft tissue extension, although magnetic resonance imaging (MRI) is the best imaging modality of full tumor extension. On gross inspection, the lesion is characteristically chocolate brown, spongy, soft, and friable. GCTs are highly vascular, often producing blood-filled cystic cavities with variable degrees of cortical expansion and disruption; however, the periosteum is rarely breached.

Diagnostic Studies: Plain radiographic films initially, followed by CT or MRI of the affected area for more complete evaluation of full local extent, total body scan to rule out additional asymptomatic bony lesions, and chest radiograph to exclude lung involvement. Biopsy is mandatory to confirm diagnosis and is achieved via core-needle or open biopsy.

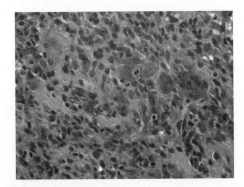

Fig. 100-1 Mitotically active polyhedral cells and scattered osteoclast-type giant cells in tenosynovial giant cell tumor. *(From Firestein GS: Kelley's Textbook of Rheumatology, 8th ed. Philadelphia, Saunders, 2008.)*

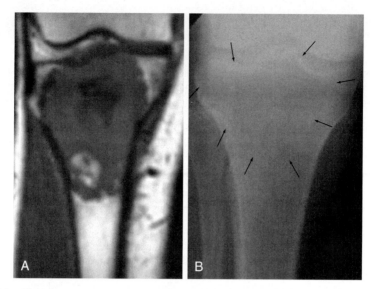

Fig. 100-2 Giant cell tumor of bone involving the proximal tibia, seen on MRI scan (**A**) and indicated by *arrows* on plain radiography (**B**). *(From Townsend CM Jr: Sabiston Textbook of Surgery, 18th ed. Philadelphia, Saunders, 2007.)*

Treatment: Curettage is the preferred treatment for most cases of GCT with a local recurrence rate of 10% to 20%. Various adjuvants such as chemical or physical agents including phenol, liquid nitrogen, bone cement, and hydrogen peroxide have been used to reduce local recurrence rates. Wide en bloc resection produces the lowest recurrence rate and is recommended for expendable bones. Radiation therapy and embolization are reserved for lesions or patients in whom surgical treatment is not feasible. Surgery should be delayed until final pathology results are available.

Definition: Extremely rare bone disorder in which normal bone dissolution is not followed by regrowth. May take place in just one bone or multiple bones. Oftentimes, bone is replaced by fibrous material or angiomatous proliferation. Gorham first reported two cases of massive osteolysis in 1954. This disease can affect axial or appendicular skeleton.

Incidence: Fewer than 200 cases have been described in the literature.

Etiology: No known etiology. Interesting theory presented by Heyden and colleagues (1977). The presence of unusually wide capillary vessels decreased flow of blood, producing local hypoxia and lowering pH, favoring the activity of various hydrolytic enzymes (acid phosphatase and leucine aminopeptidase in perivascular cells).

Age: Any age group but primarily before the age of 40.

Gender: No predilection.

Race: No predilection.

Signs and Symptoms: Symptoms vary depending on affected site. Some have a relatively abrupt onset of pain and swelling in the affected extremity, whereas others have insidious onset. Weakness and limitation of motion in the affected limb are also common. Fractures at the site of osteolysis are also a common finding. Serious complications are rare: Reports of paraplegia secondary to vertebral involvement of disease. Thoracic involvement with possible pleural involvement can compromise respiratory status. Standard blood tests are normal. The serum alkaline phosphatase may be elevated. By far, radiographic appearance is most dramatic. Definitive diagnosis is via bone biopsy.

Differential: Other causes of osteolysis (infection, cancer, inflammatory and endocrine disorders).

Imaging: In the initial lesion, radiolucent foci are seen in intramedullary or subcortical areas (similar to osteoporosis), followed by slow disappearance of bone. Can extend to contiguous bones. Regional osteolysis. May spontaneously stabilize but, more often, process continues.

Treatment: Radiation therapy, bisphosphonates, alpha-2b interferon. Surgical resection with reconstruction or radiation in moderate doses. Generally good prognosis.

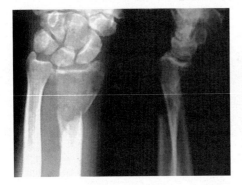

Fig. 101-1 Gorham's disease.

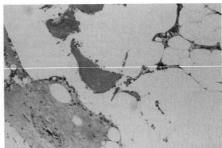

Fig. 101-2 Gorham's disease.

Definition: Gout is a metabolic disorder of uric acid causing sodium urate crystals to be deposited in systemic tissue or joints.

Incidence: Five percent of arthritis cases are gout and 840 of 100,000 people develop the disease. Approximately 2.1 million people are affected in the United States. Men are 9 times more likely to develop gout than women. It is more common in postmenopausal women. Renal pathology increases the incidence of gout.

Age: Men develop gout in their 40s and 50s. A small number of men develop gout right after puberty due to an increase in uric acid production. Uric acid levels are usually elevated for 20 years before the onset of gout.

Etiology and Pathophysiology: An abnormally high serum urate level (>0.42 mmol/L) may be due to increased purine intake, increased production of uric acid, or decreased uric acid elimination by the kidneys. Sodium urate crystal deposition leads to arthritic symptoms, including pain and immobility.

Associations: Patients with gout are 1000 times more likely to develop kidney stones and have a history of renal colic. A good number of individuals with gout also have diabetes, hypertension,

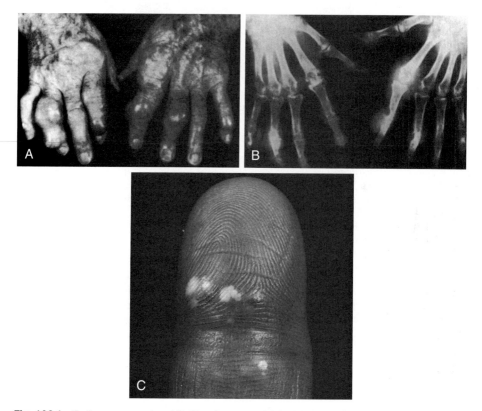

Fig. 102-1   Tophaceous gout. **A** and **B,** Chronic gouty arthritis with tophaceous destruction of bone and joints. **C,** Tophaceous deposits in the digital pad of a 28-year-old man with systemic lupus erythematosus under treatment with diuretics. A single attack of gout had occurred 2 years earlier. *(From Goldman L: Cecil Medicine, 23rd ed. Philadelphia, Saunders, 2007.)*

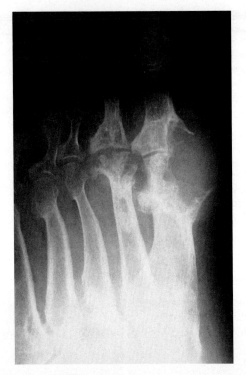

Fig. 102-2 Gout. The first metatarsal phalangeal joint is the most commonly affected. This large tophus has caused erosion at the margins of the joints; in general, however, the joint space itself is reasonably well preserved. *(From Mettler FA, Jr.: Essentials of Radiology, 2nd ed. Philadelphia, Saunders, 2005.)*

hypertriglyceridemia, and low high-density lipoproteins. However, there is no evidence that gout causes any of these disorders.

Signs and Symptoms: Although 95% of individuals with gout remain asymptomatic, symptoms include redness, inflammation, local irritation, and pain. There is maximal irritation by hour 24, followed by itchy and flaky skin.

Diagnostic Studies: The methods and techniques for diagnosis are physical examination and review of medical history, blood test, x-ray study, and arthrocentesis.

Macropathology: Gout is typically found on the helix of the ear, on fingers and toes, in the olecranon bursae, and along the olecranon.

Micropathology: Tophi, or collections of uric acid crystals, can be found in the soft tissue.

Treatment: Acute attacks of gout are treated with nonsteroidal anti-inflammatory drugs, oral colchicine, or joint aspiration and lavage. Long-term management includes lifestyle changes, reduction of uric acid levels with allopurinol, and probenecid, which prevents the reabsorption of urate.

Horizontal (Metaphyseal/Diaphyseal Growth) and Spherical (Epiphyseal Growth)

Histologic Arrangement Identical Except Metaphyseal Portion:
Reserve Zone: Storage of lipids, glycogen, and proteoglycan
• Key Diseases: Lysosomal storage disease (Gaucher's), diastrophic dwarfism, pseudoachondro-
plasia, Kniest's syndrome
Proliferative Zone: Matrix production, cellular proliferation, and longitudinal stacking of
chondrocytes
• Key Diseases: Gigantism, achondroplasia
Hypertrophic Zone: Growth and ultimately death of chondrocytes with release of calcium,
subdivided into three zones:
• Maturation Zone: Growth of chondrocytes and storage of calcium
  • Key Diseases: Mucopolysaccharidosis; Morquio's and Hurler's syndromes
• Degenerative Zone: Mitochondrial degeneration
  • Key Diseases: Mucopolysaccharidosis; Morquio's and Hurler's syndromes
• Provisional Calcification: Calcification of matrix
  • Key Diseases: Rickets, osteomalacia, slipped capital femoral epiphysis
Metaphysis: Two zones:
• Primary Spongiosa: Bone formation
  • Key Diseases: Metaphyseal chondroplasia with extension of hypertrophic zone into metaphysis
• Secondary Spongiosa: Remodeling occurs by replacement of fibrous bone with lamellar bone
  • Key Diseases: Osteopetrosis, osteogenesis imperfecta, scurvy, metaphyseal dysplasia

Periphery of the Physis

Groove of Ranvier: Supplies chondrocytes to the periphery of the growth plate to allow for
lateral growth, supplied by perichondral artery
Perichondral Ring of LaCroix: Dense fibrous band that anchors and supports the periphery of
the physis

Blood Supply

Zone Dependent:
• Epiphyseal Artery: Supplies the reserve zone, the proliferative zone, and the two upper zones of the
  hypertrophic zone. Blood supply decreases from the reserve zone to the zone of degeneration.
• Metaphyseal Artery: Supplies the secondary and primary spongiosa with a rich blood supply.

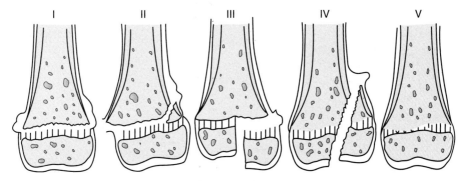

Fig. 103-1   Types of growth plate injury (I to V) as classified by Salter and Harris. *(From Salter RB, Harris
WR: Injuries involving the epiphyseal plate. J Bone Joint Surg [Am] 45:587, 1963.)*

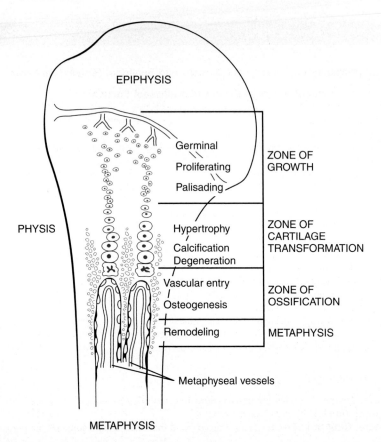

EPIPHYSIS

Germinal

Proliferating

Palisading

ZONE OF
GROWTH

PHYSIS

Hypertrophy

Calcification

Degeneration

ZONE OF
CARTILAGE
TRANSFORMATION

Vascular entry

Osteogenesis

ZONE OF
OSSIFICATION

Remodeling

METAPHYSIS

Metaphyseal vessels

METAPHYSIS

Fig. 103-2 The physics of the proximal humerus. Note that fractures through the growth plate often occur through the zone of hypertrophy and the zone of provisional calcification. *(From DeLee D, Drez D [eds]: DeLee and Drez's Orthopaedic Sports Medicine, 2nd ed. Philadelphia, Saunders, 2003.)*

Definition: Hallux rigidus is a degenerative process involving the first metatarsophalangeal (MTP) joint. Motion is restricted by periarticular osteophytes, especially in dorsiflexion.

Etiology: This condition is more common in adults than adolescents. Hallux rigidus can occur as a result of acute trauma (fracture or forced hyperextension or plantar flexion) or more often from repetitive microtrauma injuring articular cartilage. The degenerative changes result in dorsolateral osteophytes and synovitis.

Symptoms: Onset is often insidious with activity-related pain. Limitation in dorsiflexion leads to difficulties running, squatting, walking up hills, and wearing certain footwear (especially high heels). Lateral foot pain can occur due to walking in supination. Medial great toe paresthesias can occur as a result of dorsal cutaneous nerve compression between osteophytes and shoes.

Clinical Findings: On examination, the most common finding is limitation of dorsiflexion and associated pain with forced dorsiflexion. Osteophytes may be palpable, and if severe enough, may keep hallux in flexion.

Diagnostic Studies: Weight-bearing anteroposterior (AP) and lateral radiographs are usually sufficient for diagnosis when coupled with physical examination. AP radiographs reveal nonuniform narrowing of the MTP joint space and marginal osteophytes. Osteophyte proliferation may cause overestimation of degree of narrowing. Lateral views allow visualization of the degree of dorsal osteophytes and presence of loose bodies.

Classification: Hallux rigidus has three grades based on radiographic findings. There is disagreement on the usefulness of the grading system in that degenerative changes do not necessarily correlate with clinical symptoms.

Grade I: Mild hallux rigidus—joint space maintained with minimal osteophytes

Grade II: Moderate hallux rigidus—some joint space narrowing and dorsolateral osteophytes

Grade III: Severe hallux rigidus—significant joint space narrowing and extensive osteophytes

Treatment: Nonsurgical versus surgical treatment is determined based on patient's symptoms and degree of degenerative changes.

Nonsurgical: Nonsteroidal anti-inflammatory drugs and footwear modifications (e.g., deep toe box, rigid soles, metatarsal bars) to limit first MTP motion are used.

Surgical: Treatment should be directed to relieve pain; patients should be told that no surgical procedure can restore normal anatomy.

- Cheilectomy: Resection of dorsal 25% to 33% MT head; must gain 70- to 90-degree dorsiflexion; good relief of dorsal osteophyte impingement; preserves joint motion; arthrodesis if cheilectomy fails

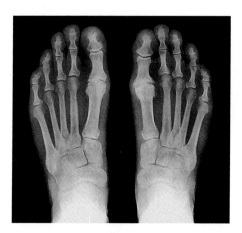

Fig. 104-1 Standing anteroposterior radiograph of both feet. This demonstrates bilateral hallux rigidus or degenerative joint disease of the hallux MTP joints. The signs are narrowing of the joint space, osteophyte formation, and sclerosis. This is more pronounced on the right. *(From Frontera WR: Essentials of Physical Medicine and Rehabilitation, 2nd ed. Philadelphia, Saunders, 2008.)*

- Osteotomy of proximal phalanx: Dorsal closing wedge osteotomy increases proximal phalanx flexion on first MT; done in conjunction with cheilectomy to gain sufficient range of motion
- Resection arthroplasty: Removal of the base of proximal phalanx to decompress the first MTP joint; can result in cock-up deformity due to instability of joint
- Arthrodesis: Definitive procedure for pain relief with severe joint narrowing; fuse 10- to 15-degree dorsiflexion recommended; complications include nonunion, malunion, arthritis of interphalangeal joint
- Interpositional arthroplasty: High complication rate and lacks superiority to arthrodesis

Definition: Deviation of the first metatarsal and lateral deviation and/or rotation of the hallux.

Etiology: Perhaps a genetic predisposition. Other sources include biomechanical instability, traumatic, and metabolic factors such as gouty and rheumatoid arthritis. Additionally, neuromuscular diseases such as Charcot-Marie-Tooth disease and multiple sclerosis have been implicated.

Incidence: Afflicts approximately 1% of the adult population in the United States.

Age: Evidence suggests an increased incidence with age.

Gender: Purported female-to-male ratio of 2:1 to 4:1.

Race: No predilection.

Signs and Symptoms: Patients may present with deep, sharp, stabbing pain with ambulation or a dull aching pain that may or may not be exacerbated with the use of certain types of footwear.

Clinical Findings: Decreased range of motion, medial prominence, abnormal hallux position, pain, and contracture.

Diagnostic Studies: Laboratory studies are indicated when metabolic disease is suspected (i.e., uric acid, sedimentation rate). Radiographs, anteroposterior, lateral, and lateral oblique are standard imaging views for diagnosis. Angles, structures, and positions should be assessed.

Classification: Root and colleagues described the pathomechanical development of hallux valgus in four stages:

Stage 1: Excessive pronation causes hypermobility of the first ray, causing the tibial sesamoid ligament to be stretched and the fibular sesamoid ligament to contract, as well as lateral subluxation of the proximal phalanx.

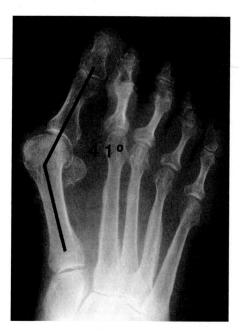

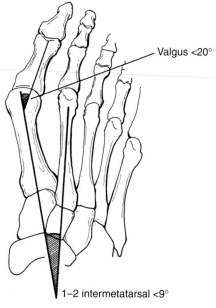

Fig. 105-1 Severe hallux valgus deformity with subluxation of first metatarsophalangeal joint. *(From DeLee D, Drez D [eds]: DeLee and Drez's Orthopaedic Sports Medicine, 2nd ed. Philadelphia, Saunders, 2003.)*

Fig. 105-2 The 1-2 intermetatarsal angle is measured by lines bisecting the axis of the first and second metatarsals. The hallux valgus angle is the angle subtended by the axis of the proximal phalanx and the first metatarsal. *(From DeLee D, Drez D [eds]: DeLee and Drez's Orthopaedic Sports Medicine, 2nd ed. Philadelphia, Saunders, 2003.)*

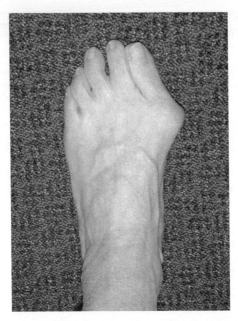

Fig. 105-3 Clinical photograph of hallux valgus deformity. *(From Firestein GS: Kelley's Textbook of Rheumatology, 8th ed. Philadelphia, Saunders, 2008.)*

Stage 2: Hallux abduction progresses, with the flexor hallucis longus and flexor hallucis brevis gaining lateral mechanical advantage.

Stage 3: Further subluxation at the first metatarsophalangeal joint occurs, with formation of metatarsus primus adductus.

Stage 4: The first metatarsophalangeal joint finally dislocates.

Treatment: Conservative and surgical treatment may be considered.

Medical: Aimed at decreasing symptoms, medical interventions include a wider toe box for shoes, nonsteroidal anti-inflammatory drugs, corticosteroid injection, and orthotic therapy.

Surgical: Exostectomy, osteotomy, resectional arthroplasty, and arthrodesis are the surgical options with the common goal to correct deformity or restore function.

Complications: Infection, nonunion, delayed wound healing, hardware failure, and numbness or tingling are some of the sequelae following surgical intervention.

Characteristics:
- Abnormal flexion posture of proximal interphalangeal (PIP) joint of one of the lesser four toes
- May be fixed or supple

Etiology:
- May involve flexure contracture of flexor digitorum longus (FDL) tendon (dynamic deformity)
- Long second metatarsal
- Bunions/hallux valgus (high heels, crowded shoes)
- Rheumatoid arthritis

Physical Examination:
- Examine for callus formation over dorsum of PIP joint
- Look for accentuation of hammer toe when standing (intrinsics relax)
- Distinction between supple/dynamic:
  - Pressure on the plantar aspect of the metatarsal heads will cause toe extension in supple hammer toes.
  - Plantar flexion of the ankle will straighten the toe. In contrast, dorsiflexion of the ankle will worsen the deformity if the hammer toe is due to contracture of the FDL tendon (dynamic).

Treatment:
Nonoperative: If recent onset, pads over corns and daily stretching of PIP joint or hammer toe; orthotics
Operative:
- Hallux valgus must be corrected before hammer toe correction.
- Mild Deformity (No Fixed Deformity): Isolated tenotomy of FDL tendon (transfer of FDL tendon over mid-portion of proximal phalanx, which serves to augment intrinsic function, metatarsal phalangeal [MTP] flexion, PIP extension).
- Moderate Deformity (Fixed PIP Flexion Contracture and Mild Extension Contracture of MTP): Girdlestone Taylor procedure or PIP arthroplasty.
- Severe Deformity (Fixed PIP Flexion and MTP Extension Contractures and/or MTP Dislocation/Subluxation): PIP arthroplasty plus release of MTP dorsal capsule, intrinsics, collateral ligaments, plus extensor tenotomy. PIP/MTP K-wire stabilization for 3 weeks.

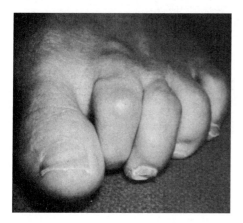

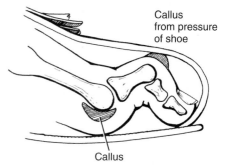

Fig. 106-1 Contracture of all the lesser toes may indicate a tightness of the flexor digitorum longus. (© *M. J. Coughlin. From DeLee D, Drez D [eds]: DeLee and Drez's Orthopaedic Sports Medicine, 2nd ed. Philadelphia, Saunders, 2003.*)

Fig. 106-2 Dorsal aspect of the proximal interphalangeal joint strikes the toe box, leading to callus formation. An intractable plantar keratosis may develop beneath the metatarsal head. (*From DeLee D, Drez D [eds]: DeLee and Drez's Orthopaedic Sports Medicine, 2nd ed. Philadelphia, Saunders, 2003.*)

The Eight Tendon Transfer Principles

1. Preoperative correction of joint contractures
2. Adequate strength of transferred muscles
   - The transferred muscle will lose one grade of strength (i.e., go from 4/5 to 3/5)
   - Avoid transferring previously denervated muscles
3. Match donor excursion—may increase amplitude of excursion by increasing the number of joints a transferred tendon crosses or with more dissection of muscle
   - Wrist flexors and extensors = 33 mm
   - Finger extensors and extensor pollicis longus (EPL) = 50 mm
   - Finger flexors = 70 mm
4. Make a straight line of pull
5. One tendon for one function
6. Use synergistic muscle groups
   - In the hand, finger flexion and wrist extension (and vice versa) are biomechanically linked. It is easier to rehabilitate if the transfers stay between the related groups.
7. Use expendable donor muscles
8. Avoid adhesion formation
   - Delay transfers until wounds are well healed and scars are soft.
   - Use natural tissue planes and avoid placing tendons under scars.

Test Taking: First ask what is missing? Then what is still available? Then remedy the two.

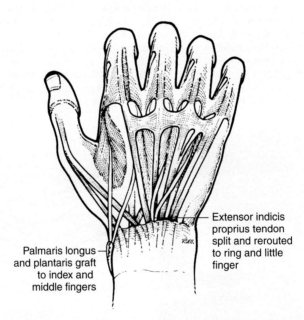

Palmaris longus and plantaris graft to index and middle fingers

Extensor indicis proprius tendon split and rerouted to ring and little finger

Fig. 107-1 Riordan transfer to restore intrinsic function of fingers. *(From Canale ST, Beaty J [eds]: Campbell's Operative Orthopaedics, 11th ed. Philadelphia, Mosby, 2007.)*

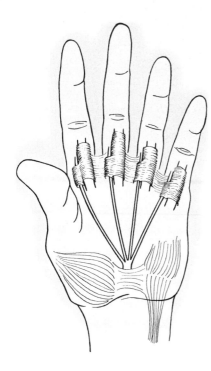

Fig. 107-2 Modification of Bunnell transfer to restore intrinsic function of fingers. *(From Canale ST, Beaty JH [eds]: Campbell's Operative Orthopaedics, 11th ed. Philadelphia, Mosby, 2007.)*

PALMAR VIEW WITH STRUCTURES PASSING THROUGH AND OVER CARPAL TUNNEL

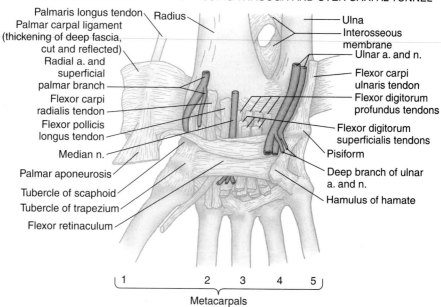

Fig. 107-3 Vascular supply to the wrist. Note the relationship of the wrist ligaments to the neurovascular supply to the wrist. *(From Marx JA: Rosen's Emergency Medicine: Concepts and Clinical Practice, 6th ed. Philadelphia, Mosby, 2006.)*

Common Tendon Transfers

Radial Nerve Dysfunction:
- Pronator teres (PT) to extensor carpi radialis brevis (ECRB) *and*
- Flexor carpi radialis (FCR) to extensor digitorum communis (EDC) *and*
- Palmaris longus (PL) to rerouted EPL

Low Median Nerve (Distal to Anterior Interosseous Nerve [AIN]) Dysfunction
- Opponensplasty
- Flexor digitorum superficialis (FDS) of ring finger to thumb *or*
- Extensor indicis proprius (EIP) to adductor pollicis brevis from volar-ulnar side *or*
- Abductor digiti minimi to adductor pollicis brevis

High Median Nerve (Proximal to AIN) Dysfunction
- Brachioradialis to flexor pollicis longus (FPL) *and*
- Suture all flexor digitorum profundus (FDP) together

Ulnar Nerve Dysfunction (Many Options)
- Extensor carpi radialis longus (ECRL) through carpal tunnel to lateral band of index through small
- *and* FDS ring to thumb adductor tubercle

Nonfunctional, Clenched, Spastic Hand:
- FDS to FDP *and* FPL Z-lengthening

Principles: No esmarch, extensile incisions, minimize exposure of vessels/nerves/tendons.

Common Bacteria	Antibiotics
Staphylococcus—primary organism in 50% to 80% of infections	Cefazolin
Mixed gram (+) and (−)—in bites, IV drug abuse	Augmentin (amoxicillin/clavulanate potassium)
Eikenella corrodens—up to ⅓ of human bites	Penicillin
Pasteurella multocida—up to ¼ of dog and cat bites	Augmentin/Unasyn (ampicillin and sulbactam)

Paronychia: Infection beneath eponychial fold, usually mixed infection, most common organism is *Staphylococcus aureus*.
Treatment:
• Usually incision and drainage, then soaks
• For chronic *Candida albicans*, atypical mycobacteria, and gram-negative cases, usually marsupialization and nail removal.
Felon: Tense pulp space infection, usually with *S. aureus*.
Treatment:
• Incision and drainage, then soaks and intravenous antibiotics
• High lateral or midvolar incisions (high risk of tip necrosis with "fish-mouth" incision)
Herpes: Can be confused with felons/paronychia.
• Most often in dental/medical personnel, organism is herpes simplex
• *Diagnosis:* Cultures of vesicular fluid, Tzanck smear
• Self-limited, *avoid* incision and drainage (risk of superinfection); acyclovir may shorten duration
Flexor Tenosynovitis: Bacterial infection of the flexor sheath, risk is of adhesion, tendon rupture
• Flexor sheaths to thumb and small finger usually contiguous with radial and ulnar bursae
• *Kanavel's Signs:* Finger held flexed, "sausage" digit, tender over sheath, pain with passive extension
• *Treatment:* Urgent, either open or limited (with catheter irrigation) decompression
• Postoperative early range of motion and soaks; low threshold for repeat operation
• Radial and ulnar bursae are extensions of sheaths to thumb and small finger
Deep Space Infections: Infections of potential spaces in the hand or forearm
• *Deep Spaces:* Dorsal subaponeurotic, thenar, midpalmar, hypothenar, Parona's space (forearm)
• *Horseshoe Abscess:* Infection of radial or ulnar bursa that connects through Parona's space
• *Collar Button Abscess:* Barbell-shaped web space infection; incision and drainage without incising web space
• Midpalmar and hypothenar space infections are rare
Septic Arthritis: *Staphylococcus aureus* and *Streptococcus* most common organisms
• Presentation, workup, and management similar to that for other septic arthritides
Animal Bites: Commonly polymicrobial
• *Most Common Organisms: Streptococcus, Staphylococcus, Pasteurella*
• *Treatment:*
  • Wound exploration and extension, if suspicion of joint, bone, or tendon sheath penetration
  • Rabies prophylaxis for wild skunk, bat, fox, coyote, raccoon, bobcat, or rabid domestic pet bites
• *Vibrio* (acute, aggressive) or *Mycobacterium marinum* (chronic, indolent) with aquatic environments

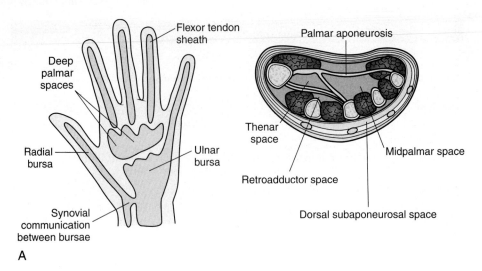

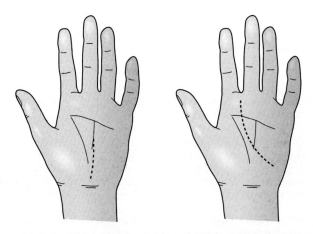

Fig. 108-1 **A,** Deep spaces of the hand and synovial bursae. Infections may be bound by these spaces or may track along anatomic dissection planes between these spaces. **B,** Incision for thenar space infection. A dorsal first webspace incision is also often required. Incision for midpalmar space abscess. *(From Townsend CM, Jr: Sabiston Textbook of Surgery, 18th ed. Philadelphia, Saunders, 2007.)*

Human Bites: Clenched fist type (metacarpal head); may involve metacarpophalangeal joint despite proximal location of wound
- May appear benign; requires incision and drainage and intravenous antibiotics (coverage for *Eikenella, Staphylococcus, Streptococcus,* and gram-negative organisms
- Assume fight/bite type injury until proved otherwise

Atypical Infections

- *Fungus:* Superficial—*Candida* in paronychia, *Trichophyton* in onychomycosis
- *Subcutaneous: Sporothrix* after rose thorn or soil injuries, treat with potassium iodine
- *Deep:* Histoplasmosis, blastomycosis, coccidioidomycosis, opportunistic infections
- *Mycobacterial: M. marinum,* in fresh and salt water; *Mycobacterium avium, Mycobacterium kansasii, Mycobacterium terrae* in soil

Injection Injuries: Frequently benign appearing, but often lead to tissue necrosis
- *Treatment:* Emergent, aggressive decompression and débridement
- Amputation rate 50% with oil-based paints

Necrotizing Fasciitis: Clostridia or Group A beta-hemolytic strep; mortality 9% to 75%
- *Treatment:* Emergent, extensive débridement, broad-spectrum antibiotics, close monitoring

Differential Diagnosis: Crystalline arthropathy, pyogenic granuloma, skin tumors (think basal cell carcinoma with chronic ulcers), metastatic disease

Most masses in the hand are benign.

In general, treatment for hand tumors is surgical excision. If malignancy is suspected, an incisional biopsy should be performed. Because excision is curative for benign soft tissue tumors, excisional biopsy is generally the treatment of choice. Benign tumors of bone are generally managed with curettage. Malignant tumors need wide excision with a 2-cm tumor-free cuff; depending on location, this may necessitate amputation.

Benign Lesions:

Ganglion Cyst: Ganglia are the most common type of soft tissue mass in the hand. Dorsal carpal ganglia are often centered near the lunate; volar carpal ganglia are often adjacent to the radial artery and may be intimately associated with it.

Mucous Cysts: Occur in the setting of degenerative arthritis and are located on the dorsal surface over the interphalangeal (IP) joints.

Cysts will transilluminate, which aids in differentiating them from soft tissue masses. Asymptomatic ganglia may be managed with periodic observation. A symptomatic lesion that is not adjacent to digital nerves or arteries may be aspirated. Persistent painful or enlarging lesions should be excised.

Giant Cell Tumor of Tendon Sheath: These are the second most common tumor of the hand; they are benign and often located over the palmar aspect of the finger. The lesion is firm and nodular. Excisional biopsy confirms diagnosis. Grossly yellow or tan lobulated mass. Histology—spindle cells, fibrous tissue, multinucleated giant cells; 10% recurrence after excision.

Lipoma: Most common solid cellular hand tumor, arises from mesenchymal primordial fatty tissue cells. Recurrence after marginal excision unlikely.

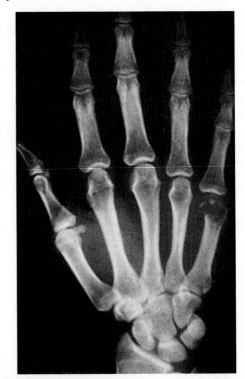

Fig. 109-1 Pathologic fracture caused by a tumor. *(From Canale ST, Beaty JH: Campbell's Operative Orthopaedics, 11th ed. Philadelphia, Mosby, 2007.*

Glomus Tumor: Pain, cold sensitivity, and point tenderness. Often located beneath the fingernail. Complete excision is curative.

Enchondroma: most common primary bone tumor of the hand. Most common location proximal metaphysis of proximal phalanx. Managed with curettage and bone grafting.

Aneurysmal Bone Cyst: Eccentric metaphyseal ballooning lesions.

Giant Cell Tumor of Bone: Curettage and bone grafting generally not sufficient—resection of bone and reconstructive surgery may be needed.

Malignant Lesions: Primary malignant tumors of the hand are very rare.

Osteogenic Sarcoma: Very rare. Necessitates wide excision.

Chondrosarcoma: Most common primary malignant bone tumor. Pain is the presenting symptom. Total resection needed.

Epithelioid Sarcoma: Commonly misdiagnosed due to benign course—present as subcutaneous firm masses. Metastasis to regional nodes and the lungs. Histology granulomatous pattern with central necrosis. Primary wide excision needed.

Squamous Cell Carcinoma: Comprises 58% to 90% of all hand malignancies and is the most common malignancy of the nail bed. Metastasis is rare. Excision with tumor-free margins of at least 0.5 cm (small lesions) to 3 cm (recurrent or fixed lesion.)

Basal Cell Carcinoma: Manifests as a raised, pearly bordered lesion. Excise with 0.5-cm free margin.

Melanoma: Any black or brown lesion beneath a fingernail must be assessed for the possibility of subungual melanoma

Metastatic Lesions: The most common sites of metastatic lesions to the hand are lung, kidney, breast, prostate, colon, and uterus. Median survival is 5 to 6 months after the identification of a metastatic lesion in the hand.

Definition: Autosomal recessive disease characterized by high intestinal iron absorption resulting in the pathologic deposition of iron in organs.

Incidence: Common among northern European descent; variable expression; exact incidence unknown, 1 to 5 per 1000.

Gender: Male-to-female ratio of 5 to 10:1.

Age: Patients typically present between 40 and 60 years of age.

Clinical Features:

Extra-articular: Lethargy, hepatomegaly, hyperpigmentation, diabetes, abdominal pain, decreased libido, testicular atrophy, osteoporosis.

Articular:

- Arthropathy of hemachromatosis: Pain and stiffness before objective enlargement of joint
  - Final stages: Limitation of motion, increased pain with use, progressive deformity, and bone spur formation.
  - Absent synovial thickening, warmth, and erythema.
  - Predominantly hands (especially metacarpophalangeal [MCP] joints) and wrists, but also common in knees, hips, ankles, feet, and shoulders
  - Chondrocalcinosis due to calcium pyrophosphate dehydrate (CPPD) or hydroxyapatite deposition

Radiographic Features: Joint space narrowing and subchondral sclerosis of MCP joints (particularly second and third), hooklike osteophytes of metacarpal head, minimal radiocarpal joint space narrowing. Subtle chondrocalcinosis in the triangular fibrocartilage complex above the ulna styloid.

Laboratory Feature: Elevated transferrin saturation and serum ferritin levels.

Diagnosis: Direct measurement of iron in liver biopsy specimen.

Treatment: Remove excess iron by phlebotomy.

- Phlebotomy generally does not alleviate symptoms of arthralgia and loss of joint mobility in patients with established arthropathy.
- Nonsteroidal anti-inflammatory drugs used for chronic arthritis.
- CPPD is treated with joint aspiration, intra-articular cortisone, and prophylaxis with colchicine.
- Arthroplasty is indicated for progressive joint destruction.

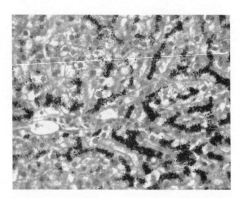

Fig. 110-1 Hereditary hemochromatosis. Hepatocellular iron deposition is blue in this Prussian blue–stained section of an early stage of the disease in which parenchymal architecture is normal. *(From Kumar V, et al: Robbins and Cotran Pathologic Basis of Disease, 7th ed. Philadelphia, Saunders, 2005.)*

228

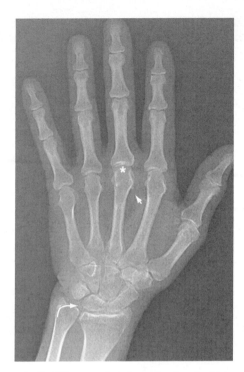

Fig. 110-2 Hemochromatosis. Hooklike osteophyte (*arrowhead*) at the third metacarpal head with cartilage loss at metacarpophalangeal joints (*Star*) and chondrocalcinosis of triangular fibrocartilage (*bent arrow*) are typical features of hemochromatosis. *(From Firestein GS: Kelley's Textbook of Rheumatology, 8th ed. Philadelphia, Saunders, 2008.)*

Definition: Hemophilia is a hereditary blood coagulation disorder causing either a deficiency or absence of one of the clotting factors.

Incidence: One in 7500 males and 1 in 25 million females are born with hemophilia. There are about 17,000 individuals in the United States with the disease. Hemophilia A is 7 times more common than hemophilia B, and 1 in 100,000 individuals are born with hemophilia C.

Age: Onset of inherited hemophilia is in vitro. Onset of acquired hemophilia is at any age; however, acquired hemophilia is typically seen in older adults and in individuals with an autoimmune disease.

Gender: Hemophilia is significantly more prevalent in males.

Etiology and Pathophysiology:
Hemophilia A is an X-linked recessive deficiency of factor VIII:C. Factor VIII:C is required for the activation of factor X in the coagulation cascade. Hemostasis is interrupted due to this deficiency. Hemophilia B is an X-linked recessive deficiency of factor IX. The etiology and pathophysiology are similar to those of hemophilia A. Hemophilia C is an autosomal recessive deficiency of factor XI, also interrupting hemostasis. Acquired hemophilia is caused by autoantibodies directed at factor VIII.

Associations: Family history plays a major role in the onset of hemophilia. In hemophilia C there is an increased frequency in Ashkenazi Jews.

Signs and Symptoms: The two major signs and symptoms of hemophilia are bleeding and bruising. Hemarthrosis and blood in the urine and stool are indicative of a more severe case of hemophilia.

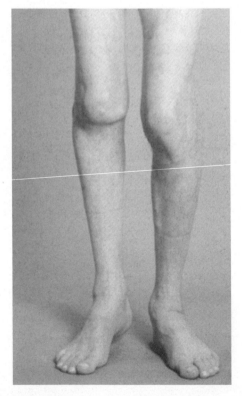

Fig. 111-1 Severe chronic arthritis in hemophilia. The knee is the most commonly affected joint. Both knees are severely deranged in this patient. Note that he is unable to stand with both feet flat on the floor. *(From Forbes CD, Jackson WF: Color Atlas and Text of Clinical Medicine, 3rd ed. London, Mosby, 2003, with permission.)*

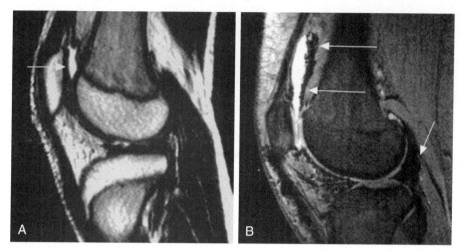

Fig. 111-2 Magnetic resonance imaging (MRI) of soft tissue changes associated with hemophilic arthropathy. **A,** Small effusion in the knee of a child with hemophilia (*arrow*). **B,** Moderate synovial hyperplasia in the knee of an adult with hemophilia (*arrows*). (*A, B, From Nuss R, Kilcoyne RE [eds]: The MRI Atlas of Hemophilic Arthropathy. New York, Professional Publishing Group, 2002. Courtesy of Professional Publishing Group, Ltd.*)

Diagnostic Studies: A routine blood workup can detect prolonged prothrombin time (PT), partial thromboplastin time (PTT), or both. Mixing studies are used to detect antibody formation against a clotting factor, and an activated PTT test may be performed to monitor the activities of factors VIII, IX, and XI.

Macropathology: An injured blood vessel of an individual with hemophilia will not complete the basic mechanisms of hemostasis and will continue to bleed out into the tissues, causing bruise formation and internal/external bleeding. Although hemarthrosis may occur in any joint, it most commonly occurs in the knees, elbows, and ankles.

Micropathology: After vascular injury, an individual with hemophilia will have low or zero blood levels of factor VIII, factor IX, or factor XI, resulting in low levels of thrombin. There are normal levels of other coagulation factors, macrophages, platelets, and tissue factors that accompany a hemostatic response.

Treatment: Treatment is dependent on the severity of the disease. Severe hemophilia is treated with replacement therapy by infusions of the deficient or absent clotting factor concentrates. Desmopressin is given in mild case hemophilia on an "as needed" basis. Other forms of treatment include immunosuppressive therapy, plasma exchange, factor VII product transfusions, recombinant activated factor VIIa transfusions, prothrombin complex concentrates (PCCs), and activated PCCs.

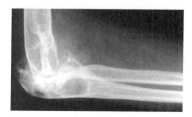

Fig. 111-3 Hemophilia. A lateral view of the elbow shows marked destruction of the joint space. Chronic bleeding within the joint has destroyed the cartilage. Similar findings may be seen with juvenile rheumatoid arthritis. (*From Mettler FA, Jr: Essentials of Radiology, 2nd ed. Philadelphia, Saunders, 2005.*)

Definition: Viral hepatitis refers to a group of diseases caused by the known hepatotropic viruses that cause inflammation of the liver, including hepatitis viruses A (HAV), B (HBV), C (HCV), D (HDV), and E (HEV). These viruses all cause acute viral hepatitis, which in some cases leads to chronic hepatitis. HAV is the most common cause of acute hepatitis in the United States; HCV is the most common cause of chronic hepatitis. There are also other viral agents, referred to as hepatitis F (HFV), hepatitis G (HGV), or other non-ABC viruses, that may cause a small percentage of acute hepatitis cases; however, there is very little information on these viruses.

Etiology: HAV is most commonly transmitted through the fecal-oral route. It may also spread via contaminated food or water or infected serum. Maternal-neonatal transmission is not established. HBV is most commonly caused by sexual contact or perinatal transmission due to contact with a mother's infected blood at the time of delivery. HBV infection is also often due to mucous membrane exposure or percutaneous exposure to infectious body fluids, which include semen, vaginal mucus, saliva, and tears. The virus is not detected in urine, stool, or sweat. HCV can be transmitted parenterally, perinatally, and sexually. It is most reliably transmitted through blood transfusions, organ transplants, and needle sharing among intravenous drug users. HDV transmission is similar to HBV transmission, although perinatal transmission rarely occurs and has not been documented in the United States. Needle sharing among intravenous drug users is thought to be the most common means of transmitting HDV. HEV is transmitted mainly by the fecal-oral route. The most common means of transmission is fecally contaminated water. Transmission by person-to-person contact is undocumented.

Incidence:

HAV: Approximately 22,700 new cases are reported annually in the United States. It is estimated that for every reported case, there are five or six unreported cases. Almost one third of adults in the United States have serologic evidence of prior HAV infection. In developing countries, infection is highly endemic; nearly 100% of the adult population has serologic evidence of past HAV disease.

HBV: Approximately 200,000 new cases occur annually in the United States. Approximately 200 million people worldwide are carriers.

HCV: Approximately 30,000 new cases occur each year in the United States. More than 170 million people are infected worldwide.

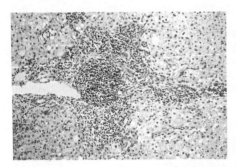

Fig. 112-1   Chronic viral hepatitis due to hepatitis C virus, showing portal tract expansion with inflammatory cells and fibrous tissue and interface hepatitis with spillover of inflammation into the adjacent parenchyma. A lymphoid aggregate is present. *(From Kumar V, et al: Robbins and Cotran Pathologic Basis of Disease, 7th ed. Philadelphia, Saunders, 2005.)*

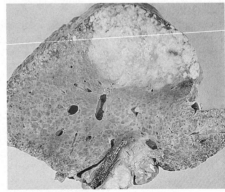

Fig. 112-2   Hepatocellular carcinoma. *(From Cohen J, Powderly W: Infectious Diseases, 2nd ed. Philadelphia, Mosby, 2004.)*

HDV: Worldwide prevalence is approximately 15 million.

HEV: Not currently endemic in the United States.

Age:

HAV: Usually acquired before the age of 2 in developing countries. In Western countries it is usually acquired between the ages of 5 and 17, but is often subclinical. The older a person is when he or she acquires HAV, the greater the chance of adverse symptoms and sequelae.

HBV: Usually acquired after the age of 12, due to the initiation of sexual contact. The earlier in life HBV is acquired, the higher the chance of developing chronic hepatitis.

HCV: Of new cases, 65% are in persons between 30 and 49 years of age. The younger a person is when HCV is acquired, the better the prognosis.

HDV: Usually acquired in adulthood.

HEV: Usually acquired between the ages of 15 and 40.

Gender: HBV—more common in males than in females. HAV, HCV, HDV, HEV—no preponderance.

Race:

HAV: Prevalence higher among American Indians, Alaskan natives, and some Hispanic groups.

HBV: Prevalence is higher among African Americans and persons of Hispanic or Asian origin. Also a higher carrier rate exists among certain subpopulations such as the Alaskan natives, Asian Pacific islanders, and Australian aborigines.

HCV: More common among minority populations.

HDV: More common among persons from the Mediterranean basin.

HEV: No racial predilection.

Signs and Symptoms:

HAV: General appearance is that of mild-to-moderate illness. Initial symptoms during the prodromal period include low-grade fever, nausea, vomiting, decreased appetite, and abdominal pain. Diarrhea may occur in young children, whereas constipation is more common in adults. In the icteric phase dark urine appears followed by pale stool. Jaundice occurs in 70% to 85% of adults but is less common in children and may be accompanied by itching. Abdominal pain occurs in approximately 40% of patients. Hepatomegaly is common and splenomegaly may occur in 10% to 20% of patients.

HBV: Generally expressed as anicteric hepatitis and is usually asymptomatic. If it is expressed as icteric hepatitis, symptoms may be similar to those of HAV.

HCV: Acute infections are generally subclinical or asymptomatic. Only 25% to 35% of patients with acute infection have nonspecific symptoms such as weakness, malaise, and anorexia. Less than one third of acutely infected patients have hepatomegaly.

HDV: Clinically hard to distinguish from other forms of hepatitis. Up to 90% of cases are subclinical. If symptomatic, they are the same as those for HBV.

HEV: During the prodromal phase, symptoms include myalgia, arthralgia, low-grade fever, anorexia, weight loss, nausea, vomiting, dehydration, and right upper quadrant tenderness.

Diagnostic Studies: No specific imaging is needed to make the diagnosis; liver biopsy may be ordered to guide management strategy. Laboratory studies are indicated to identify surface antigen or core antibodies.

Medical Treatment: Interferons, corticosteroids, and antivirals are used in treatment.

Sequelae:

HAV: Prolonged cholestasis may follow the acute infection, with frequency having a positive correlation to age.

HBV: Fulminant hepatitis is the most serious complication. Other severe complications are cirrhosis and hepatocellular carcinoma. Rare complications include pancreatitis, myocarditis, atypical pneumonia, aplastic anemia, transverse myelitis, and peripheral neuropathy.

HCV: Of persons infected with HIV, 30% to 50% are co-infected with HCV. Co-infection with HIV accelerates the clinical progression of HCV.

HDV: Complications include liver failure, hepatocellular carcinoma, and autoimmune manifestations.

HEV: Pregnancy leads to higher rates of fulminant hepatic failure.

Definition: Heterotopic ossification (HO) is bone formation in the soft tissues surrounding the joint that develops after surgery.

Etiology: An unknown trigger during the surgery seems to cause the primitive mesenchymal cells in the soft tissues surrounding the joint to differentiate into osteoprogenitor cells.

Incidence: The reported rates of HO after a total hip arthroplasty (THA) range from 2% to 90%, depending on the risk factors of the population. Symptomatic HO after total knee arthroplasty (TKA) has been reported in less than 1% of patients.

Associations: Male gender, previous history of HO in hip, ankylosing spondylitis, diffuse idiopathic skeletal hyperostosis (DISH), lateral surgical approach, and cementless femoral components seem to increase the prevalence of HO.

Age and Gender: HO is approximately twice as prevalent in men as in women with spinal cord injury. Osteoarthritic populations older than 65 years are also at an increased risk. There is no significant correlation between age and HO.

Clinical Findings: Pain or restricted range of motion resulting in functional impairment seems to be an important finding in patients with HO after THA or TKA.

Symptoms: Clinically, patients with developing HO can display local signs of inflammation, such as erythema, swelling, effusion, tenderness or pain, and loss of motion.

Signs: Limitation of motion is the most clinically relevant method of assessing the influence of HO on function after THA and TKA.

Staging (Brooker)

Class I: Consists of islands of bone within the soft tissue about the hip.

Class II: Consists of bone spurs from the pelvis or proximal end of the femur, with at least 1 cm between opposing bone surfaces.

Class III: Consists of bone spurs from the pelvis or proximal end of the femur, reducing the space between opposing bone surfaces to less than 1 cm.

Class IV: Apparent bone ankylosis of the hip.

A fifth stage, class 0, no ossification, was added later by Maloney et al.

Pathology: HO represents mature lamellar bone with trabeculae formation in soft tissue.

Investigations: X-rays and computed tomography studies can be used in identification and diagnosis of the condition.

Medical Care: Prophylaxis of high-risk patients, either with external beam radiation therapy or pharmaceutical prophylaxis with nonsteroidal anti-inflammatory drugs (NSAIDs) or other agents, has been shown to reduce the incidence of HO.

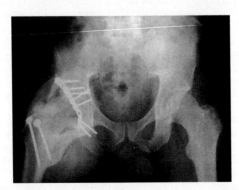

Fig. 113-1 Brooker grade IV heterotopic ossification occurred despite postoperative irradiation. *(From Canale ST, Beaty JH [eds]: Campbell's Operative Orthopaedics, 11th ed. Philadelphia, Mosby, 2007.)*

Surgical Care: Once HO becomes visible on radiographs, only surgical excision will eradicate it. Excision of HO is rarely required after THA or TKA. It is indicated only in cases of increasing pain and decreased range of motion when other causes are excluded.

Complications: Radiation for the prevention of HO carries a potential for malignant transformation. Gastrointestinal tract intolerance, platelet inhibition, and alteration of the anticoagulation profile in patients undergoing thromboembolic prophylaxis with warfarin and other antithromboembolic agents are adverse effects that must be considered with NSAID use.

Definition: High tibial osteotomy (HTO) corrects alignment of the knee, relieving pressure from the arthritic portion of the joint, and transferring it to an area of more normal cartilage. This frequently leads to pain relief and, subsequently, improved function.

Background: HTO for the treatment of medial compartment osteoarthritis has gained acceptance for two reasons. First, the osteotomy can correct the varus malalignment of the limb in question, thereby reducing the stresses passed through the medial compartment of the knee. Second, this restoration of normal limb alignment prevents the further destruction of the medial articular cartilage and further collapse into varus. The goal of HTO in the varus-aligned knee is to correct or even overcorrect the limb into valgus, which serves to redistribute the mechanical forces from the medial compartment.

Patient selection is probably the most important key to a successful outcome.

Age: Candidates for HTOs are patients with localized activity-related knee pain, varus malalignment, and medial compartment degenerative arthritis. However, young patients may be candidates as well in an effort to correct deformity and thwart total knee arthroplasty.

Types: The osteotomy can be distal to the tibial tubercle, as described by Jackson and Waugh, or proximal as described by Coventry. Three types of osteotomies can be performed:

Lateral Closing Wedge Osteotomy: In this osteotomy, a lateral wedge of bone is resected from the tibia. This is the most stable form of osteotomy and has the highest union rate. Problems arise because the limb is shortened and the distance between the tibial tubercle and patella is decreased, thereby shortening the patellar tendon.

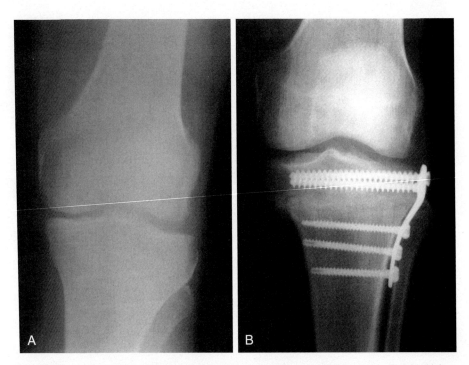

Fig. 114-1   **A,** Medial joint collapse resulting in varus deformity and medial knee pain. **B,** After high tibial osteotomy. *(Courtesy of S. Terry Canale, MD. From Canale ST, Beaty [eds] JH: Campbell's Operative Orthopaedics, 11th ed. Philadelphia, Mosby, 2007.)*

Medial Opening Wedge Osteotomy: The wedge to be opened is determined from radiographs, and the procedure is performed under fluoroscopy. Autograft and allograft are generally used to fill the opening wedge. The osteotomy is then fixed. This osteotomy lengthens the leg and moves the tibial tubercle laterally, which may lead to patellofemoral symptoms. The risk of nonunion also is higher in this osteotomy. Fixation must be significant.

Dome Osteotomy: The dome osteotomy requires a dome cut. The tibia then can be rotated into the appropriate position and fixed. This is the least stable osteotomy and requires significant fixation.

Treatment: Fixation options include simple casting, staples and casting, plate and screw fixation, and external fixation. Each of these methods has advantages and drawbacks. Staple and cast fixation is used quite commonly. There may be loss of motion when the knee is removed from the cast. Postoperative management depends on the type of fixation used. The cast and staple technique requires the patient to be immobilized for 5 to 8 weeks. Weight bearing is begun gradually and, by 10 weeks after surgery, the osteotomy should be healed and nontender, at which time, full weight bearing is resumed. With plate and screw fixation, early mobilization may be undertaken.

Prognosis: With failure defined as the performance of a total knee arthroplasty after the osteotomy, studies report the survivorship was 89% at 5 years and 75% at 10 years. If, at 1 year after the operation, the valgus angulation of the anatomic axis (femorotibial angle) is less than 8 degrees or if the patient's weight is more than 1.32 times the ideal body weight, then survivorship decreases to 38% at 5 years and to 19% at 10 years. Statistics have shown that about 65% to 75% of patients were still satisfied with the result of the tibial osteotomy 10 years after the operation.

Complications: Slight chance of infection, stiffness of the knee, nerve injury, and reflexive sympathetic dystrophy.

Hip arthroscopy allows thorough visualization of acetabular labrum, femoral head, and acetabular chondral surfaces as well as the fovea, ligamentum teres, and adjacent synovium.
- Technically demanding, with a steep learning curve; meticulous positioning and portal placement are essential for safety
- Requires special equipment and distracting tools
- Aids in diagnosis and treatment of labral tears, loose bodies, chondral lesions of the acetabulum and the femoral head, osteonecrosis, ruptured or impinging ligamentum teres, and synovial abnormalities

Acetabular Labral Tears

Acetabular labral tears are the most common cause for mechanical hip symptoms.

History:
- Progression of a minor injury seems to be the rule, as slight injury to the labrum, when subjected to repetitive motion and stress, seems to progress; not necessarily traumatic
- Athletes often recall trauma involving hip flexion, abduction, and forceful knee extension
- Labral tears associated with sudden twisting or pivoting motions
- Tears often associated with congenital or structural hip anomalies (dysplasia, slipped capita femoral epiphysis, Perthes)
- Chronic labral tears may contribute to the progression of hip osteoarthritis, in that labral disruption is part of a continuum of joint pathology that leads to degenerative joint disease

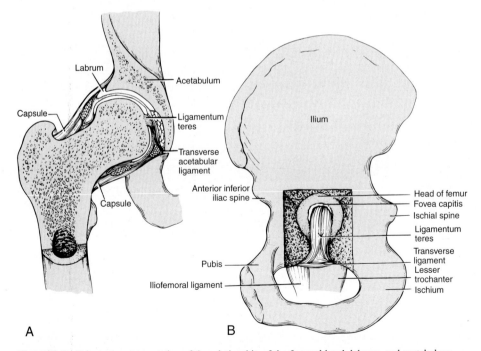

Fig. 115-1   Schematic representation of the relationship of the femoral head, labrum, and acetabulum. The labrum extends beyond the equator of the femoral head, producing excellent joint stability. (*From Browner BD: Skeletal Trauma: Basic Science, Management, and Reconstruction, 3rd ed. Philadelphia, Saunders, 2003.*)

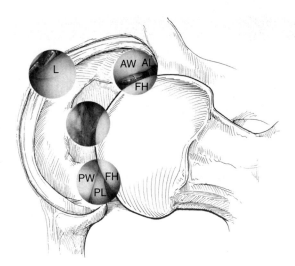

Fig. 115-2   Arthroscopic anatomy of the hip. AL, anterior labrum; AW, wall of acetabulum; FH, femoral head; L, labrum; LT, ligamentum teres; PL, posterior labrum; PW, posterior wall. *(From Miller MD, Osborne JR, Warner JJP, Fu FH [eds]: MRI-Arthroscopy Correlative Atlas. Philadelphia, Saunders, 1997, p 101.)*

Physical Examination:
- Difficult Diagnosis: Hip/anterior inguinal pain; high level of clinical suspicion is paramount.
- Catching, locking, or a painful click in the inguinal area that radiates toward the gluteus.
- McCarthy Sign: A painful click reproduced after both hips are flexed fully; the affected hip is extended, first in external rotation, then in internal rotation.

Radiographic Evaluation:
- Plain radiographs and magnetic resonance imaging (MRI) scans have a low diagnostic yield.
- Gadolinium-enhanced MRI is much more sensitive but not as accurate as hoped.

Anatomic Keys:
- Acetabular labrum has no significant influence on the weight-bearing function of the normal joint; a possible role of this peripheral structure is to seal the joint and provide stability.
- Tears are frequently anterior, at the anterior marginal attachment of the acetabulum.

Treatment:
- Hip arthroscopy is useful in patients with suspected labral pathology based on refractory hip pain with reproducible physical findings and equivocal or negative radiographic studies.
- Arthroscopic treatment involves careful and conservative débridement back to a stable base and healthy-appearing tissue; this will eliminate the source of mechanical symptoms.

Definition:

Intracapsular-Femoral Neck: Fracture between the most distal portion of the articular surface and the most proximal portion of the intertrochanteric region. Location may be subcapital, transcervical, or basicervical; may treat as intertrochanteric.

Extracapsular-Intertrochanteric: Fracture with at least one component between the greater and lesser trochanter.

Etiology: In older adults, usually from simple falls; in young persons, usually from high-energy trauma.

Incidence: More common in older adults. Incidence increasing with the aging population.

Gender: No preponderance.

Symptoms: Present with painful ambulation or the inability to bear weight.

Signs: May have a shortened and rotated lower extremity.

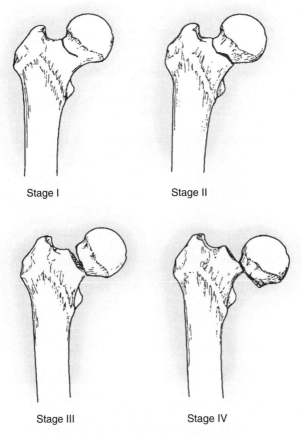

Stage I   Stage II

Stage III   Stage IV

Fig. 116-1 Garden classification of femoral neck fractures. *(From Kyle RF: Fractures of the hip. In Gustilo RB, Kyle RF, Templeman DC, eds: Fractures and Dislocations. St Louis, Mosby, 1993.)*

Classification:

Femoral Neck, Garden's Classification: Type 1, incomplete or impacted in valgus; type 2, non-displaced; type 3, incompletely displaced and in varus alignment; type 4, completely displaced.

Treatment: Depends on type of fracture.

Femoral Neck, Nondisplaced, Impacted Valgus: Cannulated screws.

Displaced: Younger than 50 years, emergent reduction, cannulated screws; older, hemiarthroplasty, unipolar vs. bipolar or total hip arthroplasty if preexisting degenerative changes.

Intertrochanteric: Stable, two and three parts, dynamic hip screw (DHS) vs. trochanteric femoral nail (TFN); unstable, four parts, subtrochanteric extension, TFN.

Reverse Obliquity: TFN, blade plate, dynamic condylar screw, *not* DHS.

Other Considerations:

Stress Fractures: Young, military recruits, runners, female athlete triad (eating disorder, menstrual dysfunction, premature osteoporosis).

Compression Side (Nondisplaced): Non–weight bearing, progress to no crutches in 6 weeks.

Tension Side: Cannulated screws.

Vascular Supply to the Femoral Head:

Medial Femoral Circumflex Artery: Enters capsule posteriorly.

Lateral Retinacular Artery: Intertrochanteric region has excellent blood supply and thus a low nonunion rate.

Definition: Horner's syndrome results from an interruption in the sympathetic nerve supply to the eye and has a high incidence of malignancy.

Incidence: Rare.

Age: May develop at any age.

Gender: Affects both men and women equally.

Race: No racial preference.

Etiology and Pathophysiology: The sympathetic nervous system innervates the eye through a three-neuron arc; Horner's syndrome occurs when this pathway is somehow disrupted.

Associations: May be hereditary, but other causes include migraines, stroke, problems with the carotid artery, cerebral hemorrhaging, tuberculosis, Pancoast tumors, or infection of the lung apex.

Signs and Symptoms: Miosis, loss or slowing of the dilator muscle, anhidrosis, loss of sweating on the affected side, ptosis, and red conjunctiva are indicators of Horner's syndrome.

Diagnostic Studies: Computed tomography scans, chest radiographs, and magnetic resonance imaging scan showing cross-sectional areas of the neck can be used to detect the underlying causes for Horner's syndrome, but the cocaine test detects Horner's syndrome itself. The 10% liquid cocaine is administered as eye drops and inhibits the reuptake of norepinephrine. A positive test occurs when the pupil dilates poorly after 30 minutes.

Micropathology: Lesions interrupt the sympathetic pathway, affecting the primary ganglionic, preganglionic, or postganglionic neuron and resulting in the symptoms of Horner's syndrome.

Macropathology: Skin or eye redness and dry skin paired with a lack of sweating may help localize the affected region.

Treatment: Treatments vary depending on the underlying cause. There is no general treatment for the disease.

Distal Humerus Fracture

A distal humerus fracture (DHF) is a fracture whose epicenter falls within the square created by epicondyle to epicondyle to the distal end of the humerus. DHF is a rare fracture that comprises only 0.5% of fractures. The mechanism of injury (MOI) is an axial load through the elbow with the joint flexed greater than 90 degrees (at 90 degrees, an axial load will produce an olecranon fracture). Neuritis results in 15% of cases of DHF that undergo open reduction and internal fixation (ORIF). Most frequently, the ulnar nerve is affected due to its vulnerable position in the cubital tunnel.

Classification: Based on the Orthopaedic Trauma Association (OTA) fracture classification in which increasing letters and numbers indicate increasing difficulty of treatment:

A	Supracondylar	A1	Epicondylar avulsion fracture
	Extra-articular	A2	Simple metaphyseal fracture
		A3	Comminuted metaphyseal fracture
B	Unicondylar	B1	Sagittal plane: lateral condylar, including capitellum
		B2	Sagittal plane: Medial condylar, including trochlea
		B3	Frontal Plane
		B31	Capitellum
		B32	Medial condylar: capitellum
C	Transcondylar	C1	Simple articular, simple metaphyseal (Fig. 118-1)
	Bicondylar or	C2	Simple articular, comminuted metaphyseal
	Intercondylar	C3	Comminuted articular

Treatment:

ORIF: Most commonly approached posteriorly by means of olecranon osteotomy.

Plate Fixation: Well-contoured plates should provide light active joint motion through the period of bone healing while minimizing tissue necrosis. Stability can be enhanced by placing plates perpendicular to each other or on separate columns; plates in the same plane are more likely to fatigue and fracture.

Fracture of the Shaft of the Humerus

Fracture of the shaft of the humerus includes fractures of the humerus that fall between the upper border of the insertion of the pectoralis major and the supracondylar ridge. Patients with this fracture present with typical symptoms of a long bone fracture, extreme tenderness at the fracture site, immobilization of affected limb, crepitation, swelling, and so on. There is no specific classification scheme and fractures are described in terms of anatomy, MOI, bone quality, age of patient, and quality of fracture lines. Six percent of humerus fractures are accompanied by radial nerve palsy due to its intimate course medial to lateral posteriorly around the humerus.

Biomechanics: Klenerman and colleagues determined that violence to the shaft is imparted directly, indirectly, or through muscular force.

Directly: Patient falls against fixed object producing transverse, butterfly, or oblique fracture.

Indirectly: Energy is absorbed through the humerus from abrupt twisting of arm, creating spiral fracture.

Muscular Force: Predictable deformities of humerus based on muscular actions of fragments.

Treatment: Because of its thick soft tissue envelope and non–weight-bearing status of the humerus, angular deformity can be tolerated. Open fractures require thorough débridement and rarely if ever are treated in a closed fashion.

243

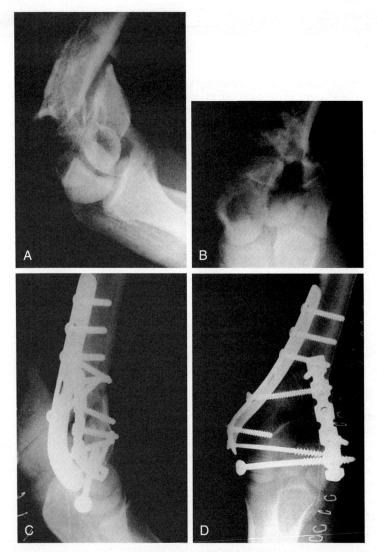

Fig. 118-1 **A and B,** Preoperative radiographs of a comminuted, high-energy distal humeral fracture. **C and D,** Postoperative radiographs showing application of the precontoured "Dupont" plate. *(From Browner BD: Skeletal Trauma: Basic Science, Management, and Reconstruction, 3rd ed. Philadelphia, Saunders, 2003.)*

Closed: Thoracobrachial immobilization (e.g., sling and swathe) provide poor realignment. Hanging arm cast is adequate for nondisplaced/minimally displaced fracture.
Operative: Needs to be considered when closed reduction cannot achieve or maintain reduction.
• Compression plating, flexible nailing, interlocking nail

Proximal Humerus Fracture (PHF)

Shoulder fractures have long been a source of controversy and confusion eliciting debate from specialists in trauma, sports medicine, and hand and upper extremities, as well as general orthopedists. Fractures occur most commonly in osteoporotic bone after a fall, but high-energy trauma as well as the strong muscular contraction of electrical shock or seizure can cause injury as well.

Biomechanics: Similar to mid shaft fractures, muscle contraction contributes to the displacement of the humeral head. The shaft is drawn anteriorly by the pectoralis major while the greater tuberosity (GT) may be pulled posterior and superior by the infraspinatus and the supraspinatus, respectively. The subscapularis draws its segment of the lesser tuberosity (LT) medially and internally.

Classification: Because of the action of the rotator cuff and the musculature of the shoulder, Neer classified proximal humerus fracture (PHF) by displacement of the four principle fragments: head, shaft, GT, and LT, with each fragment being equal to 1 cm and/or 45 degrees rotated to be considered displaced.

Treatment:

- *Nonoperative:* Nondisplaced fractures, surgical neck fractures, reduced demands, poor health, or poor rehabilitation candidate.
- *ORIF:* Options include screw fixation, tension band sutures, and even humeral head replacement for four-part PHF.

Definition: Ulnar artery thrombosis in Guyon's canal.
Etiology: Repetitive trauma to the artery may cause aneurysmal dilatation and thrombosis with associated emboli or occlusion.
Associations: Repetitive trauma to the hypothenar eminence, manual laborers, tobacco use.
Age and Gender: Male laborers in their 40s
Symptoms: Pain, cold intolerance, weakness, numbness
Signs: Absent ulnar artery flow on Allen's test, less than 10% painless pulsatile mass, nailbed changes.
Diagnostic Studies: Doppler ultrasound, color Doppler imaging (CDI), and digital pulse volume recording (PVR), magnetic resonance imaging, or angiogram.
Treatment:
• Stop tobacco products.
• Environmental and behavior modification
• Medications, such as calcium channel blockers, alpha and beta blockers
• Biofeedback
• Resection and ligation of involved segments
• Cervicothoracic sympathectomy
• Surgical reconstruction with primary repair or vein grafting

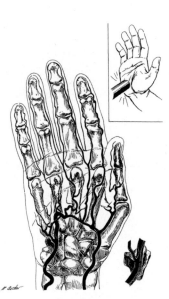

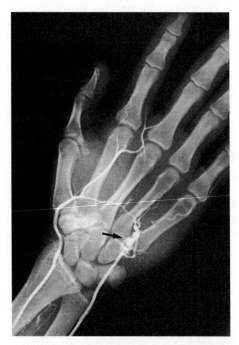

Fig. 119-1 Mechanism of ulnar artery injury in a patient with hypothenar hammer syndrome. The terminal branch of the ulnar artery is vulnerable to injury because of its close proximity to the hamate bone (inset). *(From Rutherford R: Vascular Surgery, 6th ed. Philadelphia, Saunders, 2005.)*

Fig. 119-2 Arteriogram of the hand of a carpenter. Note the aneurysm of the ulnar artery (*arrow*) because of repetitive trauma from using the hand as a hammer. *(From Rutherford R: Vascular Surgery, 6th ed. Philadelphia, Saunders, 2005)*

Incidence: There are more than 200,000 total hip arthroplasties (THAs) performed each year in the United States, with instability being one of the major complications. It occurs in 0.3% to 10% of cases after primary arthroplasty and up to 28% after revision THA. The risk of dislocation after THA diminishes as time passes.

Etiology: There are four main causes of instability: (1) positional (no radiographic abnormality); (2) component malposition (femur or acetabulum); (3) soft tissue imbalance; (4) component malposition. Several factors are associated with higher rates of dislocation, including female gender, nonunion of the trochanteric osteotomy, revision surgery, and use of a posterior approach. Patients can initiate the dislocation by either using too vigorous a range of motion, usually in external rotation, or secondary to some sort of fall or loss of balance.

Evaluation: Recurrent dislocation should be examined carefully for a definite cause. A careful history and a thorough physical examination are mandatory. Taking the hip through a full range of motion can help diagnose component-to-component impingement, inadequate offset soft tissue tension, extra-articular impingement, and other possible causes. Imaging studies are done to evaluate the abduction and anteversion of the cup and anteversion of the femoral component. However, in a small number of patients, evaluating instability can be difficult, and an identifiable etiology is never found.

Prevention: Factors important in preventing dislocation are proper placement of components, adjustment of myofascial tension, component design, and patient compliance with restrictions.

Treatment: Most dislocations after THA are single episodes that can be managed nonoperatively with closed reduction and bracing for 3 months. Long-term bracing is a possible solution for recurrent dislocation in a patient with limited goals for activity.

When these measures fail, surgical options should target the underlying etiology. Surgical treatment for recurrent instability entails component revision, use of a larger femoral head, and/or a constrained liner. Insertion of bipolar arthroplasty into the reamed acetabulum may be the best salvage procedure. Greater trochanteric advancement and soft tissue enforcement have been described but lack consistent results. Revision of the malpositioned component is the most common and effective surgical intervention. Categories of treatment of dislocations were established to correlate with the cause of the dislocation:

Category I: Successful closed reduction
Category II: Successful reoperation
Category III: Reoperation with subsequent repeat dislocations successfully treated with closed reduction
Category IV: Composed of hips that require multiple reoperations for treatment of dislocations

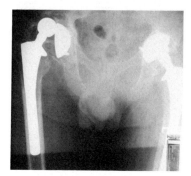

Fig. 120-1   Total hip arthroplasty may lead to hip instability.

247

Definition: Intoeing means that the feet curve inward instead of pointing straight ahead when walking or running. Intoeing is caused by one of three types of deformities: metatarsus adductus, internal tibial torsion, and increased femoral anteversion. Tibial torsion is in-turning of a child's lower leg (tibia). Femoral torsion is the in-turning of a child's upper leg (femur). Metatarsus adductus is a common birth defect in which a child's metatarsal bones bend inward from the middle of the feet. Out-toeing is when the feet are turned outward. Out-toeing causes are similar but opposite to those of intoeing. These include femoral retroversion and external tibial torsion. Femoral retroversion is common in early infancy and is caused by external rotation contracture of the hip secondary to intrauterine packing. It becomes apparent when the prewalking child stands with his or her feet turned out to nearly 90 degrees. External tibial torsion refers to a tibia that rotates outward.

Incidence: Intoeing is the most common pediatric foot problem seen in doctors' offices. Metatarsus adductus is the most common congenital foot deformity, occurring in 1 in 1000 live births. Out-toeing is less common than intoeing.

Etiology and Pathophysiology: The cause of intoeing varies with the age of the child. In the first year of life, metatarsus adductus, alone or combined with internal tibial torsion, is usually the cause. In toddlers, the cause is internal tibial torsion alone or combined with metatarsus adductus, and it may involve one or both sides. In early childhood, the cause is usually femoral anteversion, which is nearly always bilateral and symmetrical. Out-toeing results from positional confinement in utero

Association: Persistent lateral femoral torsion is associated with osteoarthrosis, increased risk of stress fracture of the lower limbs, and slipped capital femoral epiphysis. Femoral retroversion occurs more commonly in obese children.

Signs and Symptoms: In the case of intoeing, the parent reports an abnormal appearance of the foot, an awkward gait or "clumsiness" with the tendency to trip or fall. On standing

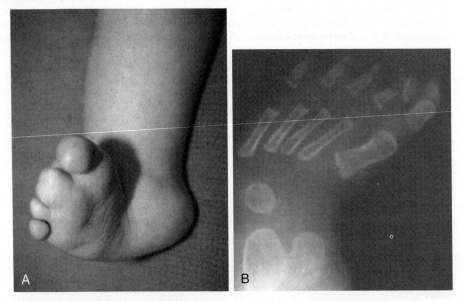

Fig. 121-1 Congenital metatarsus adductus. **A,** Severe; note deep medial transverse crease. **B,** Severe adduction as seen on radiograph. *(From Canale ST, Beaty JH [eds]: Campbell's Operative Orthopaedics, 11th ed. Philadelphia, Mosby, 2007.)*

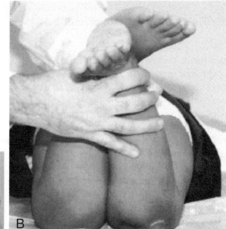
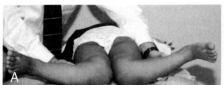

Fig. 121-2 Anteversion measured by medial rotation of hip (*A*) and lateral rotation of hip (*B*). *(From Kliegman RM: Nelson Textbook of Pediatrics, 18th ed. Philadelphia, Saunders, 2007.)*

examination of tibial torsion, the knees face forward while the ankles and feet face inward. Femoral torsion is most apparent when the child is about 5 to 6 years old. It is recognized by the medial facing of the knee, as well as the ankle and foot. Examination of metatarsus adductus reveals adduction of the forefoot with a convex lateral border. The ankle has normal motion. Out-toeing is easy to diagnose shortly after birth because the foot has an up and out appearance. In the case of femoral retroversion, physical examination reveals increased external rotation to almost 90 degrees and decreased internal rotation. External tibial torsion is usually seen between 4 and 7 years of age. The tibia rotates laterally with growth, making lateral tibial torsion worse.

Diagnostic Studies: In the case of intoeing, a structural and biomechanical examination of the lower extremities, including watching the child walk, allows for differential diagnosis and appropriate treatment recommendations. For out-toeing, an assessment known as the *rotational profile* (also called the *torsional profile*) is performed, which involves taking six different measurements of the angles of the feet, legs, and hips when the child is in various positions and when walking or running. This allows for detection of isolated abnormal angles and facilitates identification of the cause of the rotational problem. X-rays of the legs and feet are also taken to assist with definitive diagnosis and treatment planning. More sophisticated radiographic imaging techniques, such as computed tomography and magnetic resonance imaging, are sometimes performed as well.

Treatment: Intoeing is caused by three conditions, whose timing and treatment considerations vary. In tibial torsion the condition improves without treatment, usually before the age of 4. Consider surgery only if the child is at least 8 to 10 years old and the problem has persisted, causing significant walking problems. Femoral torsion gets better without treatment. Consider surgery only if the child is older than 9 years and has a very severe condition that causes a lot of tripping and an unsightly gait. The condition of metatarsus adductus improves by itself most of the time. That is why most newborns are not treated until they are at least several months old. Treatment, when necessary, usually involves applying casts or special corrective shoes; there is a high rate of success in babies ages 6 to 9 months. In most cases, the abnormalities of out-toeing improve with time. A careful physical examination, explanation of the natural history, and serial measurements are usually reassuring to the parents.

Definition: Synovial fluid and articular cartilage provide lubrication within the joint space of diarthrodial, or synovial joints. Lubrication helps protect articular cartilage from joint stresses.

Classification of Joints: A joint, or articulation, is a joining together of two or more bones. Two categories of joints include synarthrodial and diarthrodial. Synarthrodial joints permit little movement and do not contain synovium. Diarthrodial joints enable greater movement and contain synovium, synovial fluid, and a joint capsule.

Unit Load: The compressive force over articular cartilage is expressed in kilograms per cubic centimeter (kg/cm^3) of cartilage. The body uses various means, including joint lubrication, to guard the joint from surpassing the unit load and thereby injuring the cartilage.

Synovial Fluid: Secreted by the thin layer of synovium and provides low-friction and low-wear properties to articular cartilage. Synovial fluid composition varies between normal, abnormal, and artificial joints.

Articular Cartilage: Hyaline cartilage that lines the articular ends of bones. Its main functions are to absorb shocks and to lubricate the joint surface. Consists mainly of water, in addition to type II collagen, proteoglycans, and chondrocytes.

Joint Lubrication Mechanisms: Normal joints demonstrate all four mechanisms.

Boundary: An absorbed lubricant protects the joint from the surface-to-surface wear; holds greatest responsibility under sustained high loads.

Fluid Film (Squeeze-Film): Thin viscous layer of lubricant increases the surface separation; holds greatest responsibility under brief high loads.

Mixed: Combination of boundary and fluid film mechanisms.

Self-Lubrication (Weeping): Lubricant moves out in front of and beneath the rotating joint's surface. After peak stress has passed a certain point, the cartilage reabsorbs the lubricant.

Osteoarthritis (Osteoarthrosis, Degenerative Joint Disease): Most common form of arthritis. Damage to surface lining of articular cartilage after the compressive forces have surpassed the unit load. Leads to pain, swelling and stiffness, typically affecting the hands, knees, hips, and spine. Radiographic findings on x-ray study include joint space narrowing, osteophyte formation, and subchondral sclerosis and cysts. Treatment includes exercise, weight control, rest,

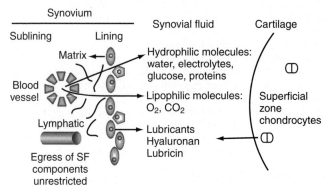

Fig. 122-1 Schematic representation of the formation of synovial fluid. Many of the soluble components and proteins in synovial fluid exit the synovial subintimal microcirculation through pores or fenestrations in the vascular endothelium, then diffuse through the interstitium before entering the joint space. Synovial permeability to most small molecules is determined by a process of free diffusion through the double barrier of endothelium and interstitium, limited mainly by the intercellular space between the synovial lining cells. Fat-soluble molecules can diffuse through, and between, cell membranes, and their passage across the synovial surface is less restricted. Additional components, including hyaluranon and lubricin, are produced by the synovial lining cells. *(From Firestein GS: Kelley's Textbook of Rheumatology, 8th ed. Philadelphia, Saunders, 2008.)*

medications (acetaminophen, nonsteroidal anti-inflammatory drugs) for pain relief, surgery (joint replacement), in addition to complementary and alternative therapies.

Role of Lubrication in Osteoarthritis Treatment: Hyaluronic acid, glucosamine, and chondroitin sulfate are major components of proteoglycans, which form the ground substance in the extracellular matrix of cartilage. Their role as nutritional supplements in osteoarthritis is currently debated. Advocates promote that they provide nutrition and enhance lubrication to the joint, thereby decreasing further damage and degeneration of the joint. Although some research has shown their benefit, further double-blinded, placebo-controlled studies with greater follow-up are required to confirm their role and mechanism in the treatment of osteoarthritis.

Definition: First described by Sir Robert Jones in 1902, the Jones fracture occurs at the base of fifth metatarsal at the metaphyseal-diaphyseal junction. It is located within 1.5 cm of the tuberosity of the fifth metatarsal and should not be confused with the more common avulsion fracture of the tuberosity. It presents a particularly challenging clinical problem, because the poor blood supply to this region results in a tendency toward delayed union. Although many of these fractures do have an acute component, many (if not most) are superimposed on chronic stress injury to the bone.

Anatomy: The proximal fifth metatarsal has been classified into three separate fracture patterns: (1) tuberosity avulsion fracture, (2) acute fracture at the metaphyseal-diaphyseal junction (acute Jones fracture), and (3) proximal diaphyseal stress fractures (chronic Jones fracture). Management and prognosis of both acute and stress fractures of the fifth metatarsal within 1.5 cm of the tuberosity depend on the type of fracture, based on Torg's classification. Type I fractures, or early union, are acute fractures that show sharp margins and no intramedullary sclerosis. Type II fractures, or delayed union, show a persistent fracture line with new periosteal bone formation and intramedullary sclerosis. Type III fractures, or nonunion, have a wide fracture line with periosteal new bone formation and complete obliteration of the medullary canal.

Clinical: Patients describe sudden pain at the base of the fifth metatarsal, with difficulty bearing weight on the foot. Often, ecchymosis and/or edema is present at the site. The mechanism of injury is described as a laterally directed force on the forefoot during plantar flexion of the ankle. Examples include pivot-shifting in football or basketball, with the heel off the ground. Risk factors include younger athletes with a high level of activity in a running or jumping sport. Those

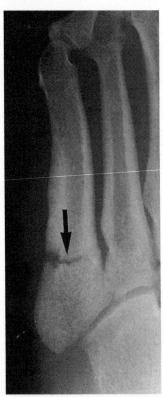

Fig. 123-1 Fracture of the proximal shaft of the fifth metatarsal ("true Jones fracture") (*arrow*). Jones originally described a fracture in this location, which he himself suffered while dancing. (*From Adam A, et al: Grainger & Allison's Diagnostic Radiology, 5th ed. Philadelphia, Churchill Livingstone, 2008.*)

with hindfoot varus of any cause also have a predilection for this fracture because of lateral column overloading.

Radiographs: X-ray study establishes the diagnosis in most cases. In addition to fracture location, which distinguishes avulsion from Jones fracture, it is important to note the characteristic features at the fracture site in order to guide treatment.

Treatment: Type I fractures are treated with a non–weight-bearing, short leg cast for 6 to 8 weeks, with progressive ambulation after cast removal. Type II fractures may also be treated with a non–weight-bearing cast, but a prolonged period may be required until union is achieved; up to one third of these fractures will go on to nonunion. In competitive athletes, these fractures are usually treated operatively. Type III fractures should be treated operatively. The surgery typically consists of internal fixation with an intramedullary screw placed from the proximal tubercle in a distal direction past the fracture site. Treatment failure after screw fixation of Jones fractures are reported to be infrequent, but have been associated with an early return to vigorous activity and a small screw size in relation to body mass.

Definition: Painful, osteonecrosis (ON) of the lunate carpal bone.

Etiology: Post-traumatic or idiopathic. Approximately 20% of lunates have a single nutrient vessel that, when damaged, may lead to ON. Ulnar length has been postulated to play a role in its development; negative ulnar variance may create higher shear stresses across the radiolunate joint leaving an at-risk lunate more susceptible to ON.

Incidence: Seventy-five percent of patients have a history of trauma with the wrist in severe dorsiflexion.

Age and Gender: Most commonly occurs unilaterally and in individuals between 15 and 40 years of age. Male manual laborers typically present with this disease.

Signs and Symptoms: Insidious onset of wrist pain localized over the dorsum of the wrist, most pronounced in dorsiflexion; decreased range of motion with extension of the wrist and mild tenderness to palpation over lunate; pain with passive dorsiflexion in the middle of the finger.

Diagnostic Studies: Radiography may not illustrate evidence of disease for up to 18 months after onset of symptoms. Magnetic resonance imaging (MRI) has replaced bone scanning and can detect early ON of the lunate.

Classification: Lichtman and Degnan's classification:

I: Radiographs, MRI scan, or bone scan positive for linear compression fracture

II: Normal lunate outline but density changes within the lunate

IIIa: Fragmentation and collapse of lunate

IIIb: Dorsal intercalated segment instability (DISI) deformity

IV: Lunate fragmentation carpal collapse; degenerative changes of radiocarpal or mid carpal joints

Natural History: Uncertain. Immobilization may preserve normal anatomy in the preadolescent and decrease inflammation in all patients; however, neither immobilization nor surgery is 100% effective in preventing collapse of the lunate. Treatment should be dictated by (1) presence or absence of negative ulnar variance and (2) stage of disease.

Medical Treatment: Immobilization and anti-inflammatory medications.

Surgical Treatment: Goal in stages I and II is to preserve anatomy, prevent collapse, and unload lunate via radial shortening or ulnar lengthening. Bone grafting with revascularization is technically difficult. In stages III and IV, lunate unloading procedures are less predictable. Silastic implants and lunate excision are associated with high complication rates. Limited intercarpal arthrodesis may be used in stage IIIb disease. Wrist arthrodesis and proximal row carpectomy are salvage options.

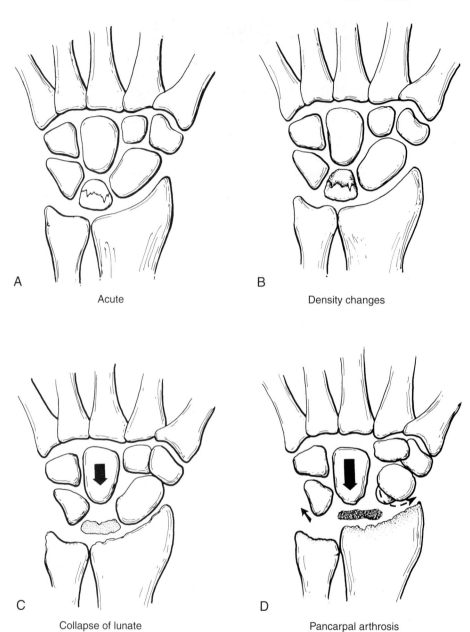

A Acute

B Density changes

C Collapse of lunate

D Pancarpal arthrosis

Fig. 124-1 Modified Stahl's classification of Kienböck's disease. **A,** Stage I: Normal-appearing lunate with a compression fracture demonstrated by a radiolucent line. **B,** Stage II: Sclerosis of the lunate. **C,** Stage III: Collapse of the lunate. **D,** Stage IV: Pancarpal arthrodesis. *(Redrawn from Lichtman DM, Alexander AH, Mack GR, Gunther SF: Kienböck's disease—update on silicone replacement arthroplasty. J Hand Surg 7:343-347, 1982. From DeLee D, Drez D: DeLee and Drez's Orthopaedic Sports Medicine, 2nd ed. Philadelphia, Saunders, 2003.)*

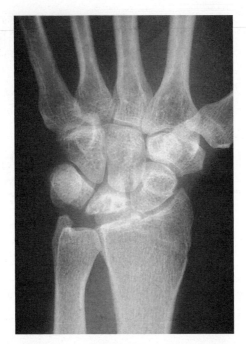

Fig. 124-2 Advanced Kienböck's disease. Cystic and sclerotic changes are present within the collapsed lunate (*arrow*). (*From Frontera WR: Essentials of Physical Medicine and Rehabilitation, 2nd ed. Philadelphia, Saunders, 2008.*)

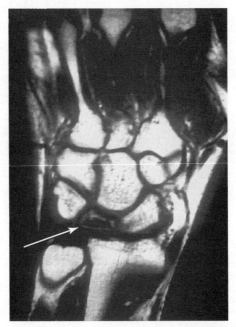

Fig. 124-3 MRI in Kienböck's disease. T1-weighted images demonstrate diffuse low signal within the lunate (*arrow*). (*From Frontera WR: Essentials of Physical Medicine and Rehabilitation, 2nd ed. Philadelphia, Saunders, 2008.*)

Definition: Medial compartmental arthritis of the knee is a degenerative condition characterized by abnormal articular cartilage in the medial part of the tibiofemoral joint.

Etiology: Osteoarthritis of the knee usually occurs secondary to mechanical factors, which include partial or complete meniscectomy, femoral osteonecrosis, lower extremity trauma, ligamentous laxity, obesity, and lower extremity malalignment.

Incidence: Osteoarthritis affects more than 16 million people in the United States (1 in 3 people). Autopsy specimens have demonstrated a 90% prevalence of articular cartilage degenerative changes in weight-bearing joints in individuals older than 40 years. Prevalence increases with age.

Pathophysiology: With removal of approximately one third of the meniscus, increased force is transferred directly to the tibial articular surface. The joint also becomes less congruent and is not able to disperse the force across the joint. Both of these factors increase contact stresses, which can lead to articular cartilage damage and subsequent osteoarthritis. Normal gait requires 67 degrees of flexion in the swing phase, 83 degrees of flexion for stair climbing, 90 degrees of flexion for descending stairs, and 93 degrees of flexion in rising from a chair.

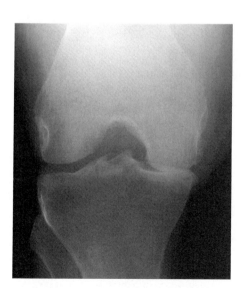

Fig. 125-1 Osteoarthritis with medial compartment cartilage narrowing shown to advantage on tunnel view. *(From Firestein GS: Kelley's Textbook of Rheumatology, 8th ed. Philadelphia, Saunders, 2008.)*

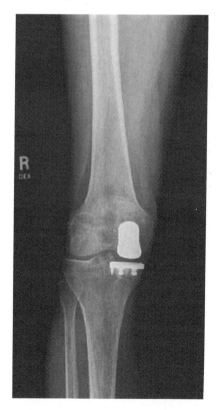

Fig. 125-2 Unicompartmental knee arthroplasty. Anteroposterior radiograph of a patient after medial unicompartmental knee replacement. Unlike total knee replacement, the opposite lateral tibiofemoral and patellofemoral compartments are not resurfaced. *(From Goldman L: Cecil Medicine, 23rd ed. Philadelphia, Saunders, 2007.)*

Biomechanics: During normal daily activities, a load of two to four times of body weight crosses the knee joint. In the normal knee, approximately two thirds of this load pass through the medial compartment.

Signs and Symptoms: A mechanical axis of 0 to 3 degrees of varus is considered to be within normal limits. Generally, a varus deviation of greater than 10 degrees is associated with symptoms of medial compartment arthritis. Medial side knee pain worsens over time, being worse in the morning and then lessening with activity. As the day progresses, so does the pain.

Anatomic Alignment: A line from the center of the femoral head to the center of the talus forms the mechanical axis. This line should pass through the center or just lateral to the center of the tibial spines. In a varus-aligned limb, the line passes well medial to the knee. Anatomic varus is represented by the angle that is formed by the intersection of the lines drawn through the long axes of the femur and tibia. Normal anatomic valgus is 5 to 7 degrees. The measure of the dysplasia of the medial or lateral condyle of the distal femur also is important. The angle is formed by the intersection of a line passed through the femoral condyles and the long axis of the femur. The angle ranges 80 to 85 degrees and is larger in varus knees. Also, measure the angle formed by a line drawn across the tibial plateau and the long axis of the tibia. This indicates metaphyseal bowing and usually is 0 to 3 degrees varus. The metaphyseal bowing offsets the slight mechanical varus angulation at the knee to provide a joint line that is horizontal to the floor.

Table 125-1. TREATMENT OPTIONS

Major Surgical Treatments	Pros	Cons
Arthroscopy	Minimally invasive; 74% with proven relief up to 14 months.	Patient Specifics: Patients with coexisting varus angulation, ACL instability, and inflammatory disease associated with poor outcomes.
Osteotomy	Corrects varus malalignment and prevents progression of OA. Keeps native knee joint.	Patient Selection: Not overweight, ROM of more than 90 degrees flexion, competent ACL/MCL. Possible shortened limb length postoperatively. Higher challenge to perform TKA at later time.
Unicompartmental knee replacement	Better range of motion, quicker recovery. Patient can be discharged on post-operative day 1, as well as begin weight bearing and full ROM. More lenient long-term restrictions. Lower complication rate than TKA.	Lateral (nonreplaced) compartment may continue to deteriorate, eventually requiring TKA within 3 to 4 years postoperatively.
Arthroplasty	Long-term treatment and benefit with a 10- to 15-year life expectancy. Treats most mechanical problems of knee, with pain relief in almost all cases.	Surgical Risks: Limited kneeling/ROM in replaced knee joint.

ACL, Anterior cruciate ligament; MCL, medial collateral ligament; OA, osteoarthritis; ROM, range of motion; TKA, total knee arthroplasty

Definition: Knee dislocation is classified according to the position of the tibia relative to the femur.

Etiology: Traumatic high-energy motor vehicle accidents or contact sports, especially motor vehicle bumper versus pedestrian or confrontational tackling. A knee dislocation is a difficult injury for the junior surgeon to diagnose. It represents a disabling and limb-threatening injury. Where doubt exists, the patient must be admitted for vascular observation and treatment, in that popliteal artery injury occurs in 35% to 45% of all knee dislocations.

Incidence: Relatively rare injury that is, however, often underdiagnosed and spontaneously reduces.

Associations: Vascular and neurologic injury.

Age and Gender: Young males, but both genders with high-energy and sporting injuries.

Clinical Findings: Large hemarthrosis, swollen and bruised, hyperextension often possible. Common peroneal palsy (20% to 40%). Popliteal artery injury, often intimal flap/tear, may not be present initially; if any doubt, defer to a vascular consult.

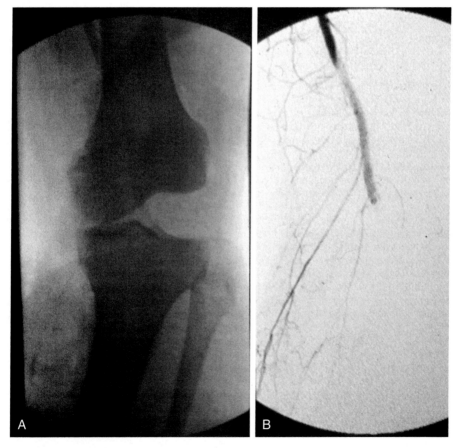

Fig. 126-1 Angiogram of the lower extremity after posterior knee dislocation. **A,** The fluoroscopic image shows significant displacement after posterior knee dislocation. **B,** Disruption of popliteal blood flow at the level of the dislocation is clearly appreciated on the angiogram. *(From Townsend CM Jr: Sabiston Textbook of Surgery, 18th ed. Philadelphia, Saunders, 2007.)*

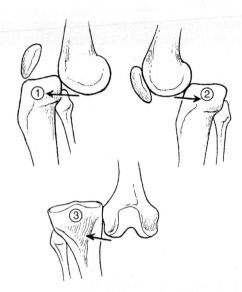

Fig. 126-2 Types of knee dislocations. Anterior (1), posterior (2), and lateral (3). *(From DePalma AF: Management of Fractures and Dislocations: An Atlas. Philadelphia, Saunders, 1970.)*

Classification: Depends on position relative to distal femur: anterior, posterior, medial, lateral or rotatory. Anterior most common and requires marked hyperextension of knee (>30 degrees).

Pathology: Various injuries of at least two and often more of the stabilizing structures of the knee are required. Seventy-one percent are said to have bicruciate ruptures. Bicruciate knee injuries cannot be distinguished from knee dislocations and should be treated with the same respect. End of the bed test, angiography, posterolateral corner injury, compartment syndrome.

Investigations: Only after reduced! Radiography: Look for congruent reduction and associated bony avulsions. Consider magnetic resonance imaging, which determines whether avulsions or ruptures occurred and assists with reconstruction planning, arteriogram, and examination under anesthesia.

Treatment: Emergent reduction of the knee, confirm reduction radiologically, and consider angiography. Early/later early repair of any avulsed structures and additional reconstruction of any cruciate injury with autograft and allograft seems to offer some benefit. After reduction, splint the lower extremity, apply ice, and keep the knee elevated. Nonsteroidal anti-inflammatory drugs, analgesics, and anxiolytics are used to treat the pain associated with dislocations.

Complications: Ongoing stiffness or instability, compartment syndrome, vascular injury, and persisting common peroneal palsy (50% of palsies remain long term). Popliteal artery injury, popliteal vein injury, peroneal nerve injury, ligamentous injury, compartment syndrome.

Knee ligament injuries are common in sports-related activities. Rupture of these ligaments upsets the balance between knee mobility and stability, resulting in abnormal kinematics and gradual damage to other structures such as menisci and articular cartilage, leading to pain and morbidity.

Anterior Cruciate Ligament (ACL)

Anatomy: The ACL is a broad ligament joining the anterior tibial plateau to posterior lateral femoral condyle. It is composed of multiple nonparallel fibers which, although not anatomically separate, act as functionally distinct fibers (i.e., anteromedial, posterolateral, and intermediate), so the tension in each bundle varies throughout the range of motion.

Biomechanics of ACL: The biomechanical function of ACL is complex in that it provides both stability and proprioceptive feedback to the knee.

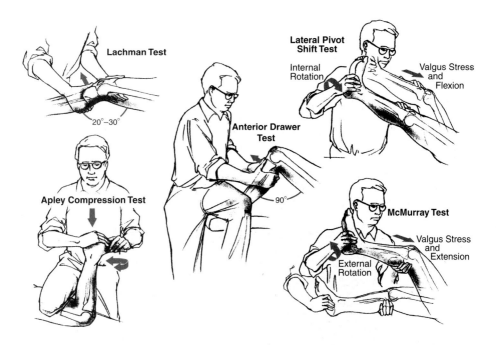

Fig. 127-1 Examination maneuvers. Right knee shown. Examination maneuvers include the Lachman, anterior drawer, lateral pivot shift, Apley compression, and McMurray tests. The Lachman test, performed to detect anterior cruciate ligament (ACL) injures, is conducted with the patient supine and the knee flexed 20-30 degrees. The anterior drawer test detects ACL injuries and is performed with the patient supine and the knee in 90 degrees of flexion. The lateral pivot shift test is performed with the patient supine, the hip flexed 45 degrees, and the knee in full extension. Internal rotation is applied to the tibia while the knee is flexed to 40 degrees under a valgus stress (pushing the outside of the knee medially). The Apley compression test, used to assess meniscal integrity, is performed with the patient prone and the examiner's knee over the patient's posterior thigh. The tibia is externally rotated while a downward compressive force is applied over the tibia. The McMurray test, used to assess meniscal integrity, is performed with the patient supine and the examiner standing on the side of the affected knee. *(From Solomon DH, Simel DL, Bates DW, et al: Does this patient have a torn meniscus or ligament of the knee? JAMA 2001;286:1610.)*

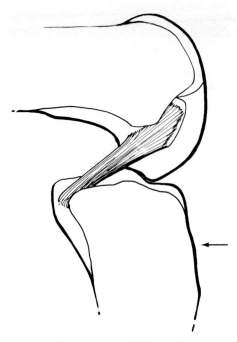

Fig. 127-2 Posterior cruciate ligament injuries are most frequently the result of a blow to the front of the flexed knee. *(From DeLee J, Drez D [eds]: DeLee and Drez's Orthopaedic Sports Medicine, 2nd ed. Philadelphia, Saunders, 2003.)*

In its stabilizing role it has four functions: (1) restrains anterior translation of the tibia; (2) prevents hyperextension of the knee; (3) acts as a secondary stabilizer to valgus stress, reinforcing the medial collateral ligament; (4) controls rotation of the tibia on the femur in femoral extension of 0 to 30 degrees.

This final role is the main clinical function of the ACL. ACL deficiency causes failure of this screw-home mechanism, resulting in subluxation of the tibia on the femur. This critical function in the range of 0 to 30 degrees is important for movements such as side-stepping and pivoting.

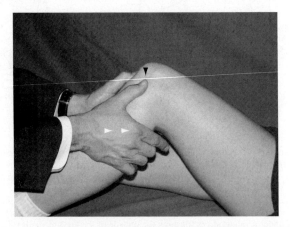

Fig. 127-3 The posterior drawer is the most sensitive test for evaluating function of the posterior cruciate ligament. The examiner's thumbs should be placed on the femoral condyles, feeling the tibial offset at the level of the joint line (*black arrowhead*). The examiner then creates a posteriorly directed force (*white arrowheads*) and the tibial step-off is reassessed. *(Courtesy of Mark R. Hutchinson, MD. From Rakel: Textbook of Family Medicine, 7th ed. Philadelphia, Saunders.)*

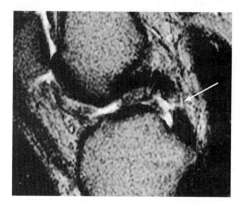

Fig. 127-4 Complete disruption of the posterior cruciate ligament (PCL). Sagittal T_2-weighted image with fat saturation through the intercondylar notch reveals high signal (*arrow*) completely traversing the midsubstance of the PCL. (*From DeLee J, Drez D [eds]: DeLee and Drez's Orthopaedic Sports Medicine, 2nd ed. Philadelphia, Saunders, 2003.*)

Mechanism of ACL Injury:
- Rapid change of direction
- Slowing down when running
- Landing from a jump (Nearly 60% of ACL injuries in female basketball players occur when landing from a jump.)
- Direct contact as in a football tackle

Sign and Symptoms: *Major Symptom:* Popping sound, followed by giving way and swelling within 2 to 12 hours due to hemarthrosis and pain while trying to stand. Pain may not be felt immediately. Pivoting of the knee on the fixed foot induces giving way and pain.

Diagnostic Tests: Examination maneuvers mimic instability. Anterior Lachman test in early examination of the traumatized knee, and anterior drawer test and pivot shift test in later examinations are helpful.

Imaging and Arthroscopy: Magnetic resonance imaging and arthroscopic examination can further delineate ACL injury and associated damage.

Treatment:
Nonoperative: Nonoperative treatment is indicated in (1) very young patients, (2) patients with overall low activity level, and (3) in patients with good overall stability of the knee despite torn ACL.

Operative: Operative reconstruction by either arthroscopic surgery and less often open surgery with use of autogenous tendons such as hamstrings and patellar tendon is the gold standard of treatment in the younger, active, and more symptomatic patients who cannot decrease their level of activity.

Rehabilitation: Programmed exercises and proper rehabilitation to strengthen the muscles and restore the full joint mobility are mandatory in both types of treatments.

Prevention: Several risk factors contribute to a higher incidence of ACL injuries among women athletes; these can be prevented by practicing and improving the motor skills. These are (1) less knee bending than men when landing from a jump; (2) turning and pivoting in a more erect position; (3) use of quadriceps when changing direction rapidly.

Posterior Cruciate Ligament (PCL)

The posterior cruciate ligament is not as commonly injured as the ACL.

Mechanism of Injury:
- Blow to the front of the knee as in a dashboard injury
- Simple misstep
- Fall on the flexed knee

Signs and Symptoms: Patients with PCL tears often do not have symptoms of instability. Many athletes return to activity without significant improvement after completing a prescribed rehabilitation program.

Treatment: Patients with bony insertion avulsion and those with symptomatic severe posterior laxity and greater than 10 mm of displacement on posterior drawer test are candidates for repair and reconstruction. Isolated PCL injury can be treated nonsurgically because they do not involve other structures.

Collateral Ligaments

Medial Collateral Ligament

Medial collateral ligament stabilizes the medial side of the knee and in contrast to cruciate ligaments has a good healing potential.

Conservative Treatment: PRICE (protect, rest, ice, compression, elevation) followed by rehabilitation and bracing and passive range of motion. For restoration of flexibility, quadriceps muscle strengthening is the treatment of choice.

Lateral Collateral Ligament

Lateral collateral ligaments have a complex structure but are fortunately rarely injured. Lateral collateral ligament injury is caused by direct blow to the medial aspect of the knee or to the anterior medial tibia with the foot planted and the knee in various degrees of flexion. An ACL injury should not be confused with other overuse lateral knee injuries (e.g., iliotibial band syndrome or biceps femoris tendonitis).

Complex Knee Ligament Injuries

Ligament injuries may be complex in more severe injuries such as knee dislocation or severely stressed knee. If multiple ligaments are torn (three or four), potential popliteal damage necessitates arterial evaluation by color Doppler sonography or arteriogram. An electromyogram (EMG) and nerve conduction velocity (NCV) test may assess for peroneal nerve injury in lateral and posterolateral ligament injury, and exploration at the time of repair or primary reconstruction is indicated.

Posterolateral complex ligament injury can be quite disabling and lead to abnormal gait due to varus thrust, hyperextension, and excessive external rotation of tibia on the femur. These injuries are best treated by complex surgical reconstructions.

Definition: Köhler disease is a type of osteochondrosis in which the navicular bone develops avascular necrosis.

Incidence: True incidence is unknown.

Age: Occurs in patients 5 to 10 years of age and its onset is most frequently between the ages of 5 and 6.

Gender: 3 to 5:1 male-to-female ratio.

Etiology and Pathophysiology: The exact etiology of Köhler disease is unknown. However, vascular incidents, trauma, and hereditary factors have been posited. It is often believed to have a vascular etiology because the navicular bone is the last tarsal bone to ossify and bears compressive stress; these conditions may compress the bone, thereby inhibiting the blood supply.

Clinical Presentation: A patient with Köhler disease will have pain, swelling, and possibly redness over the navicular bone. Limping and an inability to bear weight may also be present. The patient may walk by positioning most of his weight over the lateral aspect of the foot.

Pathology: The navicular bone develops abnormal endochondral ossification.

Diagnostic Procedures: X-ray studies and bone scans may be used to aid in the diagnosis of Köhler disease. Lateral view x-ray studies show a flat, dense, and sclerotic navicular but with irregular ossification. If pain persists for more than 6 months, magnetic resonance imaging or computed tomography should be ordered to exclude tarsal involvement.

Treatment: The goal of treatment is to free the navicular bone from mechanical stresses. This disease is treated nonsurgically by a below-the-knee cast for severe cases or soft arch supports and a medial heal wedge for mild cases. The cast, which is worn for approximately 6 to 8 weeks, should allow the patient to be weight bearing and be placed in moderate varus and equinus. This disease has an excellent prognosis in which the navicular bone fully ossifies.

Complications: Acquired talonavicular coalition following avascular necrosis of the tarsal navicular joint is an extremely rare complication.

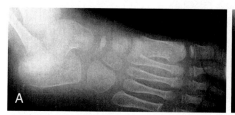 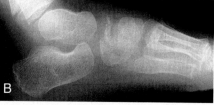

Fig. 128-1 Aseptic necrosis of the tarsal navicular. This usually occurs between the ages of 4 and 8 years and most commonly is recognized incidentally. Increased density (**A**) or irregularity (**B**) of the tarsal navicular may be found. This also is called Köhler osteonecrosis. The abnormality is almost always self-limited and requires no therapy. (*From Mettler FA, Jr: Essentials of Radiology, 2nd ed. Philadelphia, Saunders, 2005.*)

Definition: A disorder of increased natural curvature in the sagittal plane of the spine resulting in a hunchback deformity.

Etiology: Kyphosis can be congenital or postural, or result from trauma or degenerative disease. Additionally, spondylolisthesis, neurofibromatosis, Paget's disease, and tumors have been shown to cause kyphosis. Scheuermann's disease is a thoracic kyphosis of greater than 45 degrees associated with three sequential vertebrae anteriorly wedged at 5 degrees or more. Although kyphosis is idiopathic, there is evidence to suggest that Scheuermann's disease may be inherited through autosomal dominance or caused by juvenile osteoporosis.

Incidence: Between 0.04% and 10% of school-age children, depending on etiology.

Age: Occurs at any age (rare at birth). Scheuermann's disease appears during adolescence.

Gender: Debated. Both 2:1 and 1:2 male-to-female ratios have been reported.

Signs and Symptoms: "Poor posture," mild back pain, tightness in hamstrings, and in rare cases difficulty breathing. Scheuermann's disease may illicit cardiopulmonary complaints, neurologic compromise (rare), and progressive deformity.

Clinical Findings: Kyphotic curve of more than 50 degrees. Fused vertebrae in congenital cases and wedge-shaped vertebrae in Scheuermann's disease. Fracture is not uncommon.

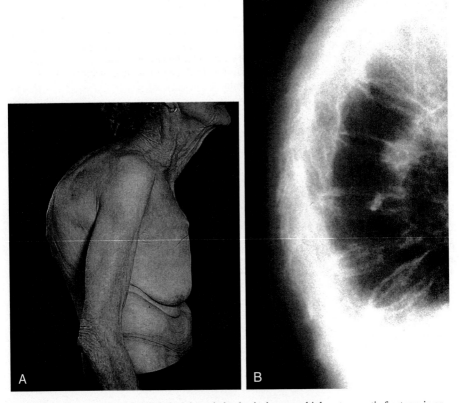

Fig. 129-1 Dowager's hump. **A,** Marked thoracic kyphosis due to multiple osteoporotic fractures in an elderly woman. **B,** Corresponding radiograph. *(From Hochberg MC, Silman AJ, Smolen JS, Weinblatt ME, Weisman MH [eds]: Rheumatology, 3rd ed, St. Louis, 2003, Mosby.)*

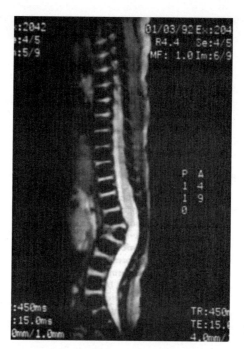

Fig. 129-2 MRI of type I congenital kyphosis. Failure of formation of anterior vertebral body is shown, but growth potential of involved vertebra cannot be determined. Note pressure on dural sac. *(From Warner WC: Kyphosis. In Morrissy RT, Weinstein SL [eds]: Lovell and Winter's Pediatric Orthopaedics, 6th ed, Philadelphia, 2006, Lippincott Williams & Wilkins.)*

Staging: Mild kyphosis improves when individual stops growing, whereas severe kyphosis gets worse with age.

Medical Treatment: None if asymptomatic. Physical therapy, anti-inflammatory medication, and braces can treat symptoms in mild kyphosis as well as Scheuermann's disease. Controversies are many; generally in cases of kyphosis greater than 70 degrees, surgical treatment yields better outcomes.

Surgical Treatment: Congenital kyphosis requires correction at an early age. Scheuermann's disease may require surgery from a posterior, anterior, or combined approach.

Studies: Computed tomographic scan, magnetic resonance imaging, bending films, and x-ray study.

Sequelae: Reasonable pain relief and resumption of normal activities can be expected postoperatively. Scoliosis is commonly seen as additional (compensatory) curve that appears in the nonoperative treatment groups. Scheuermann's disease can cause disk herniation and compression fractures that may result in paraparesis.

Complications: Round-back deformity, decreased lung capacity, disabling back pain, leg weakness or paralysis. Extensive surgical procedures for Scheuermann's disease can have complications including death, neurologic compromise, and hardware failure. Also, pseudarthrosis and pulmonary, chest tube, and thoracotomy complications can occur as can blood clots, pulmonary emboli, wound infections, dural tears, and positional and anesthetic complications.

Definition: Legg-Calvé-Perthes disease (LCPD) was first described in 1909 as an idiopathic avascular necrosis of the femoral head.

Etiology: An idiopathic disorder, but some risk factors have been identified including gender, socioeconomic group, inguinal hernia, and the presence of genitourinary tract anomalies. There is a family history in 6% of patients.

Incidence: One in 1200 children younger than 15 is affected. LCPD is bilateral in 10% to 20% of patients.

Age: It is most commonly seen in patients 3 to 12 years of age.

Gender: Male-to-female ratio is 3 to 5:1.

Race: This disease is more common in whites.

Signs and Symptoms: The patient usually presents with a limp and with groin, thigh, or knee pain. Range of motion of the affected hip is limited, especially abduction and internal rotation. Muscle spasm and muscular atrophy that have resulted over time from disuse can be found during physical examination. Patients often have delayed bone age and no history of trauma.

Diagnostic Studies: Plain and frog-leg hip x-ray studies are very useful in the diagnosis. Computed tomography scan and magnetic resonance imaging are two additional imaging techniques used in the evaluation of the disorder.

Catterall Classification:

Group I: Involvement only of the anterior epiphysis (therefore seen only on the frog-leg lateral film).

Group II: Central segment fragmentation and collapse. However, the lateral rim is intact and thus protects the central involved area.

Group III: The lateral head is also involved or fragmented and only the medial portion is spared. The loss of lateral support worsens the prognosis.

Group IV: The entire head is involved.

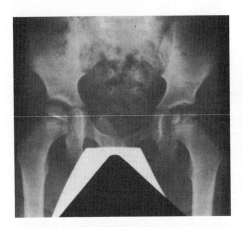

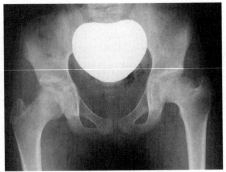

Fig. 130-1 Radiograph of a 5-year-old boy who had chronic groin pain and a limp while playing soccer. Legg-Calvé-Perthes disease frequently manifests with activity-related pain. *(From DeLee D, Drez D: DeLee and Drez's Orthopaedic Sports Medicine, 2nd ed. Philadelphia, Saunders, 2003.)*

Fig. 130-2 Legg-Calvé-Perthes disease at 17 months. Note the metachronous nature of the disease. *(From Adam A, et al: Grainger & Allison's Diagnostic Radiology, 5th ed. Philadelphia, Churchill Livingstone, 2008.)*

Pathology: After interruption of blood flow to the femoral head, bone infarction occurs in the capital femoral epiphysis. Deformity of the femoral head results from secondary epiphyseal growth plate changes due to subchondral fracture. There are four stages of LCPD:
1. Femoral head becomes more dense with possible fracture of supporting bone
2. Fragmentation and reabsorption of bone
3. Reossification when new bone has regrown
4. Healing, when new bone reshapes

Medical Treatment: Nonsteroidal anti-inflammatory drugs, non–weight-bearing for pain control, casting, traction, and bracing as well as range-of-motion physical therapy exercises.

Surgical Treatment: Tenotomy, various osteotomies including femoral varus and acetabular.

Prognosis: Progressive loss of movement with age, adduction contracture, and higher stages in the radiographic assessment are poor prognostic factors.

Complications: Permanent distortion of the femoral head and degenerative joint disease.

Definition: Leiomyosarcoma is classified as an aggressive malignant soft tissue sarcoma. It develops in smooth muscle tissues. It is the most common type of genitourinary sarcoma in older patients. It most often develops in the retroperitoneum but can also develop in the extremities. Leiomyosarcoma has a high rate of recurrence and metastasis. It is important to determine whether the tumor is cutaneous or deep because the two behave very differently. Cutaneous leiomyosarcoma usually is more benign, whereas deep leiomyosarcoma is very aggressive and resistant to many types of treatment.

Incidence: Occurs at a rate of approximately 1.4 cases per 100,000 patients.

Age: Mainly in adults between 50 and 60 years of age.

Gender: The male-to-female ratio is approximately 2:1.

Race: No known differences.

Etiology and Pathophysiology: The following translocations have been linked to the development of leiomyosarcoma: t(12:14) and 12q15.

Associations: Leiomyosarcoma has an increased likelihood of local invasion and metastasis.

Signs and Symptoms: Leiomyosarcoma has rather vague symptoms, allowing it to mature gradually. If the tumor is cutaneous, it manifests as small, solitary nodules. If the tumor is deep, it tends to arise near medium to large veins. Rarely, leiomyosarcoma can be found near large vascularized structures. In these cases, the tumor obstructs the vessel leading to decreased outflow. This occurs most frequently in the pulmonary artery.

Diagnostic Studies: Diagnosis is based on the presence of smooth muscle actin and desmin by immunochemistry. Imaging from computed tomography scans and magnetic resonance imaging scans can be very useful when contrast materials are used.

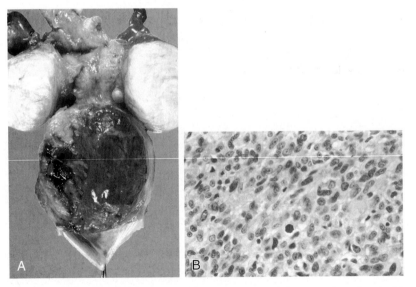

Fig. 131-1   Leiomyosarcoma. **A,** A large hemorrhagic tumor mass distends the lower corpus and is flanked by two leiomyomas. **B,** The tumor cells are irregular in size and have hyperchromatic nuclei. *(From Kumar V, et al: Robbins and Cotran Pathologic Basis of Disease, 7th ed. Philadelphia, Saunders, 2005.)*

Micropathology: Typically elongated cells with abundant cytoplasm can be seen. Multinucleated giant cells can occur as well. It is also possible for epithelioid changes to occur, such as a cell becoming rounded with concomitant clear cell changes in the neoplasm.

Macropathology: Leiomyosarcoma is most often discovered by chance; however, abdominal cramping, bloating, or vaginal bleeding is possible due to the growth of the tumor.

Treatment: The keystone treatment is complete resection. Chemotherapy has not been shown to be beneficial in some cases.

Definition: Limb length discrepancy (LLD) is a difference in anatomic or functional leg lengths.

Incidence: Approximately 90% of the general population has some anatomic leg length asymmetry. This anatomic average is approximately 5 mm, often with a longer left leg. Between 5% and 40% of all total hip replacement surgeries result in some limb length discrepancy.

Age: Anatomic limb length discrepancy occurs throughout the course of development and growth, but due to the nature of joint replacement, it is more frequently seen in patients in middle age or older.

Gender: Distribution between the genders is equal.

Associations: LLD is a common complication following total hip arthroplasty. It can also be representative of congenital dysplasia of the hip or pelvis, resulting in uneven anatomy and limb length inequality. Lower back pain, scoliosis, and change in gait pattern are the most common associations with LLD. In younger patients, LLD can be symptomatic of Legg-Calvé-Perthes disease.

Signs and Symptoms: There has yet to be complete agreement as to what constitutes clinically significant LLD. Generally, LLD of greater than 1 inch (2.54 cm) is considered to be significant. With LLD of greater than 1 inch, common symptoms include lower back pain, changes in gait, pelvic torsion, flexion in the knee of the long leg, and postural distortion. LLD of less than 1 inch is asymptomatic.

Diagnostic Studies: Radiographic measurements are the most reliable method of LLD detection. The most accurate of measurements are taken by x-ray study while controlling for distortion and magnification and measuring from the intersection of the horizontal line across the pelvis and the region of the lesser trochanter.

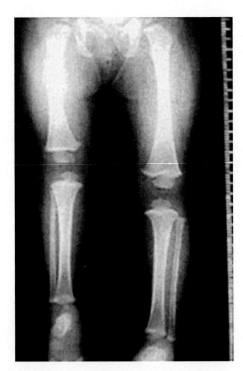

Fig. 132-1   Scanogram to demonstrate exact leg-length discrepancy. *(From Kliegman RM, et al: Nelson Textbook of Pediatrics, 18th ed. Philadelphia, Saunders, 2007.)*

Macropathology: LLD is most often a result of pelvic asymmetry.

Treatment: Asymptomatic LLD usually goes untreated, because it does not affect functionality or quality of life. Clinically significant LLDs are most often treated with shoe lifts to reach equality of the legs. In rare cases when the discrepancy between limb lengths is too large to be treated with shoe lifts and causes great discomfort or affects quality of life, surgical therapy can be undertaken.

Definition: Lipomas are benign tumors of connective tissue composed of a well-encapsulated nodule of fat and may contain fibrous tissue.

Incidence: Most common benign mesenchymal tumor.

Age: Lipomas can occur at any age, but usually arise in early adulthood.

Gender: Solitary lipomas occur predominately in middle-aged women. Multiple lipomas are seen more frequently in men.

Etiology and Pathophysiology: The etiology of lipomas is generally unknown. Some solitary cutaneous lipomas display clonal alterations on chromosome bands 12q13-15. Lipomas differ biochemically from normal fat by demonstrating increased levels of lipoprotein lipase.

Associations: Lipomas frequently occur with onset of obesity in people of middle age.

Signs and Symptoms: The majority of lipomas are asymptomatic. Clinically, they are soft, circumscribed, moveable masses that are painless and grow slowly. Symptoms vary depending on the location of the lipoma. Associated pain and multiple tumors are indicative of a more serious multiple lipoma or liposarcoma.

Diagnostic Studies: On plain radiographs, larger lipomas appear as discrete radiolucent areas within soft tissue. Magnetic resonance imaging and tomography imaging can be used to identify soft tissue tumors composed of fat, but they do not distinguish between lipomas and liposarcomas.

Macropathology: Lipomas may develop in virtually all organs throughout the body. They arise from fatty tissue between the skin and deep fascia. Lipomas are lobulated, are of rubbery consistency, and are not attached to the overlying skin. The neck, back, and proximal extremities are affected most commonly.

Micropathology: Lipomas are composed of mature adipocytes that differ biochemically from normal fat by demonstrating increased levels of lipoprotein lipase. Some lipomas have a prominent vascular pattern and can be called *angiolipomas*.

Treatment: Lipomas are removed for cosmetic reasons, histology evaluations to rule out malignancy (presence of liposarcomas), when they become symptomatic, or when they grow to larger than 5 cm. The standard treatment is marginal resection. The method of surgical therapy depends on the location of the tumor. Biopsies are important in large lipomas or those tethered to fascia to rule out a liposarcoma.

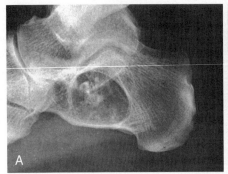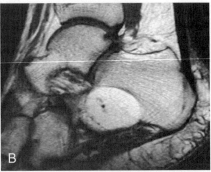

Fig. 133-1 Intraosseous lipoma of the calcaneus. **A,** Lateral radiograph showing a geographic, calcified lytic lesion. **B,** Sagittal T1-weighted spin-echo MRI showing the hyperintense fatty nature of the lesion. *(From Adam A, et al: Grainger & Allison's Diagnostic Radiology, 5th ed. Philadelphia, Churchill Livingstone, 2008.)*

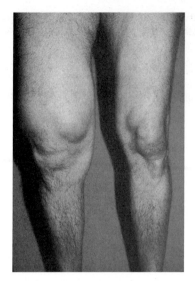

Fig. 133-2 Lipoma arborescens manifesting as a suprapatellar mass. *(From Firestein GS: Kelley's Textbook of Rheumatology, 8th ed. Philadelphia, Saunders, 2008.)*

Definition: A malignant tumor that develops from fat cells of mesenchymal origin, in which the bulk of the tumor differentiates into adipose tissue.

Incidence: The annual number of reported cases in the United States is roughly 5000, which accounts for less than 20% of all soft tissue sarcomas. The reported incidence is far less in the pediatric population.

Etiology: Trauma has been implicated; however, no true cause has been established.

Age: The average age at presentation is 50 years.

Gender: Slightly more common in males than females.

Race: No predilection.

Signs and Symptoms: Most commonly located on the extremities, retroperitoneal area, or inguinal area. Most patients experience no symptoms until the size of the tumor impacts local structures, resulting in pain or tenderness. Additional symptoms include numbness, decrease in function, and swelling. A well-circumscribed mass is the presenting manifestation in most cases.

Classifications:

World Health Organization Classification: (1) well differentiated, which includes the adipocytic, sclerosing, and inflammatory subtypes; (2) de-differentiated; (3) myxoid; (4) round cell; (5) pleomorphic.

Micropatholgy: Histologically, the tumors exhibit moderate-sized cells with variable cytoplasmic fat formation set in a myxoid background. They typically demonstrate a rich capillary network; however, fat formation and cellularity are variable.

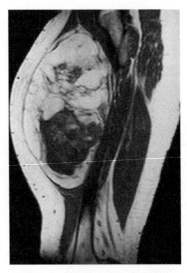

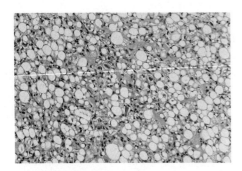

Fig. 134-1   Liposarcoma showing irregular fat cells with atypical nuclei. *(From Regezi JA, et al: Oral Pathology: Clinical Pathologic Correlations, 5th ed. Philadelphia, Saunders, 2008.)*

Fig. 134-2   Low-grade liposarcoma. Sagittal T1-weighted MR image of the thigh showing a heterogeneous mass. The cephalic portion is hyperintense, typical of simple lipoma, whereas the caudal component is isointense with muscle, much more suggestive of sarcoma. *(From Adam A, et al: Grainger & Allison's Diagnostic Radiology, 5th ed. Philadelphia, Churchill Livingstone, 2008.)*

Macropathology: May interrupt organ function or compromise neurovascular structures.

Diagnostic Studies: An x-ray study, ultrasound, computed tomography scan, positron-emission tomography scan, or magnetic resonance imaging may be used to evaluate the mass. In addition, angiography as well as cytogenetic testing is used to assist with the diagnosis. Following an open biopsy, histologic and immunohistochemical testing should be conducted.

Treatment: Responses to chemotherapy are not well documented; some advocate radiation therapy as a valuable adjunct to surgery. Wide surgical excision of the tumor is the recommended treatment strategy.

Complications: Typical complications following chemotherapy, radiation, and surgical interventions should be considered before any treatment. The morbidity and mortality rates are contingent on the location and histologic classification of the liposarcoma.

Definition: Lisfranc injury indicates an injury to the normal alignment of the cuneiforms and metatarsal joints with the loss of their normal spatial relationships.

Homolateral: All five metatarsals are displaced in the same direction.

Divergent: Metatarsals are displaced in sagittal and coronal planes.

Incidence: Injuries to the Lisfranc joints occur in less than 1% of all foot fractures.

Etiology: Lisfranc fracture occurs because the second metatarsal is the longest metatarsal proximally, so it is often fixed at its base, with the other metatarsals dislocated. As well, if the dorsal capsule of the Lisfranc joint is lacking sufficient reinforcement to support the load, it will collapse, resulting in dorsal fracture dislocation of the metatarsal bases.

Associations: A Lisfranc dislocation may be a fracture of the base of the second metatarsal, cuboid fracture, a fracture of the shafts of metatarsals, navicular compression fractures, longitudinal stress injuries, and rupture of the posterior tibial tendon.

Signs and Symptoms: Lisfranc fracture-dislocations are often mistaken for sprains. The top of the foot may be bruised, swollen, and painful. If the injury is severe, the patient may not be able to put any weight on the foot. Lisfranc injuries are often difficult to identify on x-ray studies.

Diagnostic Studies: Accurate diagnosis requires a physical examination to determine the amount of swelling, the location of the bruising, and the areas of tenderness. When Lisfranc fracture is suspected, radiographs of the foot are obtained. In some patients, it is necessary to proceed to more sophisticated scanning techniques including computed tomography or magnetic resonance imaging. It is possible to have a scan that is interpreted as normal, even when the joints are unstable and partially dislocated.

Treatment: If there is significant separation of the bones, a surgical open reduction or internal fixation is done to stabilize the bones and joints.

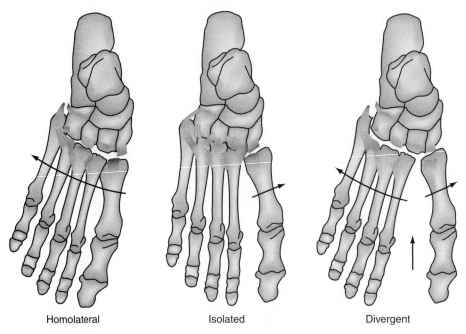

Homolateral   Isolated   Divergent

Fig. 135-1   Classification of Lisfranc injuries. The ligamentous anatomy of the Lisfranc complex is also depicted. *(From Hardcastle PH, et al: Injuries to the tarsometatarsal joint: Incidence, classification and treatment. J Bone Joint Surg [Br] 64:349, 1982.)*

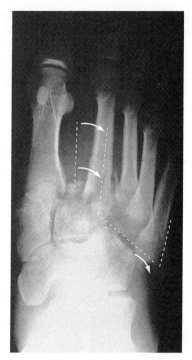

Fig. 135-2 Lisfranc fracture/dislocation. In this fracture/dislocation, the second through fifth metatarsals are fractured and/or subluxed laterally (*arrows*). (*From Mettler FA, Jr: Essentials of Radiology. Philadelphia, Saunders, 2005.*)

Definition: Pain in the lower back, which may or may not have a radicular component; pain that lasts beyond 3 months and is associated with significant impairment is defined as chronic low back pain.

Etiology: Broad in scope given the multifactorial etiology. Diskogenic pain is believed to arise from afferent pain fibers in the outer one third of the annulus fibrosis, and is associated with phospholipase A_2-regulated arachidonic acid cascade, which results in tissue injury and edema. Fracture (traumatic or pathologic) may cause pain arising from the bone. Neurogenic pain is associated with nerve root irritation from either mechanical compression or inflammation. The facet joints are extensively innervated by pain fibers. Spinal musculature may cause pain from mechanical pressure or stretch, anaerobic exercise, or ischemia. Sacroiliac joint dysfunction and chronic stress of the spinal ligaments are also associated with low back pain. Low back pain is of an idiopathic etiology in up to 85% of presenting patients.

Associations: Associated risk factors include tobacco history (50 pack per year), alcohol abuse, obesity, and osteoporosis.

Incidence: The lifetime incidence in the general population is estimated to be 70%. It is the most expensive benign condition in industrialized society and accounts for more than 15 million patient visits to physicians' offices per year in the United States. Low back pain (LBP) has an incidence of 5% per year and a prevalence of 60% to 90% in the general population.

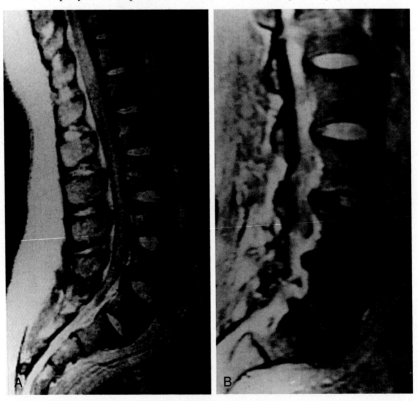

Fig. 136-1   MRI of lumbar spine. **A,** Normal T2-weighted image. **B,** T2-weighted image showing degenerative bulging or herniated discs, or both, at L3-4, L4-5, and L5-S1. *(From Canale ST, Beaty JH [eds]: Campbell's Operative Orthopaedics, 11th ed. Philadelphia, Mosby, 2007.)*

Age: Incidence is 50% by age 20, increasing to 80% by 60 years of age.

Clinical Findings: Straight leg raise test is associated with radicular pain. Facet joint pain may be exacerbated with extension. Pain associated with spinal muscles may be exacerbated by mechanical pressure or stretch. Sacroiliac pathology may be elicited with palpation of the posterior inferior iliac spine, buttock, thigh, or groin.

Signs and Symptoms: The history and physical examination remain the most important source of diagnostic information. Onset of symptoms, relation to work or other injury, history of litigation related to pain, the location of pain and exacerbating/alleviating factors, as well as the time of day when pain is most prominent must be determined. While symptoms may be diffuse and multifactorial, there are associated "red flags" that may alert to significant pathology. Fever, weight loss, trauma, age older than 50 years, failure of conservative management, alcohol or drug abuse, history of cancer, osteoporosis, progressive neurologic deficit, and history of immunosuppression all require careful evaluation.

Diagnostic Studies: Diagnostic studies are used to exclude or further evaluate severe disease. In the absence of "red flag" symptoms, imaging studies are generally not necessary at the initial evaluation and should be reserved for follow-up evaluation after the failure of several weeks of conservative management. Initial studies (if indicated) are plain films. Further studies should be geared to establish a pathoanatomic diagnosis. Magnetic resonance imaging (MRI) is useful to assess neural compression and disk degeneration. Facet injections have questionable efficacy, both as a provocative test and for pain control. Provocative diskography may be used to assess disk pathology, but its role in predicting surgical outcome is controversial. Computed tomography myelography provides comparable information with MRI for evaluating spinal stenosis, but is invasive in nature. Electromyography may be indicated in the setting of leg pain.

Surgical Care: The role of surgery in back pain is highly controversial. The majority of patients will improve with conservative management. Patients with established mechanical instability or identified neurologic compression that corresponds to physical findings may benefit from operative decompression and stabilization. Stabilization aims to eliminate the disk space as a pain source, whereas decompression seeks to alleviate radicular symptoms. Decompression may be direct or indirect, and fusion may be anterior, posterior, or circumferential. Anterior decompression provides better access to the disk space and indirect decompression of nerve roots via distraction and restoration of disk height. Posterolateral and posterior interbody fusions provide direct decompression of the nerve roots but more limited access to the disk space. Pedicle screw instrumentation has been demonstrated to result in higher fusion success; whether this higher fusion rate correlates to improved clinical response is controversial. Revision and complicated cases may require combined anterior and posterior stabilization. Emerging technology such as disk replacement may play a role in the future; at this time, clinical data are limited. Surgical intervention in the absence of defined pathophysiology is likely to have a suboptimal result.

Definition: The lower cervical spine (subaxial C-spine) is comprised of vertebrae C3 to C7. Injuries in this region of the spine can have devastating outcomes due to the proximity of the bone and soft tissue structures to the spinal cord.

Etiology: Motor vehicle accidents (MVAs) and associated head traumas from both violent and recreational activities constitute the large majority of C-spine injuries. Ground level falls (GLFs) are a significant cause in older adults.

Incidence: In trauma cases, the reported incidence of C-spine injuries ranges from 2% to 4.6%. In patients with confirmed C-spine injuries, nearly 40% suffer some level of neurologic damage. However, in approximately 10% of spinal cord injuries there is no evidence of spinal column damage.

Age: Bimodal distribution with a peak at 15 to 24 years of age and another peak at older than 55 years of age. The former is more often due to MVAs and inflicted head trauma while the latter is primarily the result of GLFs.

Gender: In the 15- to 24-year-old age group, males have a greater risk of incurring C-spine injuries because of more dangerous behavior. In the older population, females are at greater risk, most likely because of weakened osteoporotic bone.

Signs, Symptoms, and Clinical Findings: A thorough history should be taken with particular attention to the timing and mechanism of the injury. The mechanism can be characterized according to Allen-Ferguson: pure compression; compression-flexion; distraction-flexion, and compression-extension. Flexion injury with posterior disruption may result in unilateral or bilateral facet dislocation and 25% or 50% canal compromise, respectively. Complaints of tingling, paresthesias, or pain must be noted as well as any bony step-offs. Decreased motor function, changes in sensation to light touch or proprioception, or abnormal deep tendon reflexes (DTRs) should be evaluated. The primary DTRs include biceps (C5), brachioradialis (C6), triceps (C7), quadriceps (L3-4), and gastrocs (S1). Next, the presence of pathologic reflexes indicating

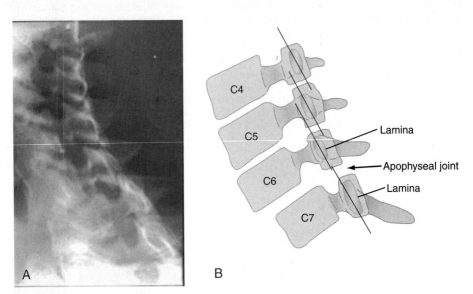

Fig. 137-1 Unilateral facet dislocation. Mechanism: flexion and rotation. Stability: stable. **A** and **B**, Oblique view of unilateral facet dislocation with the lamina of C6 projecting into the neural foramina. *(From Marx JA: Rosen's Emergency Medicine: Concepts and Clinical Practice, 6th ed. Philadelphia, Mosby, 2006.)*

upper motor neuron damage must be assessed: Clonus, Hoffmann's sign, and Babinski are most commonly tested. Finally, anal sphincter tone, anal wink, and bulbocavernosus reflex and sacral sparing help determine the completeness of the spinal cord injury.

Micropathology: In older adults, osteoporosis causes a change in the microarchitecture of bone. With constant stress on the spine, compression fractures of the spine are some of the most common fractures associated with osteoporosis.

Medical Treatment: There is no specific medical treatment other than pain control and cervical collar support for lower C-spine fractures. With associated spinal cord injury, steroids can be used as a practice option to minimize local edema and possibly decrease secondary injury; however, if presentation is greater than 8 hours after the injury, steroid use is no longer recommended.

Surgical Treatment: The initial surgical management focuses on spinal realignment using traction. Reduction of bilaterally locked facets in a neurologically incomplete patient improves neurologic recovery. Once realignment is achieved and instability persists, surgery may be necessary via anterior and/or posterior decompression and fusion.

Imaging Studies: Lateral C-spine radiograph is the standard for evaluating subaxial cervical injuries with an emphasis on visualizing the cervicothoracic junction. A computed tomography scan is particularly helpful to identify posterior column injuries such as lamina or facet fractures. Magnetic resonance imaging is useful in demonstrating spinal cord injury, ligamentous instability, and disk herniations.

Complications: Complications secondary to lower cervical spine injuries include difficulty realigning the spine and reducing the dislocation. This may require open reduction, while neurologic deterioration can occur. Neural complications include nerve root or vertebral artery injury and autonomic dysreflexia. This can manifest as severe headache, nausea, chills, anxiety, sweating, and malignant hypertension.

Outcome and Prognosis: The prognosis for patients who suffer any C-spine injury primarily depends on the severity of spinal cord damage. Outcomes of spinal column fractures/dislocations are generally excellent, with only a slight decrease in mobility if cervical fusion is required. However, injury to the spinal cord is still irreversible and can result in devastating outcomes.

Definition: The lumbosacral plexus is a network of nerves derived from lumbar and sacral roots with each one of them dividing into anterior and posterior branches. Their communications are called *lumbar plexus* (compare: brachial plexus). The anterior branches supply the flexor muscles of thigh and leg and posterior branches supply the extensor and abductor muscles.

Etiology: Problems with lumbosacral plexus can occur due to trauma at the pelvic level that damages the roots or nerves, and can be due to birth defects/trauma or lumbosacral (carcinomatous) neuropathy. Carcinoma of the intestines, bladder, or prostate can invade the lumbosacral plexus. Other masses (e.g., benign tumors, abscess, or hematoma) may also cause plexus disorders by direct pressure on any roots or trunks.

Incidence: Birth trauma and damage to the lumbosacral plexus is very rare. If injury occurs, the L4-5 portions of the plexus are most involved. Overall occurrence of lumbar plexus disorders is unknown.

Signs and Symptoms: Pain in the lower back and leg, as well as weakness in part or all of the leg. The weakness may be limited to movements of the foot or calf, or the whole leg may become paralyzed. Recovery depends on the cause. Plexus injury due to an autoimmune reaction may resolve slowly (several months); damage due to an accident may never fully recover.

Clinical Findings: The lumbar plexus provides innervations to back-buttock, abdomen, groin, thighs, knees, and calves. The sacral plexus provides innervations to the pelvis, buttocks, genitals, thighs, calves, and feet. When there is dysfunction to the plexus, areas affected can be traced by dermatomes (numb/pain) or individual muscle dysfunction. Nerve root compression is due to intraspinal pathology

Staging: No definite staging but if compressed and left untreated, it can cause long-term irreversible nerve damage, possibly paralysis.

Medical Treatment: Treatment varies depending on the cause of plexus malfunction. Corticosteroids are prescribed in the acute stage of an autoimmune reaction or inflammation/compression. Very

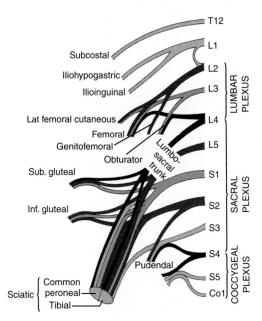

Fig. 138-1 Diagrammatic representation of the lumbosacral nervous plexus *(From Wein AS, et al: Campbell-Walsh Urology, 9th ed. Philadelphia, Saunders, 2007.)*

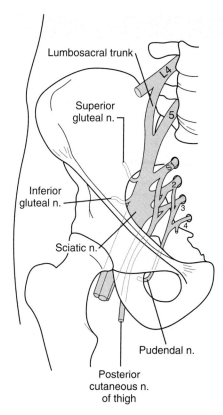

Fig. 138-2 The sacral plexus. The lumbosacral trunk is the connection between the lumbar and sacral plexus. *(From Haymaker N, Woodhall B: Peripheral Nerve Injuries. Philadelphia, Saunders, 1953.)*

limited benefit has been proven. Stretch injury needs time; transection needs operative repair with mixed results.

Surgical Treatment: If damage is caused by cancer near the plexus, it may be treated with radiation therapy or chemotherapy. Occasionally, surgical removal of compressive masses may be indicated. Traumatic transection needs open repair.

Studies: Electromyography nerve conduction studies can aid in locating the reason for malfunction. Computed tomography or magnetic resonance imaging can show pelvic masses as well as show the plexus (large nerves) itself.

Sequelae: Permanent dysfunction can occur, and as with any peripheral nerve dysfunction, healing takes time. Transection of large nerves has an overall poor prognosis.

Complications: Permanent limb dysfunction; joint stiffness and injury from loss of protective sensation.

Definition: Loss of extensor tendon continuity at the level of the distal interphalangeal joint, causing the joint to rest at the flexion position.

Etiology: It is commonly an athletic injury caused by sudden forced flexion of the extended finger at the distal interphalangeal joint. It can happen after a crushing work-related accident or after a deep cut on the extensor surface of the affected finger.

Incidence: It is often seen in young to middle-aged males. The long, ring, and small fingers of the dominant hand are mostly involved. Women with this injury tend to be older.

Signs and Symptoms: Immediately after injury, the patient is unable to actively extend the finger but passive range of motion is almost complete. The patient experiences pain, swelling, and redness over the involved joint. In examination, the finger is in flexion position and tenderness over the involved joint can be elicited after acute injury.

Diagnostic Studies: Posteroanterior, oblique, and lateral radiographs of the affected finger to assess the joint alignment and possible foreign bodies in the area after cuts and bony injuries are recommended.

Pathology: Acute deformities are those occurring within 4 weeks of the injury, and chronic deformities are defined as those occurring after 4 weeks. This injury is classified by Doyle into four groups:

Type I: Closed or blunt trauma with loss of tendon continuity with or without a small avulsion fracture.

Type II: Laceration at or proximal to the distal interphalangeal joint with loss of tendon continuity.

Type III: Deep abrasion with loss of skin, subcutaneous cover, and tendon substance.

Type IV:

    A. Transepiphyseal plate fracture in children

    B. Hyperflexion injury with fracture of articular surface of 20% to 50%

    C. Hyperextension injury with fracture of the articular surface, usually greater than 50% and with early or late volar subluxation of the distal phalanx

Treatment: Nonsurgical treatment in the form of immobilization with splint is the standard of care for the type I and closed mallet fractures involving less than one third of the articular surface with no subluxation. Surgical treatment is an option for some open injuries and injuries accompanied by volar subluxation of the distal phalanx.

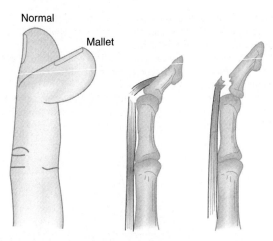

Normal

Mallet

Fig. 139-1   Mallet finger occurs with loss of extensor function to the distal phalanx. This may be caused by a tear of the tendon itself or an avulsion fracture of the dorsal base of the distal phalanx. *(From Marx JA: Rosen's Emergency Medicine: Concepts and Clinical Practice, 6th ed. Philadelphia, Mosby, 2006.)*

Definition: Marfan syndrome is an autosomal dominant connective tissue disorder that results in abnormal fibrillin-1, a glycoprotein of microfibrils.

Incidence: It occurs in approximately 1 in 10,000 individuals.

Age: Diagnosed at any age, however, several symptoms such as protrusio acetabuli and increase in extremity length are more noticeable in mature patients than in children.

Gender: No gender predilection is known.

Etiology and Pathophysiology: A mutation in the fibrillin-1 gene of chromosome 15q21.1 causes Marfan syndrome.

Clinical Presentation: Pyeritz and McKusick divided the Marfan traits into major signs and minor signs. The major signs include aortic enlargement, thoracic pectus excavatum, scoliosis, and ectopia lentis. The minor signs include arachnodactylia, tall stature, mitral valve prolapse, ligamentous laxity, myopia, as well as a positive thumb, wrist, and knee sign. Marfan syndrome has a wide variety of symptoms that affect various organs; however, the cardiac problems, such as dysrhythmia and aortic dissection, are the most problematic. Patients may have pain in the joints, lower back due to dural ectasia, or sudden thoracic pain due to aortic dissection. Pes planus, protrusio acetabuli, which may decrease hip range of motion, and abnormally long limbs may also be present.

Micropathology: The fibrillin-1 gene, also known as *FBN1*, is necessary for the production of fibrillin-1 monomers. A mutation of this gene prevents the formation of microfibrils, which results in abnormal connective tissues.

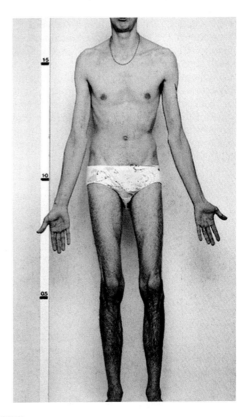

Fig. 140-1 External phenotype of patients with Marfan syndrome, showing long extremities and digits, tall stature, and pectus carinatum. *(Used with permission from Mediscan, Medical-On-Line-Ltd, London. From Libby P: Braunwald's Heart Disease: A Textbook of Cardiovascular Medicine, 8th ed. Philadelphia, Saunders, 2007.)*

287

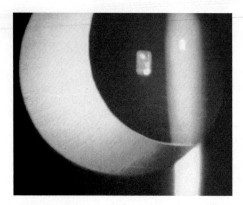

Fig. 140-2 Subluxation of the lens in Marfan syndrome. *(From Kliegman RM, et al: Nelson Textbook of Pediatrics, 18th ed. Philadelphia, Saunders, 2007.)*

Classifications: Marfan syndrome can be diagnosed using the older Berlin criteria or the more recent Ghent criteria. The Berlin criteria focus symptoms of the skeletal system and two other systems, whereas the Ghent criteria include family history and require two major criteria and the involvement of three organ systems.

Diagnostic Studies: Molecular studies can detect fibrillin-1 mutations. Chest radiography, echocardiography, aortography, and magnetic resonance imaging (MRI) can be used to detect aortic dissection. MRI can detect dural ectasia. Radiographs may be used to detect orthopedic abnormalities, such as protrusio acetabuli.

Treatment: Pes planus can be treated with orthotics or arch supporting shoes. Bracing may be used to treat scoliosis; however, surgery may be necessary in severe cases. Beta blockers can delay aortic expansion, although surgery may be warranted as a corrective measure.

Complications: Complications affecting the aorta are the primary cause of death. Aortic dissection can result in lethal hemorrhage, acute aortic valvular insufficiency, mitral insufficiency, or pericardial tamponade. Mitral valve prolapse may cause clinically significant mitral regurgitation, the most common cause of death in children with Marfan syndrome. Following surgical interventions, bacterial endocarditis may occur. Additionally, severe pectus excavatum can compromise cardiac and pulmonary function. Retinal detachment has also been described as a complication.

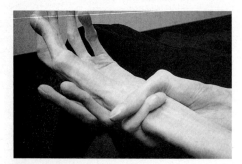

Fig. 140-3 "Wrist sign": when the wrist is grasped by the contralateral hand, the thumb overlaps the terminal phalanx of the 5th digit. *(From Zitelli BJ: Picture of the month. Arch Pediatr Adolesc Med 2005;159:721-723.)*

Anatomy: Formed by the median (C5-7) and lateral (C8, T1) cords, the median nerve follows the brachial artery to mid humerus before running in a groove between the brachialis and biceps, crossing the antecubital fossa, underneath the bicipital aponeurosis, beside the biceps tendon and pronator teres. In the forearm, the median nerve lies between the flexor digitorum superficialis (FDS) and profundus (FDP), giving off the anterior interosseus nerve (AIN) and muscular branches (FDS, flexor carpi radialis [FCR], pronator teres [PT]). It emerges in the distal forearm on the ulnar aspect of the FCR (radial to FDS). The palmar cutaneous branches before the canal. The terminal motor serves the abductor pollicis brevis (APB), oponens pollicis (OP), flexor pollicis brevis (FPB), and the first and second lumbricals. The terminal sensory branches serve palmar thumb, 2, 3, and half of fourth fingers. *Martin Gruber anastomosis* (10% to 15%) has ulnar motor branches running with median nerve before branching to ulnar nerve distally. *Riche-Cannieu anastomosis* involves connections between the deep ulnar and median nerve in the hand.

Anterior Interosseous Syndrome

The AIN arises from the median nerve at a variable point as it passes between two heads of the PT, descends vertically in front of the interosseous membrane between the FDP and flexor pollicis longus (FPL), supplying these two muscles, and finally terminates in the pronator quadratus near the wrist joint.

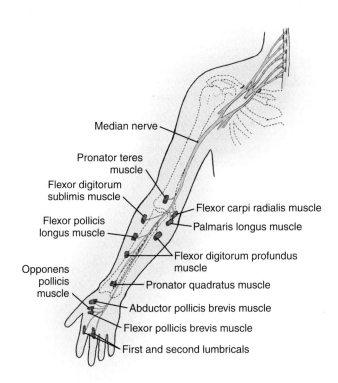

Fig. 141-1   Origin, course, and distribution of median nerve. *(From Canale ST, Beaty JH [eds]: Campbell's Operative Orthopaedics, 11th ed. Philadelphia, Mosby, 2007.)*

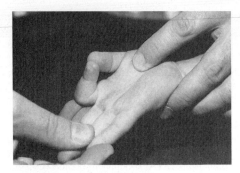

Fig. 141-2 The ability to form an "O" with the index finger and thumb, with palpable contraction of the thenar muscles, indicates an intact median nerve. *(From Grosfeld JL: Pediatric Surgery, 6th ed. Philadelphia, Mosby, 2006.)*

Etiology: Compression via tendinous bands, a deep head of the pronator teres, accessory muscles (including the Gantzer muscle, which is the accessory head of the FPL), aberrant radial artery branches, and fractures.

Clinical: Vague pain in the proximal forearm and weakness of the FPL and FDP to the index finger. Affected persons cannot form a circle by pinching their thumb and index finger (i.e., hyperextension of the index distal interphalangeal joint and thumb interphalangeal joint). No sensory involvement.

Treatment: Nonsurgical treatment includes rest, anti-inflammatory medications, and splints. Surgical treatment includes exploration of the median nerve, release of the lacertus fibrosus and division superficially more or less to the deep heads of the pronator teres, and ligation of crossing vessels.

Pronator Syndrome

Etiology: Compression near the lacertus fibrosus (bicipital aponeurosis, superficial forearm fascia), the Struthers ligament (thickened or aberrant origin of pronator teres from distal humerus), the pronator teres, and the FDS.

Clinical: Volar forearm pain worse with activity and relieved by rest; decreased sensation in median nerve distribution, thenar weakness; and a positive Tinel's sign in the proximal forearm.

Treatment: Conservative with rest and anti-inflammatory medications. Surgical treatment includes exploration of the median nerve in the proximal forearm, an incision distal and more or less proximal to the antecubital fossa in a zigzag fashion across the joint, and the release of all sites of possible compression.

Carpal Tunnel Syndrome

Most common compression syndrome at the wrist. Peak incidence at 40 to 60 years. Female-to-male ratio is 3:1; may become bilateral. Incidence reported at 1 to 3 cases per 1000 per year in the United States. Prevalence in high-risk occupations is as high as 500 per 1000.

Etiology: Nerve compression may result in ischemia, focal demyelination, decrease in axonal caliber, and finally axonal loss. Causes—accessory muscles (manus)/lumbricals, tenosynovitis, rheumatoid arthritis, type 1 diabetes mellitus, pregnancy, a ganglion, foreign or loose bodies, repetitive motion, carpal fractures or dislocations, or a persistent median artery.

Clinical: Decreased sensation, paresthesias, and tingling; worsened symptoms with repetitive use; night awakening; radiation up the forearm; a positive Tinel's or Phalen's sign; and thenar muscle wasting in advanced cases.

Studies: Electromyography or a nerve conduction velocity study, thyroid, glucose, sedimentation rate, complete blood count.

Treatment: Nonsurgical measures include wrist splinting in a neutral position to minimize intratunnel pressures at night due to posture; anti-inflammatory medications; steroid injections for transient relief; and activity modification. Surgical therapy is indicated in refractory cases. Focus on release of the volar transverse carpal ligament via open approach or endoscopic approach without injury to the palmar cutaneous, thenar, or main branch of the median nerve.

Anatomy: The meniscus is a specialized intra-articular fibrocartilaginous structure of the knee. It functions as a load-bearing and shock-absorbing structure, absorbing up to 50% of the weight distributed across the knee. It also acts with the ligamentous structures to help stabilize the knee joint. The medial meniscus is C-shaped, whereas the lateral meniscus is O-shaped. They are divided into three regions: the anterior horn, the body, and the posterior horn. The menisci are triangular in cross section, with an average thickness of 3 to 5 mm. Both are anchored to the tibial plateau via coronary ligaments and are attached superiorly to the femur via meniscofemoral ligaments. The mid aspect of the medial meniscus is firmly attached to the deep medial collateral ligament, whereas there is no attachment from the lateral meniscus to the adjacent lateral collateral ligament. The menisci have only a limited peripheral blood supply that originates from the lateral and medial geniculate arteries. In adults, the peripheral 3 mm of the menisci as well as the anterior and posterior horns are well vascularized, the zone from 3 to 5 mm has variable vascularity, whereas anything greater than 5 mm from the meniscosynovial junction are generally avascular. As a result of this avascularity, a torn meniscus does not have the ability to heal itself unless there is just a small tear confined to the peripheral vascular zone. Similarly, the nerve supply providing pain and sensation to the meniscus is also limited to the zone where the blood vessels are located.

Meniscus Tears: There are two different mechanisms for tearing a meniscus: traumatic and degenerative. Traumatic tears usually result from a twisting injury or a blow to the side of the knee that subjects the meniscus to tension, compression, and shear. Degenerative tears occur as the meniscus gradually becomes less compliant and elastic over time and then may fail with only minimal trauma. A meniscal tear can occur in almost any location; however, tears confined to the anterior horn are unusual. Typically tears begin in the posterior horn and then extend forward into the middle body. *Bucket handle tears* describe a vertical longitudinal tear of the meniscus with displacement of the inner margin; they are more common in younger patients who have also suffered an anterior cruciate ligament tear.

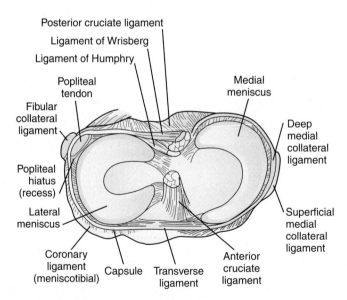

Fig. 142-1   Medial and lateral meniscus anatomy as viewed from above. *(From Rakel R: Textbook of Family Medicine, 7th ed. Philadelphia, Saunders, 2007.)*

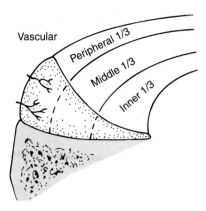

Fig. 144-2 Meniscal tear sites in relation to diameter of the radius. *(From Browner BD: Skeletal Trauma: Basic Science, Management, and Reconstruction, 3rd ed. Philadelphia, Saunders, 2003.)*

Signs and Symptoms: Pain and swelling in the affect knee are common. Sometimes the knee will become "locked" in a flexed position and will be quite painful with attempts to straighten it. This is often caused by the mechanical blockage from a torn fragment that acts as a wedge to prevent the joint surfaces from moving. In addition to history and physical examination, magnetic resonance imaging is highly accurate in diagnosing a tear.

Treatment: Outpatient arthroscopic surgery is the treatment of choice. Based on the location and geometry of the tear, the decision is made to either remove or repair the tear. Most meniscal tears need to be removed because they involve areas of avascular tissue. This involves cutting and sucking out the torn portions, while the remaining meniscal rim is then contoured to provide a gradual tapered transition. However, if the tear is confined to the zone of meniscal blood supply, it may be possible to directly repair the meniscus. The role of the repair is to hold the meniscus together long enough for it to heal firmly.

Primary bone cancer occurs predominantly among children and adolescents and is rare. By contrast, metastatic bone cancer, particularly from carcinomas of the breast, lung, prostate, kidney, and thyroid, is much more common.

Carcinomas of the breast, lungs, and prostate have a high prevalence and likely account for more than 80% of cases of metastatic bone disease. The distribution of bone metastases is predominantly to the axial skeleton—particularly the spine, pelvis, and ribs—rather than to the appendicular skeleton, although lesions in the humeri and femora are also common.

Mechanism of Metastasis

The predominant distribution of bone metastases in the axial skeleton, in which most of the red bone marrow is situated, suggests that the slow blood flow at these sites could assist in the attachment of metastatic cells.

The vertebral-venous plexus is an extensive network of valveless vessels carrying blood under low pressure and continually subjected to arrest and reversal of flow. Bypassed blood flow

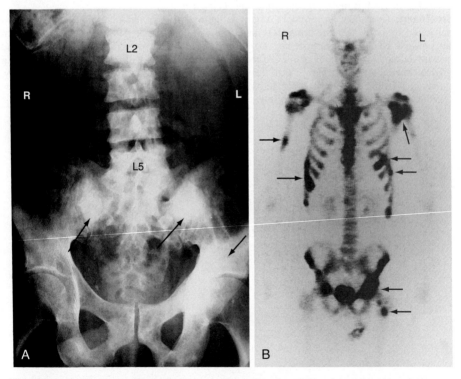

Fig. 143-1 Metastatic prostate cancer. **A,** An anteroposterior view of the pelvis and lumbar spine demonstrates multiple areas of increased density (*arrows*) in a patchy distribution. Vertebrae L2 and L5 also are abnormally white or increased in density. **B,** A nuclear medicine whole-body bone scan most commonly shows the metastatic deposits as areas of increased activity (*arrows*). (*From Mettler FA, Jr: Essentials of Radiology, 2nd ed. Philadelphia, Saunders, 2005.*)

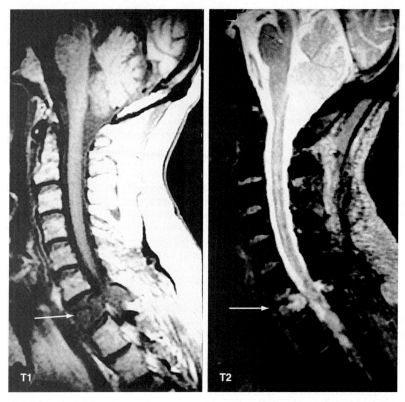

Fig. 143-2 Tumor involvement of the cervical spine. In this patient with lymphoma and neurologic deficit, a sagittal magnetic resonance image of the cervical spine demonstrates complete replacement of the marrow of C7, seen as a dark area on the T1 image (*arrow*). The T2 image also shows the tumor as a white area (*arrow*) narrowing the spinal canal and compressing the spinal cord. (*From Mettler FA, Jr: Essentials of Radiology, 2nd ed. Philadelphia, Saunders, 2005.*)

through this network provides a possible explanation for propensity of certain cancers such as breast and prostate to have a predilection for bone metastasis.

Physiology of Bone Metastasis—Imbalance in Bone Remodeling

Bone consists primarily of type I collagen, which consists of helical fibrils of tropocollagen molecules arranged in a ring structure. Bone is a metabolically active structure that is continually being absorbed and reformed. Multinucleated giant cells called *osteoclasts,* derived from granulocyte-macrophage precursors, resorb bone while *osteoblasts,* derived from mesenchymal fibroblast-like cells, build bone back up. A complex interaction between osteoblasts and osteoclasts is regulated by hormones, paracrine growth factors, and cytokines. In normal, fully developed bone, 5% to 15% is involved in remodeling. In this situation, bone resorption and reformation are balanced, resulting in no net changes in bone density over time.

Metastatic tumor cells are believed to upset the balance of remodeling in various ways. Osteolytic damage is mediated largely by stimulation of osteoclasts via tumor-derived cytokines as well as intermediary cells, including immune cells and osteoblasts.

Recent studies have demonstrated the production of cell signaling factors, which affect osteoclast activity in various primary tumor types such as breast, lung, and squamous cell carcinomas. Multiple avenues in which malignant cells can affect bone remodeling both directly and indirectly have been described.

Diagnosis and Treatment: Metastatic involvement of the skeleton typically affects multiple sites and causes pain, bony tenderness, and increasing disability. Diagnosis is typically made using imaging scan.

The isotope bone scan is a sensitive test to detect the presence of skeletal pathology but gives little information about its nature. Structural information on skeletal damage from metastatic bone disease is best obtained by skeletal radiography supplemented by computerized tomography or magnetic resonance imaging.

Treatment for metastatic bone disease requires individualized care and is dependent upon comorbidities, histologic characteristics of the primary tumor, expected life span of the patient, patient's activity level, and pain. Antitumor treatments, such as radiation therapy, endocrine therapy, cytotoxic chemotherapy, and targeted radioisotope therapy, all have roles in palliating metastatic bone disease. Drug regimens including bisphosphonates inhibit osteoclast activity and have become important agents for the treatment of metastatic bone disease, because they relieve symptoms, enable bone healing, and delay complications. Early indications of response of bone metastases to treatment can be obtained by monitoring biochemical markers, including the bone isoenzyme of alkaline phosphatase, osteocalcin, and pyridinium cross-linking amino acids.

Patients with metastasis to weight-bearing bones often require special considerations versus patients with metastasis to upper extremity or non–weight-bearing structures. Classification systems (e.g., the Mirels scoring system) have been described in an attempt to predict impending fracture and estimate the need for operative management. The Mirels system evaluates attributes of a metastatic lesion such as size, location, and type as well as a measure of pain. Additional factors that are important to consider are the presence of other comorbidities, the histologic characteristics of the primary tumor, the expected life span of the patient, and the patient's activity level. Operative management is often indicated for pathologic fracture in lower extremity long bones. However, pathologic fractures have different biologic characteristics from normal fractures and do not reliably heal. Strategies for orthopedic management of metastatic disease must take these characteristics into account and may require the need for alterations in operative management. Recent studies have shown promising data in management with the use of unconventional implants (including long stems), cement fixation and augmentation, and adjuvant therapy.

Definition: MFH is the most common soft tissue sarcoma of the extremities. Four main subtypes of MFH have been identified: (1) storiform-pleomorphic MFH, (2) myxoid MFH, (3) giant cell MFH, and (4) xanthomatous MFH.

Incidence: MFH occurs at a rate of approximately 1260 to 1440 new cases per year (18% of all soft tissue sarcomas).

Age: Peak occurrence is during the seventh decade of life.

Gender: The ratio of males-to-females is 2:1.

Race: More common in Caucasian patients.

Etiology and Pathophysiology: The following translocations have been linked to the development of MFH: 1q11, 3p12, 11p11, and 19p13.

Associations: Rare cases of MFH have arisen following hip arthroplasty. It has also been established that radiotherapy increases the likelihood of MFH developing. As with all extremity sarcomas, MFH has a high tendency to metastasize to the lungs. MFH has also been associated with non-Hodgkin's lymphoma, Hodgkin's lymphoma, multiple myeloma, and malignant histiocytosis.

Signs and Symptoms: MFH manifests as a painless mass, usually in the lower extremities following minor injury.

Diagnostic Studies: Diagnosis is established only following a biopsy of the lump to rule out other types of soft tissue sarcoma. Depending on the size of the tumor, either an excisional (<5 cm) or an incisional (≥5 cm) biopsy is performed. Physicians can use any type of imaging technique to see the tumor growth in that each has its own advantages. Radiographs allow for the defining of tumor size and extent of invasion/metastasis. Computed tomography scans provide a three-dimensional image of the tumor. Magnetic resonance imaging scans give a view of multiple planes and allow for the differentiation between tumor and adjacent structures. Scintigrams with technetium (Tc-99m) and gallium (Ga-67) are also used to define location and size of the tumor.

Micropathology: The presence of many large, multinucleate giant cells is characteristic of this tumor.

Macropathology: A large painless lump is the most common clinical presentation.

Treatment: The primary choice for treatment is a complete surgical excision of the tumor. Other treatment options include radiation and chemotherapy. Unfortunately, due to the aggressiveness of MFH, many patients experience recurrences.

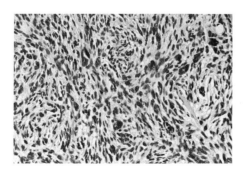

Fig. 144-1 Malignant fibrous histiocytoma revealing fascicles of plump spindle cells in a swirling (storiform) pattern, typical but not pathognomonic of this neoplasm. *(Courtesy of Dr. J. Corson, Brigham and Women's Hospital, Boston, MA. From Kumar V, et al: Robbins and Cotran Pathologic Basis of Disease, 7th ed. Philadelphia, Saunders, 2005.)*

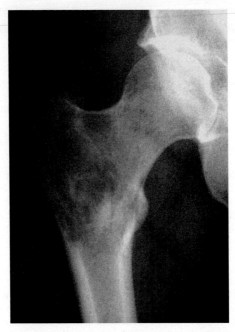

Fig. 144-2   Malignant fibrous histiocytoma. AP radiograph of the proximal femur showing a moth-eaten destructive lesion with no characteristic features. *(From Adam A, et al: Grainger & Allison's Diagnostic Radiology, 5th ed. Philadelphia, Churchill Livingstone, 2008.)*

Definition: Tendency of an object to deform along an axis when opposing forces are applied along that axis. More simply, it is the stiffness of a given material. It can determine the behavior of materials under load. It is the critical factor in load-sharing capacity. The modulus itself is determined by dividing the stress at failure by the strain at failure.

Yield Point: Transition point from the elastic to plastic range.

Ultimate Strength: Maximum strength obtained by material.

Breaking Point: Point where material fractures.

Plastic Deformation: Change in length after removing the load.

Relative Values: Comparison of the modulus of elasticity for orthopaedic materials, with ceramic the most stiff and cartilage the least.

Al_2O_3 (ceramic)
Co-Cr-Mo (alloy)
Stainless steel
Titanium
Cortical bone
Matrix polymers
PMMA
Polyethylene
Cancellous bone
Tendon/ligament
Cartilage

The importance of this concept can best be seen in stress shielding. Factors affecting stress shielding include stem stiffness, porous coating, and metal alloy. Stem stiffness is related to the modulus, degree of porous coating, and stem geometry.

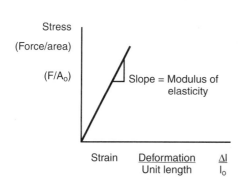

Fig. 145-1 Stress versus strain diagram showing modulus of elasticity. *(From Lemons JE, Natiella J: Biomaterials, biocompatibilitys and peri-implant considerations. Dent Clin North Am 30:3, 1986.)*

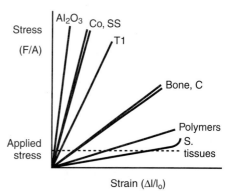

Fig. 145-2 Elastic moduli relationships and an applied interfacial stress. *(From McKinney RV, Lemons JE [eds]: The Dental Implant: Clinical and Biological Response to Oral Tissues. Littleton, Mass, PSG Publishing, 1983.)*

299

Definition: The original definition of a Monteggia fracture was a fracture in the proximal third of the ulna along with dislocation of the radial head. This definition has been expanded to include all ulna fractures with dislocation of the radial head. Monteggia fractures are classified as four types based on the concept that the apex of the fracture is in the same direction as the dislocation of the radial head.

Incidence: Less than 5% of forearm fractures are classified as Monteggia fractures.

Etiology and Pathophysiology: Monteggia fractures may be the result of a direct blow to the forearm and hyperpronation injuries.

Clinical Presentation: Monteggia fractures manifest with elbow pain, especially during forearm rotation and elbow flexion. Patients often present with swelling, crepitus, deformity, paresthesia, and numbness. The dislocated radial head is sometimes palpable. In children, Monteggia fractures may manifest with plastic deformation.

Diagnostic Procedures: The fractured ulna and dislocation of the proximal radioulnar joint are visible in radiographs. The radioulnar joint should be radiographed in orthogonal planes, in intervals of 90 degrees, to visualize the dislocation. If a line drawn through the center of the radial

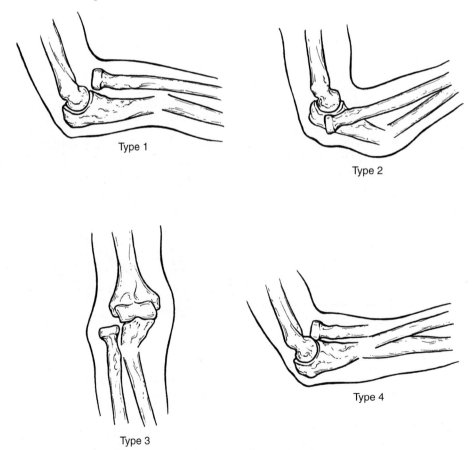

Fig. 146-1 Monteggia fracture classification. *(From Olney BW, Menelaus MB: Monteggia and equivalent lesions in childhood. J Pediatr Orthop 9:219–223, 1989.)*

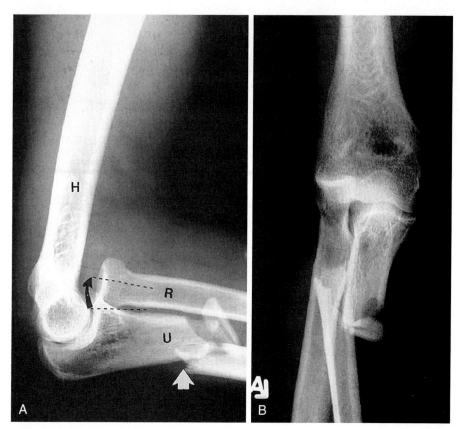

Fig. 146-2 Monteggia fracture/dislocation. **A,** The lateral view of the elbow shows a fracture of the ulna that occurs at the direct point of impact (*large white arrow*) and dislocation of the radial head from its normal position (*curved black arrow*). **B,** On the anteroposterior projection, the ulnar fracture is clearly identified, but the radial head dislocation is impossible to see. *(From Mettler FA, Jr: Essentials of Radiology, 2nd ed. Philadelphia, Saunders, 2005.)*

head and down the central axis of the radius does not pass through the middle of the capitellum, then the radial head is dislocated or subluxed.

Treatment: The treatment of Monteggia fractures depends on the age of the patient and the classification of the fracture. The dislocated radial head should be reduced within a few hours of the injury. In adults, the ulna is usually stabilized by an open reduction and internal fixation. In children, the ulna is usually stabilized by a long-arm splint with 90-degree flexion at the elbow. However, open reduction is necessary when closed reduction is not adequate.

Table 146-1. CLASSIFICATION (BADO)

Type I	There is a fracture in the ulna diaphysis and the radial head is dislocated anteriorly.
Type II	There is a fracture in the ulna diaphysis and the radial head is dislocated posteriorly.
Type III	The ulna is fractured in the metaphysis and the radial head is dislocated laterally.
Type IV	There is a fracture of the proximal third of the ulna and radius. The radius is dislocated anteriorly.

Definition: A neuroma is a growth (benign tumor) that arises in nerve cells. A Morton's neuroma is a swollen, inflamed nerve located between the bones at the ball of the foot (usually either the second or the third spacing from the base of the great toe).

Incidence: The most common neuroma in the foot is a Morton's neuroma.

Gender: The incidence of Morton's neuroma is 8 to 10 times greater in women than in men.

Etiology and Pathophysiology: The etiology of Morton's neuroma is generally unknown. The condition seems to occur in response to irritation, pressure, or injury to one of the digital nerves leading to the toes. The growth of thickened nerve tissue (neuroma) is part of the body's response to the irritation or injury. Factors that appear to contribute to Morton's neuroma include wearing high-heeled shoes or shoes that are tight and participating in high-impact athletic activities.

Associations: People with certain foot deformities—bunions, hammertoes, flatfeet, or more flexible feet—are at higher risk for developing a neuroma.

Signs and Symptoms: A Morton's neuroma usually causes burning pain, numbness, or tingling at the base of the second, third, or fourth toes. Pain also can spread from the ball of the foot out to the tips of the toes. In some cases, there also is the sensation of a lump, a fold of sock, or a "hot pebble" between the toes.

Diagnostic Studies: The diagnosis of a Morton's neuroma can usually be made by a physical examination of the feet. The foot is usually tender when the involved area is compressed and symptoms of pain and sometimes tingling can be elicited when the sides of the foot are squeezed. Magnetic resonance imaging or ultrasound testing can be used to confirm the diagnosis if necessary.

Treatment: Symptoms of a Morton's neuroma can be completely resolved with simple treatments, such as resting the foot, wearing better fitting shoes, using nonsteroidal anti-inflammatory medications, or wearing custom foot orthoses. More rapid relief of symptoms can follow a local cortisone injection. Surgical removal of the growth may be necessary if other treatments fail to provide pain relief. The surgical procedure removes both the neuroma and the nerve, which can leave permanent numbness in the affected toes.

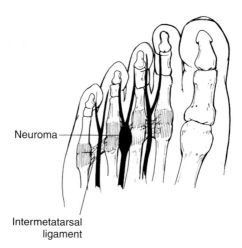

Neuroma

Intermetatarsal ligament

Fig. 147-1 Interdigital neuroma, plantar view. *(From DeLee D, Drez D [eds]: DeLee and Drez's Orthopaedic Sports Medicine, 2nd ed. Philadelphia, Saunders, 2003.)*

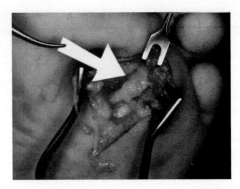

Fig. 147-2 Interdigital neuroma. Plantar incision for "recurrent" interdigital neuroma with communicating nerve entering neuroma (*arrow*). *(From Canale ST, Beaty JH [eds]: Campbell's Operative Orthopaedics, 11th ed. Philadelphia, Mosby, 2007.)*

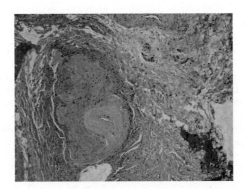

Fig. 147-3 Pathologic findings of interdigital neuroma. Interdigital nerve is greatly thickened by perineural fibrous tissue (hematoxylin and eosin stain). *(Courtesy of Bruce Webber, MD. From Canale ST, Beaty JH [eds]: Campbell's Operative Orthopaedics, 11th ed. Philadelphia, Mosby, 2007.)*

Definition: A strong magnetic field is first applied to align a portion of hydrogen nuclei, which naturally spin like magnetic dipoles within the body. The hydrogen nuclei then become excited when radio waves called *pulses* are applied selectively to move them out of alignment. A magnetic resonance image is generated by capturing and amplifying the radio waves emitted from the nuclei as they return to alignment after the pulse.

Characteristics:

Advantages:
- Exquisite images of the central nervous system and stationary soft tissues, such as muscles, ligaments, and tendons
- No ionizing radiation exposure

Disadvantages:
- Patient motion artifacts
- Inability to bring ferromagnetic objects near magnet
- High cost

Common Applications:
- Brain and spinal cord diseases or injury
- Ligamentous and muscular injury
- Detection of tumors
- Examination of organs requiring high-quality images

Basic Types of Images:

T_1-*Weighted:*
- High-signal (bright)—fat, bone marrow, subacute hemorrhage, slow-flowing blood, proteinaceous fluid, melanin
- Low-signal (dark)—cerebrospinal fluid (CSF), bile, flowing blood, bone, air

T_2-*Weighted:*
- High-signal (bright)—CSF, bile
- Low-signal (dark)—bone, flowing blood, acute or subacute hematoma, air

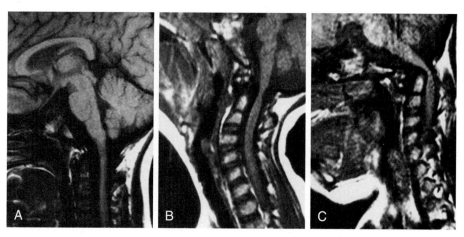

Fig. 148-1 A, This magnetic resonance imaging (MRI) study shows a normal canal, the odontoid, the cord, and the remaining space available to the cord. **B,** Extension MRI scan in a patient with Down syndrome demonstrating the odontoid, mild constriction of the cord at that level, and the space available to the cord. **C,** Flexion MRI scan demonstrating forward translation of C1 relative to the odontoid and tenting of the cord over the odontoid as the space available to the cord is compromised. *(From Green NE, Swiontkowski MF: Skeletal Trauma in Children, 3rd ed. Philadelphia, Saunders, 2003.)*

305

Table 148-1. SYMBOL STRENGTH FOR T_1- VERSUS T_2-WEIGHTED IMAGES

	T1-Weighted	T2-Weighted
Fat	High	Moderate
Tendons	Low	Low
Ligaments	Low	Low
Fascial layers	Low	Low
Cortical bone	Low	Low
Muscle	Moderate	Moderate
Normal marrow	High	Moderate
Soft tissue sarcomas	Low	High
Fluid (ganglions, effusions)	Low	High
Pigmented villonodular synovitis*	Very Low	Very Low

* Signal dropout (very low signal on gradient echo sequences).

Definition: Multiple myeloma (MM) is a malignant disease of plasma cells that manifests as lytic bone lesions and monoclonal protein in the blood or urine.

Etiology: The exact cause of MM is unknown, although monoclonal gammopathy of unknown significance (MGUS) is a precursor, and radiation exposure increases the risk. No clear-cut familial predisposition exists.

Incidence: It is the most common primary bone tumor. The incidence is 4 per 100,000.

Age: Mean age at diagnosis is 68 years. Occurrence in patients younger than 40 years of age is uncommon.

Gender and Race: Incidence is higher in African Americans and lower in Asians than in Caucasians. Men are more frequently affected.

Signs and Symptoms: Common clinical presentations include fatigue and bone pain with or without fractures or infection. Hypercalcemia, renal insufficiency, hyperviscosity syndrome, compression of the spinal cord, radicular pain, and bleeding have also been noted.

Diagnostic Studies: Diagnosis of MM can be made with greater than 10% abnormal plasma cells in a bone marrow biopsy specimen. Diagnosis can also be made with histologic evidence of plasmacytoma and either the presence of serum monoclonal protein (M protein) of at least 3 g/dL, urine M protein of at least 1 g/dL, or osteolytic lesions. Serum protein electrophoresis will reveal localized spikes in the α or γ regions

Macropathology: MM most commonly involves the spine, followed by the ribs and pelvis. Four distinct forms have been described: (1) solitary lesion (plasmacytoma), (2) diffuse lesions with discrete margins and uniform size (myelomatosis), (3) diffuse skeletal osteopenia, and (4) bone sclerotic lesions (sclerosing myeloma).

Micropathology: Bone marrow biopsy reveals sheets of plasma cells that have abundant cytoplasm and a perinuclear halo. Amyloid deposition can be abundant.

Imaging: Skeletal radiography reveals punched out or expansile lesions, diffuse osteopenia, osteosclerosis, or fractures. ^{99}Tc bone scan underestimates the extent of the disease because of

Diagnosis

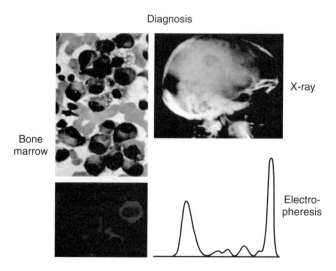

X-ray

Bone marrow

Electro-pheresis

Fig. 149-1 Common diagnostic features in multiple myeloma: light-chain restricted plasma cells in a bone marrow aspirate; multiple lytic lesions in a skull radiograph; large monoclonal spike in the γ-globulin area in serum electrophoresis. *(From Hoffman R: Hematology: Basic Principles and Practice, 5th ed. Philadelphia, Churchill Livingstone, 2008.)*

lack of osteoblastic response. On magnetic resonance imaging, MM lesions are seen as hypointensities on T1-weighted imaging, hyperintensities on short tau inversion recovery, and enhancement on gadolinium-enhanced fat-suppressed T1-weighted-images.

Treatment: Chemotherapy consists of melphalan and prednisolone or vincristine and Adriamycin accompanied by peripheral stem cell rescue. Thalidomide can decrease microvessel density and inhibit angiogenesis in the bone marrow. Bortezomib, a proteasome inhibitor, inhibits the degradation of proteins that regulate the progression of the stem cycle. Bisphosphonates (zoledronic acid) are potent osteoclast inhibitors that decrease bone resorption; their antimyeloma activity has been suggested to occur via the expansion of suppressor T cells. With vertebral involvement, decompression, vertebroplasty, or kyphoplasty is required. Open reduction and internal fixation with methacrylate, cemented total joint, or hemiarthroplasty followed by radiation should be considered.

Muscle Structure and Organization

- Consists of fibers organized in bundles of connective tissue
  - Epimysium—surrounds individual muscle bundles
  - Perimysium—surrounds muscle fascicle
  - Endomysium—surrounds individual muscle fiber
- Musculotendinous junction—weakest area where tears most frequently occur

Muscle Fiber Constitution

- Multiple peripheral nuclei
- Sarcoplasm/sarcoplasmic reticulum (SR)
  - Network of flattened tubules surrounding sarcomeres
  - Stores and releases calcium during muscle contraction
  - T tubules transmit electrical impulses from the sarcolemma inward
  - Cisternae store large Ca^+ concentrations for release into sarcomere during contraction
- Contractile elements—myofilaments
  - Thin myofilaments are composed of actin, tropomyosin, and troponin
  - Thick myofilaments consist of bundles of approximately 200 myosin molecules
- Rich in glycogen, myoglobin, and mitochondria

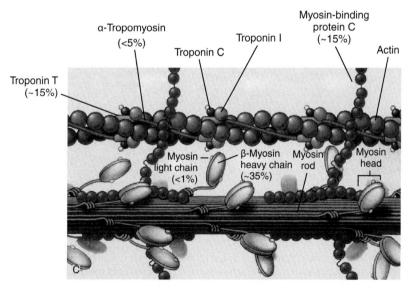

Fig. 150-1 Hypertrophic cardiomyopathy with asymmetrical septal hypertrophy. Schematic structure of the sarcomere of cardiac muscle, highlighting proteins in which mutations cause defective contraction, hypertrophy, and myocyte disarray in hypertrophic cardiomyopathy. The frequency of a particular gene mutation is indicated as a percentage of all cases of HCM; most common are mutations in the β-myosin heavy chain. Normal contraction of the sarcomere involves myosin-actin interaction initiated by calcium binding to troponin C, I, and T and α-tropomyosin. Actin stimulates ATPase activity in the myosin head and produces force along the actin filaments. Myocyte-binding protein C modulates contraction. *(From Spirito P, et al: The management of hypertrophic cardiomyopathy. N Engl J Med 336:775, 1997.)*

309

SKELETAL MUSCLE

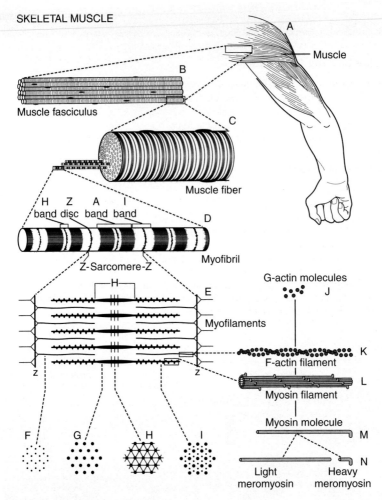

Fig. 150-2 Histologic and molecular structure of skeletal muscle. E represents a longitudinal section of a sarcomere showing the arrangement of the myofilaments actin (thin filaments) and myosin with projecting bridges (thick filaments). F, G, H, and I are cross-sections through the sarcomere showing the arrangements of the thin and thick filaments at the sites indicated. *(From Bloom W, Fawcett DW: A Textbook of Histology. Philadelphia, Saunders, 1968.)*

Sarcomere

- Smallest contractile unit of muscle composed of thin and thick filaments
  - Each thick filament is surrounded by a hexagonal array of 6 thin filaments. Each thin filament is surrounded by a triangular array of thick filaments
- During contraction thin filaments slide along thick filaments, causing increasing overlap and shortening of muscle fiber (Box 150-1)

Box 150-1

Z line—delineates sarcomere
I band—thin myofilaments composed of actin, tropomyosin, and troponin
H band—thick myofilaments composed of myosin
A band—overlap between thin and thick filaments

Muscle Fiber Contraction

- Electrical impulse travels down nerve to the neuromuscular junction
- Depolarization of motor end plate at terminal axon causes Ca^{++} to enter, and then bind with and release Ach across synapse
- SR is depolarized, causing it to release Ca^{++}, which enters sarcomere and causes contraction
- Ca^{++} binds to troponin, causing conformational change on tropomyosin, exposing myosin-binding sites on actin
- Cross-bridge formation—ATPase splits ATP into ADP + P, which energizes myosin head and causes it to bind with myosin-binding sites on actin
- Power stroke—energized cross-bridge triggers a pivoting motion of the myosin head, which causes thin actin myofilaments to slide past thick myosin myofilaments toward the center of the A bands
- During the power stroke, ADP and P are released from the myosin cross-bridge
- ATP attaches to the myosin head again, allowing it to detach from actin
  - Isotonic—constant resistance through arc of motion
  - Isokinetic—constant velocity through arc of motion; best for maximizing strength
- Isometric—muscle actively held at fixed length
  - Force generated dependent on length and degree of overlap of thin and thick filaments
  - Causes muscle hypertrophy but minimal effect on endurance
- Eccentric—muscle actively lengthening
  - External force on the muscle is greater than the force that the muscle can generate
  - Absolute tensions achieved are very high relative to the muscle's maximum tetanic tension generating capacity
  - Greatest potential for muscle injury

Definition: Noninflammatory inherited disorders with progressive muscle weakness. Duchenne muscular dystrophy (DMD) is the most common muscular dystrophy (MD) of childhood. This incurable disease is characterized by muscle wasting and loss of walking ability leading to complete wheelchair dependence by 13 years of age.

Etiology: Defect in gene coding for dystrophin on the short arm of X chromosome (Xp21.2). Dystrophin is a large, elaborate protein complex that links actin cytoskeleton to extracellular matrix in muscle. Duchenne is a fatal X-linked recessive dystrophy resulting from frameshift mutation of the dystrophin gene and results in complete absence of dystrophin protein. Other types of MD include facioscapulohumeral (FMD) and myotonic (MMD). Becker (BMD) is a less common and less severe X-linked recessive MD resulting from in-frame mutations in the dystrophin gene and results in truncated dystrophin protein, in reduced quantities, that retains some structural function.

Associations: In most patients with MD, cardiac muscle is involved, resulting in sinus tachycardia and right ventricle hypertrophy. Mild mental retardation is common. Once in a wheelchair, nearly all patients develop scoliosis. FMD causes progressive weakness in facial muscles as well as in muscles of the arms and legs. MMD is characterized by prolonged muscle spasm in the fingers and facial muscles, a floppy-footed high-stepping gait, and cataracts, among other disturbances.

Incidence: DMD is the most common inherited muscle disease, affecting 1 in 3500 boys. The other most common forms are FMD and MMD.

Age and Gender: DMD onset is between 2 and 6 years of age and it progresses rapidly. Most boys become unable to walk at 12, and by 20 are dead or have to use a respirator to breathe. BMD onset is between 2 and 16 years; BMD progresses slowly and patients have a longer life expectancy. FMD manifests in adolescence, and MMD varies in the age of onset.

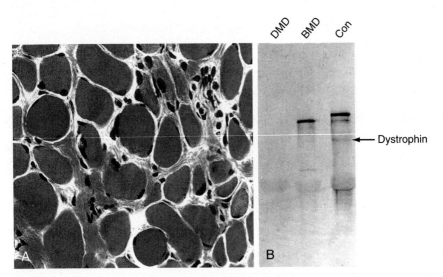

Fig. 151-1 **A,** Duchenne muscular dystrophy (DMD) showing variation in muscle fiber size, increased endomysial connective tissue, and regenerating fibers. **B,** Western blot showing absence of dystrophin in DMD and altered dystrophin size in Becker muscular dystrophy (BMD) compared with control (Con). *(Courtesy of Dr. L. Kunkel, Children's Hospital, Boston, MA. From Kumar V, et al: Robbins and Cotran Pathologic Basis of Disease, 7th ed. Philadelphia, Saunders, 2005.)*

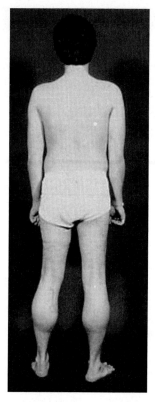

Fig. 151-2 Becker muscular dystrophy in a 24-year-old male. There is dystrophy of the shoulder girdle and calf pseudohypertrophy. *(Courtesy of Robert M. Pascuzzi, MD. From Libby PL, et al: Braunwald's Heart Disease: A Textbook of Cardiovascular Medicine, 8th ed. Philadelphia, Saunders, 2007.)*

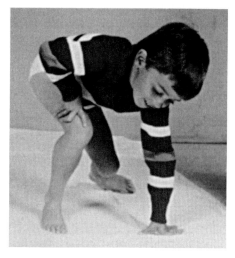

Fig. 151-3 Gower's sign. A boy with hip girdle weakness due to Duchenne muscular dystrophy. *(From Kliegman RM, et al: Nelson Textbook of Pediatrics, 18th ed. Philadelphia, Saunders, 2007.)*

Clinical Findings: Progressive proximal muscle weakness and joint contractures of upper and lower extremities are common findings. Clumsy walking, decreased motor skills, lumbar lordosis, calf pseudohypertrophy, and a positive Gower's sign are typically noted. The first muscle affected is the gluteus maximus (hip extensors).

Diagnostic Studies: Laboratory studies demonstrate markedly elevated CPK (leaks from damaged muscle). Muscle biopsy reveals an absence of the dystrophin protein. Electromyogram and nerve conduction velocity tests can distinguish between myopathy and neuropathy.

Pathology: Gene mutation results in synthesis of an unstable protein that is degraded rapidly. Sarcolemma is injured when muscle contracts, resulting in inflammation, necrosis, and replacement by fat and fibrous tissue.

Treatment: Prolongation of walking is a major aim of treatment. Moderate exercise programs and physical therapy minimize contractures. Rehabilitative devices and orthotics help maintain mobility and independence as long as possible. Surgery is indicated for releasing contractures and spinal fusion with segmental instrumentation (usually T2-L5 or sacrum) is indicated for scoliosis that develops once the patient is wheelchair-bound (curve approximately 30 degrees). Fusion improves sitting balance and quality of life, but does *not* improve pulmonary function or increase longevity. Respiratory therapy becomes essential as the disease progresses. Prednisone may prevent progressive weakness in the short term, but it has significant side effects. Cardiac abnormalities may require a pacemaker.

Definition: Necrotizing fasciitis is a rare and often fatal soft tissue infection involving the superficial fascial layers of the extremities, abdomen, or perineum.

Etiology: Group A *Streptococcus* is the most common bacterial isolate, although a polymicrobial infection with a variety of gram-positive, gram-negative, aerobic, and anaerobic bacteria is more common.

Associations: Typically begins with trauma, although the inciting event may be as innocuous as a simple contusion, minor burn, or insect bite. Necrotizing fasciitis may occur in any anatomic location; however, the extremities are most often affected. This condition mostly occurs in patients who have diabetes or use intravenous drugs.

Incidence: Even though there is no consensus among infectious disease and epidemiology experts, there are a few reports documenting an increasing incidence of necrotizing fasciitis. However, other authors believe that the numerical increase is due to heightened awareness and better reporting, rather than a true increase in incidence.

Age and Gender: Even though this disease process does not discriminate among age or gender, it does target the immunocompromised or frail patient.

Clinical Findings: Soft tissue infections encompass a wide spectrum of disease entities, ranging from the superficial to the deep and from the merely inconvenient to those that are life threatening. Necrotizing fasciitis can be distinguished from simple cellulitis by the presence of edema beyond the area of erythema, rapid development of bullae and ecchymosis, gangrenous skin, fluctuance, crepitus, and severe pain.

Symptoms: Early clinical findings of necrotizing fasciitis may be limited to pain, mild swelling, and redness.

Signs: Systemic signs of necrotizing fasciitis may include those associated with septicemia, such as hypotension, acidosis, leukocytosis, tachycardia, hyperthermia, or even more worrisome, hypothermia.

Diagnostic Studies: Laboratory evaluation should include complete blood count, electrolyte panel, coagulation levels, and liver function tests. Radiographic evaluation is not normally indicated in the workup of soft tissue infections, but can be helpful if air is seen in the soft tissues. Computed tomography may be even more sensitive than plain radiography for detecting air in the soft tissues.

Pathology: The characteristic histologic findings in necrotizing fasciitis are necrosis of the superficial fascia with blood vessel thrombosis and suppuration. The presence of inflammatory cells distinguishes necrotizing fasciitis from infections like clostridial myonecrosis.

Treatment: Initial resuscitation with fluid replacement and restoration of blood pressure is critical. Intravenous antibiotics should also be administered in conjunction with surgical débridement. Early and extensive débridement of all involved skin and fascia is mandatory. Careful postoperative monitoring is necessary, and patients who are not improving should have a second-look operation with repeat débridement. Skin grafts are usually required after the infection has been controlled.

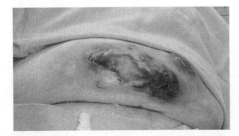

Fig. 152-1 Necrotizing fasciitis. Advanced stage of necrotizing fasciitis showing skin necrosis. *(From Williams MV, et al: Comprehensive Hospital Medicine. Philadelphia, Saunders, 2007.)*

Peripheral nerve endings are abundant in the skin, muscle, and joints. Five basic sensory receptor endings exist in the human body: thermoreceptors detect changes in temperature; mechanoreceptors respond to physical deformation; nociceptors respond to pain, photoreceptors/electromagnetic receptors are the visual receptors of the retina; chemoreceptors detect smell, taste, internal stimuli such as pH, and metabolic concentrations. Nerve endings can be classified as encapsulated or nonencapsulated, and by their adaptation times. Slowly adapting receptors change little in response to a stimulus, whereas rapidly adapting receptors change a great deal. Mechanoreceptors are the most varied receptors and lie at the interfaces between bones.

Encapsulated Receptors

Pacinian Corpuscles
Pacinian corpuscles are located throughout the body in various areas including the dermis, subcutaneous tissue, joint capsules, pleura, peritoneum, nipples, and external genitalia. They can be further classified into small and large. In joints, small pacinian corpuscles lie in mechanically strained areas such as between the synovial and fibrous layers near the insertion of the capsule. They have thin, gapless perineural capsules. Large pacinian corpuscles lie within the adipose tissue at the surface of the joint capsule. The capsules of large pacinian corpuscles have up to 30 layers of flat perineural cells. One myelinated nerve fiber ends within the capsule of the receptor. These very sensitive receptors are rapidly adapting and perceive rapidly changing mechanical stimuli. A series of impulses from a pacinian corpuscle is interpreted as vibration.

Meissner's Corpuscles
These elongated, encapsulated endings are located in the dermal papillae of hairless skin, just below the epidermis. Flattened Schwann cells are transversely located around the long axis of the corpuscle, which is perpendicular to the skin's surface. A few myelinated fibers innervate the deep end of the corpuscle. The fibers within the corpuscle decrease in size and branch out between the layers of Schwann cells. They are rapidly adapting, and a continuous impulse is interpreted as more than one individual impulse. It is important to note that the number of Meissner's corpuscles significantly decreases throughout an individual's lifetime.

Ruffini Endings
Ruffini endings are located in the dermis, subcutaneous tissues, and connective tissues. In joints, they are located in the fibrous layer and ligaments of the capsule. Large or small Ruffini endings may have one of three capsule variants: no capsule, a capsule with connective tissue, or a gapped, incomplete perineural capsule. Small Ruffini endings are frequently without a perineural capsule, and are difficult to distinguish from unmyelinated fibers. Large Ruffini endings frequently exist in groups of three or more. Ruffini endings are supplied by myelinated afferent nerve fibers, and the axons of these fibers lose their myelin sheath inside. The endings do not respond well to stimuli from the plane of the tissue, but are activated by stimuli applied perpendicularly. The slowly adapting endings respond well when skin is stretched. In the joint, they are responsible for the limits of angular excursion and detect changes in bone position.

Nonencapsulated Endings

Merkel's Endings
Merkel's endings are found in hairless skin. They exist in clusters known as *Merkel's discs*, or tactile domes. They can be classified as disc-shaped expansions of sensory fiber endings, and they lie close to Merkel's cells. Merkel's cells are associated at the synaptic endings of the sensory terminal. Although their specific role is currently unknown, Merkel's cells are thought to transmit information about mechanical stimuli to the nerve endings. Merkel's endings are innervated by a single nerve fiber. They are specialized to perceive sensations of maintained pressure and the degree of pressure being exerted.

Free Nerve Endings

Free nerve endings are the most abundant type of nerve endings. They lie near blood vessels between epithelial layers of the skin, the cornea, the alimentary tract, and in connective tissues. In joints, they are found between the synovial and fibrous layers, and within the fibrous layer itself. They can be myelinated or unmyelinated, although they are most frequently partially ensheathed by Schwann cells. Free nerve endings are formed by branching terminations of sensory fibers in the skin. The endings are slightly thickened. Although mechanoreceptors, thermoreceptors, and nociceptors are all examples of free endings, nociceptors are the most common type.

Nociceptors can be polymodal; that is, they can have more than one adequate stimulus. Most nociceptors respond to heat and cold, mechanical stimuli, and chemicals associated with tissue damage or disease. Polymodal nociceptors are more commonly known as *unmyelinated free nerve endings*. They also may be silent; that is, they are dormant until tissue damage or disease activates their sensitivity.

Muscle Nerve Endings

Muscle Spindles

There are two types of sensory endings in the muscle spindle. *Primary endings* are located at the center of the intrafusal fibers and consist of a single, large nerve fiber that branches out. Because of their appearance, primary nerve endings are also referred to as *annulospiral endings*. *Secondary endings* exist on nuclear chain fibers near the primary endings. They consist of smaller nerve fibers that branch out. The branching pattern of secondary nerve endings is different than that of primary nerve endings. Secondary endings are also known as *flower-spray endings*. Annulospiral and flower-spray endings respond to stretch.

Golgi Tendon Organs

Golgi tendon organs are structurally similar to Ruffini endings. They have a thin capsule, and are surrounded in different directions by collagenous fibers. Golgi tendon organs detect muscle tension. The Golgi tendon organs detect tension from the squeezing of adjacent fibers.

Visceral Nerve Endings

Most visceral receptors are supplied by thinly myelinated fibers. Free nerve endings ramify in tissues of visceral organs in complex patterns. Typically visceral nerve endings consist of either mechanoreceptors (e.g., in the walls of hollow organs), chemoreceptors, or nociceptors. Visceral nociceptors can cause extreme pain when stimulated.

Joint Nerve Endings

As mentioned previously, joints have an abundance of nerve endings. Hinge or condylar joints, for example, have a specifically large amount of endings in the flexion of the capsule. Joint afferents frequently respond in more than one axis of rotation. There are typically three encapsulated types of joint receptors. These resemble pacinian corpuscles, Ruffini endings, and Golgi tendon organs. There is also a nonencapsulated type of nerve ending that is thought to be a nociceptor specific for pain associated with movement. Most joint nerve endings are slowly adapting and detect position and movement. Some, however, are rapidly adapting. Despite the slowly adapting nerve endings that exist in joints, muscle receptors are specifically important in the detection of position and movement. Joint receptors are not as important.

Nerves are composed of neural and connective tissue. In myelinated axons, each nerve fiber is surrounded by the endoneurium. Groups of nerve fibers are enclosed by the perineurium to form fascicles, groups of which are surrounded by the internal and external epineurium.

Nervous System: Consists of two regions—the central nervous system, which includes the brain and spinal cord, and the peripheral nervous system, consisting of nerves made up of neurons that carry information to and from the central nervous system. Most nerves connect to the central nervous system through the spinal cord, with the exception of the 12 cranial nerves.

Clinical Importance: Damage to nerves can be caused by physical injury, swelling (e.g., carpal tunnel syndrome), autoimmune diseases (e.g., Guillain-Barré syndrome), infection (neuritis), diabetes, or failure of the blood vessels surrounding the nerve. Pinched nerves occur when pressure is placed on a nerve, usually from swelling due to an injury or pregnancy. This is accompanied by pain, numbness, weakness, or paralysis. These symptoms may be felt in areas far from the actual site of damage, because signaling is defective from all parts of the area where the nerve receives input, not just the site of the damage.

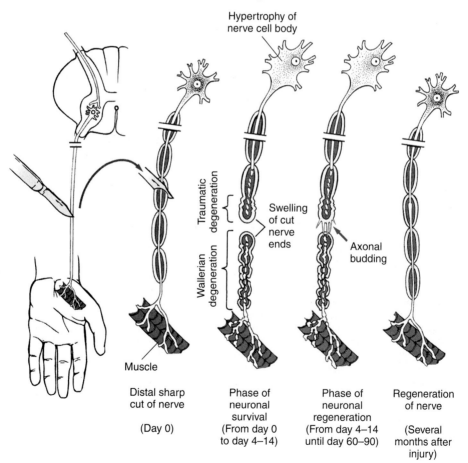

Fig. 154-1   Physiologic changes in regeneration of peripheral motor nerve axon after division with sharp object. *(From Canale ST, Beaty JH [eds]: Campbell's Operative Orthopaedics, 11th ed. Philadelphia, Mosby, 2007.)*

317

Clinical: Injury to motor nerves results in a loss of muscle function, and injury to sensory nerves results in a loss of sensation to the affected nerve's sensory distribution and/or neuromatous or causalgia pain.

Nerve Injury: Injury following bone and joint operations is one of the main causes of iatrogenic peripheral nerve injury. Most nerve injuries are secondary to tension, suture compression, or iatrogenic laceration.

Nerve injury can be associated with fractures and fracture-dislocations. The probability of nerve injury is doubled with fracture associated with shoulder dislocation. Approximately 95% of peripheral nerve injuries associated with a fracture occur in the upper extremity. The most common form is radial nerve injuries associated with humeral fractures. The most common injury resulting from dislocations or fracture-dislocation of the elbow seems to be ulnar nerve neurapraxia, which spontaneously resolves after a closed reduction. Radial nerve palsy after fracture of the humerus is the most common nerve lesion in long bone fractures.

Neural injury is more common with dislocations, which result in stretch injuries to the nerve, occurring in 18% or more of knee dislocations and 13% of posterior hip dislocations. Nerve injury is common in dislocations of the shoulder, with an incidence rate of 48%.

Classification of Nerve Injury: Described by Seddon in 1943, comprising neurapraxia, axonotmesis, and neurotmesis, and by Sunderland in 1951, who expanded this classification system to 5 degrees of increasing severity. Classification is based on the damage sustained by the nerve components, nerve functionality, and the ability for spontaneous recovery.

First-Degree Injury: Neurapraxia or "stretch injuries" involves a reduction or temporary conduction block across a segment of a nerve with axonal continuity conserved. More specifically, it is dysfunction and/or paralysis without loss of nerve sheath continuity and peripheral wallerian degeneration. Nerve conduction is preserved both proximal and distal to the lesion but not across the lesion. Complete recovery occurs within 12 weeks.

Second-Degree Injury: Axonotmesis results from a more severe trauma or compression, causing wallerian degeneration distal to the level of injury and proximal axonal degeneration to at least the next node of Ranvier. The endoneurial tubes remain intact; therefore, recovery is complete with axons reinnervating their original motor and sensory targets.

Third-Degree Injury: Neurotmesis is the most severe grade of peripheral nerve injury. It occurs when the axon, myelin, endoneurial tubes, and connective tissue components are damaged, disrupted, and/or transected, despite the preservation of the perineurium. Recovery through axonal regeneration cannot occur as intraneural fibrosis occurs.

Fourth-Degree Injury: Nerve fasciculi (i.e., axon, endoneurium, perineurium) are damaged but nerve sheath continuity is preserved. However, there is a large area of intraneural scarring at the site of injury, which precludes any axons from advancing distal to the level of nerve injury. There is no improvement in function, so surgery is used to restore neural continuity.

Fifth-Degree Injury: A neurotmesis lesion, where the endoneurium, perineurium, and epineurium, which make up the entire nerve trunk, are completely divided. Substantial perineural hemorrhage and scarring occur. Surgery is required to restore neural continuity.

Diagnostic Tests: Electrodiagnostic tests are useful in detecting nerve injury and/or nerve compression and in identifying early stages of recovery. Electromyography is performed at least 4 weeks following nerve injury, because testing done before that time may yield false-negative findings, because muscle fibrillations are not yet apparent.

Etiology: Anatomic positions of the radial, median, and ulnar nerves, including their branches, predispose them to injury with specific types of fracture. Examples are radial nerve palsies with a Holstein-Lewis distal one third humeral shaft fracture, posterior interosseous nerve injury with a Monteggia fracture-dislocation, ulnar nerve and/or anterior interosseous nerve injuries with elbow dislocations, median nerve and/or radial nerve injuries with supracondylar and medial epicondyle fracture in children, and ulnar nerve injury at the cubital tunnel.

Dysfunction of peripheral nerves results from damage to the neuron, to the Schwann cells, or to the myelin sheath. Damaged nerves cannot transmit impulses in normal fashion. Many mechanisms of injury to peripheral nerves exist, including mechanical, crush and percussion, blunt or penetrating trauma, traction, and frostbite.

Surgery: A direct repair is performed in lacerations with clean sharp injuries to the nerve. In more crushing or avulsion injuries, the nerve ends are reapproximated so that motor and sensory topography can be aligned. In the vast majority of gunshot wounds, the nerve is not divided and therefore has good potential for neurologic recovery.

Nerve Repair: Reconstruction of nerve continuity can be performed with direct repair, wherein the two ends of the nerve are directly coapted. The repair is executed without tension; otherwise, nerve grafting should be done. If the adjacent joint must be flexed or extended to permit coaptation of the distal and proximal ends of the nerve, a nerve graft should be used.

Nerve Graft: Recommended in cases in which a gap is present between the proximal and distal end of the nerve. When a large nerve gap is present, the sural nerve is used due to the large length of nerve graft material that can be obtained. For shorter nerve gaps, the anterior branch of the medial antebrachial cutaneous nerve is used because the donor site scar is minimal and the resultant sensory loss is on the anterior aspect of the forearm.

Nerve Transfer: The concept of a nerve-to-nerve transfer permits a normal, neighboring, noncritical nerve to be coapted to the distal end of the injured nerve. This is particularly useful when a large nerve gap is present and/or for proximal nerve injuries.

Complications: Following acute nerve injury, various pain syndromes can develop. Partial nerve injuries of mixed motor and sensory function can lead to causalgia. Paralysis can complicate nerve injury and at times cannot be repaired. If physical therapy is not started promptly after surgery, denervation can develop, resulting in muscle atrophy and fibrosis, joint stiffness, motor end plate atrophy, and trophic skin changes. There is also the risk of downgrading function by further injuring the nerve, particularly in mixed nerve injuries.

Outcome and Prognosis: With restoration of nerve continuity, axons may regenerate and thus reinnervate the motor end plates and sensory receptors. The outcome and prognosis vary among the different types of injuries and the type and timing of therapy. In traumatic hip dislocations and fracture dislocations, at least partial return of nerve function is expected in 60% to 70% of patients. Surgical delays in excess of 5 months dramatically decrease the rate of functional return. Neuropraxic injuries usually are reversible, and patients recover within days to weeks. In axonotmesis, axons regenerate and recovery usually occurs over months. In neurotmesis, regeneration occurs but function rarely returns to normal. Intraoperative care with proper axial orientation of fascicles, proper coaptation, suture material, hemostasis, and suture line tension leads to better outcomes. Neural injuries associated with fractures have a greater than 80% incidence rate of spontaneous resolution. Recovery is less common with neural injuries secondary to dislocations.

Definition: A group of disorders characterized by an autosomal dominant pattern of inheritance and by disordered growth of ectodermal tissues, and which is part of a group of disorders called *phakomatoses* (neurocutaneous syndrome). There are two distinct clinical types: neurofibromatosis 1 (NF1), which accounts for approximately 95% of cases, and neurofibromatosis 2 (NF2).

Neurofibromatosis 1 (von Recklinghausen's disease): Characterized by pigmented skin patches (café au lait spots) and subcutaneous neurofibromas combined with peripheral nerve tumors and a variety of others dysplastic abnormalities of the skin, most notably in tissue derived from the embryonic neural crest, nervous system, bones, endocrine organs, and blood vessels. Tumors may occur in the spinal canal, where they may press on the spinal cord. They sometimes become malignant, giving rise to neurofibrosarcomas.

Neurofibromatosis 2: Characterized by bilateral acoustic neuromas (vestibular schwannoma or neurofibroma), other central nervous system tumors, juvenile posterior subcapsular cataract, and other benign intracranial tumors including meningiomas, ependymomas, spinal neurofibromas, and gliomas.

Epidemiology and Incidence: Both types of neurofibromatosis are relatively rare.

NF1: 1 in 4000 births. It is inherited as an autosomal dominant trait, but about 50% of cases arise as mutations.

NF2: 1 in 40,000 live births.

Age: Lifelong condition. The café au lait spots are usually present at birth, whereas the subcutaneous neurofibromas and Lisch nodules start to develop in childhood or early adolescence. NF2 usually manifests clinically in the first or second decade of life.

Gender: Both genders are equally affected.

Pathology: The peripheral nerve tumors are of two types—schwannomas and neurofibromas. Both types of tumors occasionally become malignant.

Etiology and Genetics: Neurofibromatosis is an autosomal dominant, genetically transmitted condition. The *NF1* gene is large, and many different mutations occur. In NF1, there is mutation of the tumor suppressor genes located on the long arm of human chromosome 17 in the region 17q11.2, whereas in *NF2*, the mutation is on chromosome 22 in the region 22q12. In NF1, neurofibromin is the defective gene product and in NF2 schwannomin is the defective gene product.

Associated Disorders: Fibrous dysplasia, acoustic neuroma, cranial nerve neoplasms, such as optic nerve gliomas, pheochromocytomas, astrocytomas, glioblastomas, and meningiomas. There is also an association of vascular stenoses (renal, cerebral or pulmonic) and NF1.

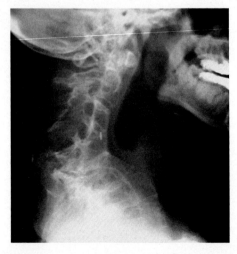

Fig. 155-1 Cervical spine deformity in a patient with neurofibromatosis. *(From Canale ST, Beaty JH [eds]: Campbell's Operative Orthopaedics, 11th ed. Philadelphia, Mosby, 2007.)*

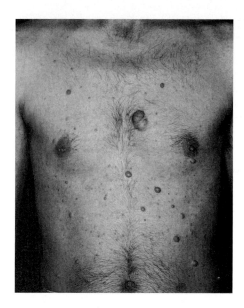

Fig. 155-2 Von Recklinghausen's neurofibroma-
tosis. Adult patient with hundreds of neurofibromas.
*(From Habif TP: Clinical Dermatology, 4th ed.
Philadelphia, Mosby, 2004.)*

Symptoms and Clinical Manifestations in NF1: The pigmented spots are irregular in shape
with relatively even borders, vary in size, are of brownish coffee color (café au lait) and are most
prominent over the trunk. There is freckling in the axilla or groin (Crowe's sign) and multiple
flesh-colored skin lesions that appear in early adolescence. The tumors are usually multiple and
vary in size from minute lesions to large tumors. The majority are smoothly rounded or lobulated,
and can sometimes be seen or felt along the course of peripheral nerves. Often they sink into the
subcutaneous fat on gentle pressure. Subcutaneous swellings appear in early adolescence. These
can be in the form of subcutaneous neurofibromas (firm nodules arising from the peripheral
nerves) and plexiform neurofibromas (lesions involving the skin and the subcutaneous tissues).
These may grow a lot, leading to grotesque overgrowth of soft tissue and bone in a limb or around
the orbit. It usually affects the face, scalp, neck, and chest, and the number of lesions increases
with age. Tumors of the spinal nerve roots may compress the spinal cord and at the same time
extend though the intervertebral foramen to form a large mass in the posterior mediastinum
(dumbbell tumors). Stenosis of the aqueduct of Sylvius with obstructive hydrocephalus is at times
observed. Lisch nodules (melanocytic hamartomas of the iris) can be seen as whitish, yellow, or
brown spots in individuals with light-colored irises.
Symptoms and Clinical Manifestations in NF2: Minimal cutaneous manifestations, no
skeletal malformations, deafness.
Focal Neurologic Signs: Both types of neurofibromatosis are associated with intracranial and
intraspinal neoplasms. The patients may therefore present with signs and symptoms of spinal
cord compression, cauda equina syndrome, increased intracranial pressure, or any other
manifestation of a central nervous system neoplasm. Scoliosis is seen in up to 50% of patients.
Learning disability and a low IQ are present in some patients.
Diagnostic Studies: Plain x-rays of the skull and long bones may reveal bony changes
associated with NF. Chest x-ray checks for appearance of honeycomb lung. Computed tomography
scan or magnetic resonance imaging of the brain, spine, and internal acoustic meatus may be
needed if signs and symptoms are suggestive of central nervous system lesions or acoustic
neuroma. Excisional biopsy of subcutaneous nodule, slit-lamp examination of the iris,
electroencephalogram, and IQ tests are also used.

Treatment: There is no specific treatment and no "cure" for neurofibromatosis.

Surgery: To confirm the nature of a subcutaneous nodule, for cosmetic reasons, to excise a trouble-some peripheral lesion, or to excise or debulk an intracranial or intraspinal lesion.

Medications: Used for neuropathic pain. Most of these are anticonvulsants (usually phenytoin, carbamazepine, and gabapentin), but pure analgesics can be used on an occasional basis.

Radiation Therapy: To treat associated intracranial lesions that are unsuitable for surgical excision.

Chemotherapy: For associated neoplasms that are not suitable for surgical excision.

Radiotherapy: A combination of carboplatin and vincristine.

Definition: Severe, progressive arthropathy associated with nerve damage to a joint. Disease process involves injury to the joint (often unrecognized by patient), repetitive stress, hyperemia, bone fragmentation, and joint subluxation. This process eventually results in the progressive destruction of bone and soft tissues around the joint. Weight-bearing joints are most often involved, usually the feet, ankles, knees, and hips.

Etiology: Any condition that causes a sensory or autonomic neuropathy can lead to a Charcot joint, including diabetes, syphilis, syringomyelia, chronic alcoholism, spinal cord injury, Charcot-Marie-Tooth disease, and congenital insensitivity to pain. Diabetes is considered to be the most common cause.

Incidence: Among diabetics: 0.1% to 6.8%; tabes dorsalis: 5% to 10%; syringomyelia, 20% to 40%

Age: Among diabetics: ages 40 to 59 most often affected; secondary to tabes dorsalis, most patients older than age 60; rare in children.

Race: Complications (including amputation) are more prevalent among African Americans, Mexican Americans, and Asian Americans.

Signs and Symptoms: Charcot arthropathy almost always manifests with signs of inflammation. Profound unilateral swelling, an increase in local skin temperature, erythema, joint effusion, and bone resorption in an insensate foot are usually present. Neurologic signs include decreased vibratory sense, absence of deep pain sensation, and decreased proprioception. Pain can be present in more than 75% of patients; however, the severity of pain is significantly less than would be expected. Instability and loss of joint function also may be present. Approximately 40% of patients also have concomitant ulceration, thereby complicating the diagnosis and raising concern for osteomyelitis.

Differential: Osteomyelitis, infectious arthritis, acute gout, cellulitis, deep venous thrombosis.

Workup: X-ray study establishes the diagnosis in most cases, which may show varying degrees of bone destruction, fragmentation, and subluxation. Aspiration of joint fluid rules out infection, as does obtaining a complete blood count. Magnetic resonance imaging or a technetium bone scan rules out osteomyelitis. A blunt sterile bone probe evaluates for possible osteomyelitis.

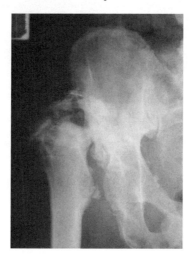

Fig. 156-1   Neuropathic arthropathy of the right hip. There are destruction and fragmentation of the right femoral head leading to bony dislocation and disorganization of the joint. The underlying cause in this patient was syphilis. *(From Adam A, et al: Grainger & Allison's Diagnostic Radiology, 5th ed. Churchill Livingstone, 2008.)*

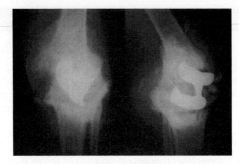

Fig. 156-2 Fourteen years after total knee arthroplasty, radiographs show almost vertical rotation of femoral component and complete destruction of polyethylene tibial component. (Courtesy of Andrew H. Crenshaw, Jr., MD.) *(From Canale ST & Beaty JH: Campbell's Operative Orthopaedics, 11th ed. Mosby, 2007.)*

Treatment: The current mainstay of therapy is immobilization and non–weight bearing on the affected extremity, along with management of the underlying neurologic disorder. Bracing or casting is usually the first choice for most Charcot joints. If the foot is affected, a total contact cast is often used for 3 to 6 months. Surgery may be needed in cases of advanced joint destruction. Surgical means include osteotomies, arthrodesis, open reduction and internal fixation, and amputation. The key to treatment is prevention, because early diagnosis and treatment help minimize joint destruction.

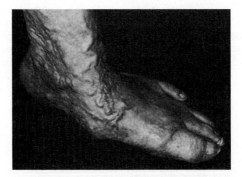

Fig. 156-3 Feet show most severe complications of diabetes—dry, scaly skin; swelling; and venous shunting from autosympathectomy. Fifth toe is dislocated at metatarsophalangeal joint. Great toe is clawed secondary to intrinsic muscle paralysis. *(From Canale ST & Beaty JH: Campbell's Operative Orthopaedics, 11th ed. Mosby, 2007.)*

Nonsteroidal Anti-Inflammatory Drugs (NSAIDs): Inhibit cyclooxygenase. One of the two major enzymes responsible for the conversion of arachidonic acid to inflammatory mediators. NSAIDs decrease the breakdown of the blood–aqueous barrier and reduce the formation of aqueous humor proteins and prostaglandin 2.

In addition to reducing the fever and pain of inflammation, NSAIDs also inhibit clotting. They do this by interfering with the synthesis of thromboxane A2 in platelets.

The use of NSAIDs is often responsible for gastrointestinal ulceration and serious complications such as perforation and bleeding. It is estimated that in the United States 16,500 NSAID-related deaths occur yearly because of gastrointestinal complications. Symptoms include gastrointestinal upset, sometimes requiring treatment with an H2 blocker or a proton pump inhibitor. This side effect arises from the fact that NSAIDs are unselective cyclooxygenase inhibitors, blocking both COX-1 and -2 isoenzymes. COX-1 effects lead to a decrease in epithelial mucus production, bicarbonate secretion, mucosal blood flow, and epithelial proliferation and therefore leave the gastrointestinal tract vulnerable.

Prostaglandins: Derived from arachidonic acid via the cyclooxygenase pathway, are important mediators in gastroprotection, platelet function, and renal function. They also modulate immune function via the lymphocyte. They are mediators of the vascular phases of inflammation and are potent vasodilators. They increase vascular permeability.

Arachidonic Acid Pathway: Constitutes one of the main mechanisms for the production of pain and inflammation, as well as controlling homeostatic function.

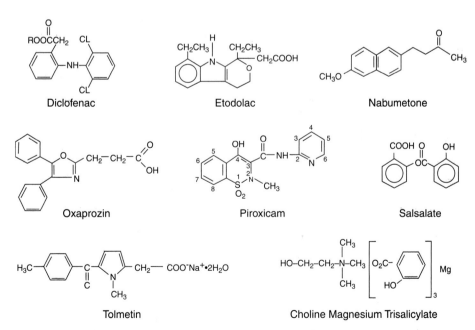

Fig. 157-1 Structures of several different NSAIDs, revealing the wide variation in chemical structures of the compounds that are grouped into this one therapeutic class. *(From Benzon HT, et al: Raj's Practical Management of Pain, 4th ed. Philadelphia, Mosby, 2008.)*

Sir John Vane first proposed that the major therapeutic action of aspirin and other NSAIDs was from the inhibition of the enzyme cyclooxygenase. The anti-inflammatory potencies of the different NSAIDs were proportional to their action as cyclooxygenase inhibitors. It was also shown that cyclooxygenase inhibition produced toxic side effects. NSAIDs cause erosive gastritis from the effects of reduction of PGE2 in the gastric mucosa. The renal toxicity is also related to the action of cyclooxygenase inhibition.

The leukotrienes catalyze the addition of molecular oxygen to specific double bonds in polyunsaturated fatty acids. The most important lipoxygenases are the 5-lipoxygenases. Products of the 5-lipoxygenase pathway are important mediators of inflammation. They cause vasoconstriction but increase microvascular permeability. They are important mediators of bronchial asthma. They cause leukocyte adherence to the vascular endothelium and activate the leukocytes to secrete their enzymes. They contract smooth muscle in the bronchi and blood vessels.

Polyunsaturated fatty acids, such as omega-3 fatty acids, compete with linoleic acid in the arachidonic acid pathway, thereby reducing the metabolism of arachidonic acid to prostaglandin E2 and thromboxane A2, which are both important in mediating inflammation.

Definition: A disorder resulting in separation of the odontoid process from the axis body. First described in 1863 (postmortem specimen) and called os odontoideum in 1886 by Giacomini.
Orthotopic: Os odontoideum results in the dens being positioned anatomically.
Dystopic: Os odontoideum results in the dens being in any nonanatomic position.

Etiology: Initially thought of as being a congenital failure of fusion; more likely etiology is trauma resulting in the fracture of a developing odontoid synchondrosis before its closure. The free dens are carried away from the axis by the alar ligaments while development continues. In the case of congenital fusion failure, this is called *ossiculum terminale*.

Incidence: Rare, but exact frequency is unknown. Cases usually identified when patient becomes symptomatic. Increased in patients with Morquio's syndrome, epiphyseal dysplasia, or Down syndrome.

Age: Birth to 6 years (then synchondrosis should be closed). Pain and neurologic symptoms can occur from the second decade to the end of the fifth decade.

Gender: Unknown.

Signs and Symptoms: Largely asymptomatic and discovered incidentally by radiography. Local neck pain, neck instability, neurovascular (vertebral artery compression), and neurologic symptoms (myelopathy with weakness and ataxia) are thought to be associated with dystopic os odontoideum and less with the orthotopic version.

Clinical Findings: No specific findings. Upper spinal cord and brainstem examinations are mandatory during a careful neurologic examination. Gait evaluation and Romberg testing can identify os odontoideum. Unusual bony projection on the dens anterior surface, C1-2 instability, spinal cord compression, soft tissue masses, vertebral artery compromise, as well as spinal canal diameter and associated osseous anomalies.

Medical Treatment: None if asymptomatic; supportive if axial neck pain alone; traction; physical therapy with cervical collar; nonsteroidal anti-inflammatory drugs for flare-ups.

Surgical Treatment: Rare for axial neck pain alone; usually for significant motion on plain radiograph, neurovascular or neurologic involvement, and/or persistent disability despite proper nonoperative management. Stabilization in children is recommended until beyond 6 to 7 years of age.

Indications for Surgical Fusion: Posteroanterior dens–C1 ring interval (PADI) less than 13 mm; sagittal translation of C1 on C2 during flexion-extension views of greater than 5 mm; rotational instability greater than 20 degrees.

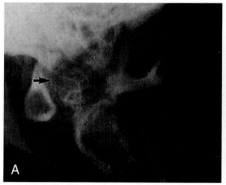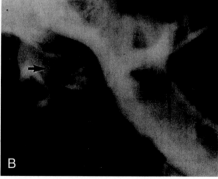

Fig. 158-1 Os odontoideum (os mobile) (*arrows*) and atlanto-axial instability: cervical myelogram, lateral projections. There was no history of trauma. The pattern of instability, with posterior atlanto-axial subluxation in extension (**B**), reduced in flexion (**A**), is common. *(From Adam A, et al: Grainger & Allison's Diagnostic Radiology, 5th ed. Philadelphia, Churchill Livingstone, 2008.)*

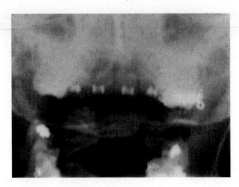

Fig. 158-2 Open-mouth odontoid radiograph. *(From Canale ST, Beaty JH [eds]: Campbell's Operative Orthopaedics, 11th ed. Philadelphia, Mosby, 2007.)*

Procedure: Posterior C1-C2 fusion, Magerl transarticular screws or wiring, or excision of fragment (and stabilization). Surgical procedures are often followed by halo immobilization if not rigid. Posterior C1–ring deficits are commonly seen, limiting surgical options. Reduction should be obtained, and if impossible, occipitocervical fusion might be necessary.

Studies: X-ray, computed tomography, and magnetic resonance imaging.

Sequelae: Transient neurologic signs resolve usually quickly, and most patients with myelopathy do not experience neurologic deterioration after surgical stabilization; however, large series are not available for review.

Complications: Complications from nonoperative management include neurologic deterioration due to progressive instability. Surgical complications include progressive neurologic deficit during reduction maneuvers or when attempted fusion results in pseudarthrosis. Vascular injuries due to hardware placement are rare. A higher risk for adverse events is present in highly unstable and fixed dislocations, in cases of ongoing cord compression, or in inherited ligamentous laxity. Generally, patients with instability fare well after surgery.

Incidence: It is estimated that about 85% of individuals older than 65 years will show radiographic evidence of osteoarthritis (OA).

Age: Alterations in collagen and proteoglycans that decrease the tensile strength of the joint cartilage are thought to describe the dramatic increase in OA after 50 years.

Race: Some variation exists between the races; Native Americans have been reported to be afflicted with this disorder more commonly than the general population. In people older than 65 years of age, OA is more common in whites than African Americans.

Gender: In people older than 55 years of age, OA occurs more often among women than men; in people younger than 45 years of age, however, OA occurs more often among men.

Pathogenesis: OA typically develops slowly and progresses over several years. Usually, the pain slowly worsens over time, but it may stabilize in some patients. In OA, the normal cartilage remodeling process is altered. Chondrocytes release abnormal amounts of catabolic enzymes, which degrade the matrix molecules (proteoglycan, type II collagen, elastin, and fibronectin). The newly formed proteoglycan aggregate is smaller and may not aggregate. Loss of cartilage results in the loss of joint space. Cystic degeneration can also be caused from trauma due to either osseous necrosis secondary to chronic impaction or the intrusion of synovial fluid.

Signs and Symptoms: Decreased range of motion, crepitus, stiffness, and pain. Joint malalignment may also be clinically visible.

Diagnostic Studies: C-reactive protein, erythrocyte sedimentation rate, complete blood count are usually normal; radiographic findings may be normal in the early stages of the disease because cartilage is not directly visualized. Eventually, cartilage loss manifests as joint space narrowing. Subchondral bony sclerosis, subchondral cysts, osteophytes, and erosions may or may not be seen on x-ray. Weight bearing radiographs are preferred for evaluation of the osteoarthritic knee to depict deformities, as well as to provide an accurate assessment of joint space narrowing. Magnetic resonance imaging can also illustrate findings from x-rays; however, they remain cost prohibitive as a primary study. Computed tomography and ultrasonography play a minor role, while scintigraphic studies are of limited use for the diagnosis of osteoarthritis because an increased uptake of the radiotracer can also be seen in several other hypervascular articular diseases.

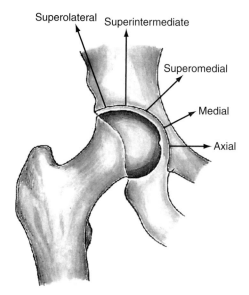

Fig. 159-1   Patterns of osteoarthritis (OA) of the hip. *(From Harris ED Jr: Kelley's Textbook of Rheumatology, 7th ed. Philadelphia, Saunders, 2005.)*

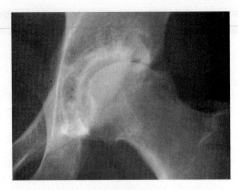

Fig. 159-2 Osteoarthritis. There is an acetabular subchondral cyst, and subchondral sclerosis is maximal on the acetabular side of the joint in this individual. Marginal osteophytes are seen medially and laterally. *(From Adam A, et al: Grainger & Allison's Diagnostic Radiology, 5th ed. Philadelphia, Churchill Livingstone, 2008.)*

Medical Treatment: Analgesics, anti-inflammatories, supplements (glucosamine, hyaluronic acid, chondroitin), corticosteroid injections (no more than every 3 months).

Surgical Treatment: Final treatment when all else fails and when the patient cannot tolerate pain or dysfunction any longer. Osteotomy, débridement, arthrodesis, arthroscopy, and finally total joint arthroplasty comprise current treatment modalities.

Definition: Generally known as bone-forming cells.

Cell Lineage: Mesenchymal cell line → Preosteoblasts → (Signals include bone morphogenetic proteins, multiple growth factors) Osteoblasts.

Function: Make *osteoid*, a precursor to bone made mostly of collagen type 1. They are polarized and aligned linearly on previously formed bone.

Bone Apposition: Osteoid is secreted between the cell and formed bone. Calcium salts are deposited. Communication with osteocytes by rank ligand.

Alkaline Phosphatase: Secreted by osteoblasts. Thought to play a role in mineralization of osteoid. Levels increased during bone formation (fracture, tumor), and is a clinical marker for bone activity.

Osteoblastic Cells. May circulate in serum during bone formation.

Osteocytes: Osteoblast surrounded by matrix. The new function is maintenance of the metabolic environment of the matrix rather than osteoid formation. Osteocytes reside in lacunae, communicating with other osteocytes via canaliculi by gap junctions.

Parathyroid Hormone: Stimulates calcium and phosphate release to serum. PTH receptors on osteoblasts not osteoclasts. Osteoblasts signal osteoclasts, which lead to increased bone resorption and mobilization of calcium and phosphate.

Estrogen: Estrogen receptors on osteoblasts. Clinically important in osteoporosis in postmenopausal women.

Nonsteroidal Anti-inflammatory Drugs: Suppress proliferation and induce cell death in vitro. Can cause poor bone healing postoperatively in vivo.

Osteoporosis: Abnormal bone remodeling. Osteoclasts remove more than osteoblasts create.

Osteomalacia: Normal osteoid, abnormal mineralization.

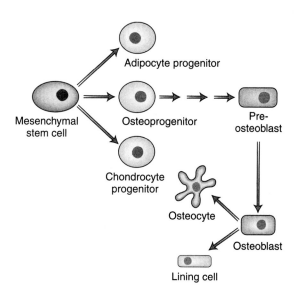

Fig. 160-1   Osteoblast lineage. All precursors of osteoblasts can proliferate; osteoblasts are transformed to osteocytes and lining cells without further proliferation. Some data suggest that lining cells might revert to osteoblast function after parathyroid hormone stimulation. At each stage in the lineage, apoptotic cell death is probably an alternative fate. *(From Kronenberg HM, et al: Williams Textbook of Endocrinology, 11th ed. Philadelphia, Saunders, 2008.)*

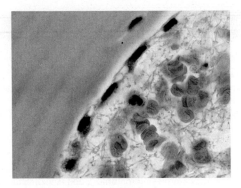

Fig. 160-2   Osteoblast. Frequently found in pediatric patients, osteoblasts line the bone trabeculae. In smears they appear as cells with eccentrically placed nuclei, resembling plasma cells, but the cytoplasmic clearing is more centrally located and not in the Golgi area like in plasma cells (×1000). *(From McPherson RA, Pincus MR: Henry's Clinical Diagnosis and Management by Laboratory Methods, 21st ed. Philadelphia, Saunders, 2006.)*

Definition: Localized injury or condition affecting an articular surface that involves separation of a segment of cartilage and subchondral bone. Lesions are found primarily in the ankle, knee, and elbow joints.

Etiology: Lesions described as osteochondritis dissecans (OCD) can be caused by several factors. Various theories about its etiology have been proposed, but none has been universally accepted. However, the essential mechanisms responsible for OCD are thought to be divided into constitutional or hereditary, vascular, and traumatic.

Associations: An association of OCD has been found with a variety of inherited conditions, including dwarfism, tibia vara, Legg-Calvé-Perthes disease, and Stickler's syndrome. The classic OCD lesion is found on the lateral aspect of the medial femoral condyle.

Incidence: OCD of the knee has been estimated at between 0.02% and 0.03% based on a survey of knee radiographs, and at 1.2%, based on knee arthroscopy.

Age and Gender: The highest rates appear among patients between 10 and 15 years of age. Male-to-female ratio historically is approximately 2:1. Bilateral lesions, typically in different phases of development, are reported in between 15% and 30% of cases. Various classification schemes have been proposed, based on location of the lesion, age of the patient, and description of the lesion. Skeletal age at onset of symptoms appears to be the most important determinant of prognosis and remains an essential factor, directing the timing and nature of treatment.

Clinical Findings: Insidious onset of pain. Anecdotal but consistent reports suggest an association between periods of increased activity and episodes of swelling and effusion.

Symptoms: Pain, swelling, and effusion generalized to the affected joint are hallmark complaints of OCD. In patients with more advanced OCD lesions, persistent swelling and effusion may be accompanied by catching, locking, or giving way. In late stage disease, the sensation of a loose body is often described.

Signs: Physical examination may reveal crepitus and tenderness of the affected joint. If the lesion is found in the lateral aspect of the medial femoral condyle, the patient may walk with the leg externally rotated in an attempt to avoid impingement of the condyle.

Diagnostic Studies: Characterizing the lesion type and assessing growth plate status typically begins by making standard weight bearing anteroposterior and lateral radiographs of both knees. Magnetic resonance imaging is extremely useful for evaluating the presence and stage of the lesion.

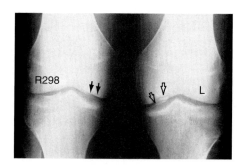

Fig. 161-1 Bilateral, asymmetrical osteochondritis dissecans with a healed right lesion (*small arrows*) and an unhealed, unstable left lesion (*open arrows*) in a 17-year-old tennis player. (*From DeLee D, Drez D [eds]: DeLee and Drez's Orthopaedic Sports Medicine, 2nd ed. Philadelphia, Saunders, 2003.*)

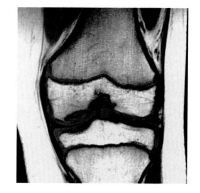

Fig. 161-2 Osteochondritis dissecans. A coronal MRI image of an osteochondritis dissecans (OCD) lesion of the medial femoral condyle. (*From Frontera WR: Clinical Sports Medicine: Medical Management and Rehabilitation. Philadelphia, Saunders, 2006.*)

333

Treatment: OCD in younger patients with open physes may not require surgical treatment and may improve with activity modification. OCD in adults and lesions refractory to conservative care may require surgical intervention. Options include arthroscopic drilling, fixation with Kirschner wires, and special screws for in situ lesions. Incompletely detached lesions usually resolve well with removal of underlying fibrous tissue, some form of chondroplasty, and possibly osteochondral allograft replacement for larger lesions.

Definition: *Osteochondrodysplasia* is a general term for a disorder of the development (dysplasia) of bone ("osteo") and cartilage ("chondro"). Dwarfism is a commonly used term for disproportionately short stature, although a more medically appropriate term for this disorder is *skeletal dysplasia* (osteochondrodysplasia). The four most common skeletal dysplasias are thanatophoric dysplasia, achondroplasia, osteogenesis imperfecta, and achondrogenesis.

Incidence: In the United States, the overall incidence of osteochondrodysplasia is approximately 1 case per 4000 to 5000 births. It has been suggested that the true incidence may be twice as high, because many skeletal dysplasias do not manifest until short stature, joint symptoms, or other complications arise during childhood. Lethal skeletal dysplasias are estimated to occur in 0.95 per 10,000 deliveries.

Age: Osteochondrodysplasias usually are detected in the newborn period or during infancy. Some disorders may not manifest until later in childhood.

Gender: Males are primarily affected in X-linked recessive disorders. X-linked dominant disorders may be lethal in males. Otherwise, males and females usually are affected equally by osteochondrodysplasia.

Etiology and Pathophysiology: Skeletal dysplasia is a heterogeneous group of disorders characterized by abnormalities of cartilage and bone growth. Their modes of inheritance are heterogeneous, that is, autosomal recessive, autosomal dominant, X-linked recessive, or X-linked dominant.

Signs and Symptoms: The distinguishing symptom of osteochondrodysplasia is abnormally and significantly shorter stature with respect to other persons in the same age cohort, and especially in adults who have reached their final heights.

Diagnostic Studies: Unusually short stature for a child's age is usually what brings the child to medical attention. Skeletal dysplasia ("dwarfism") is usually suspected because of obvious physical features (e.g., unusual configuration of face or shape of skull), because of an obviously

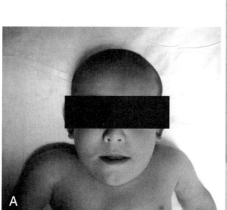
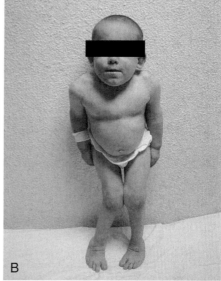

Fig. 162-1   Osteochondrodysplasia. *(From Dormans J: Core Knowledge in Orthopaedics: Pediatric Orthopaedics. St. Louis, Mosby, 2005.)*

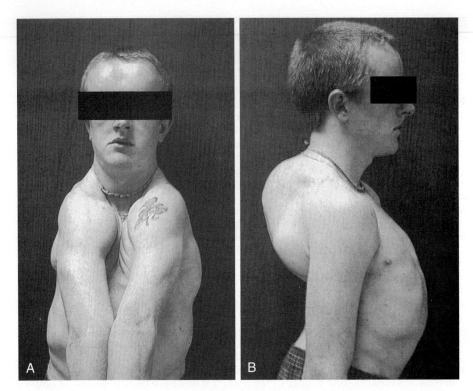

Fig. 162-2 Osteochondrodysplasia. *(From Dormans J: Core Knowledge in Orthopaedics: Pediatric Orthopaedics. St. Louis, Mosby, 2005.)*

affected parent, or because body measurements (arm span, upper to lower segment ratio) indicate disproportion. Bone x-rays are often the key to diagnosis of a specific osteochondrodysplasia, but they are not the key diagnosis. Most children with suspected skeletal dysplasias will be referred to a genetics clinic for diagnostic confirmation and genetic counseling.

Treatment: Treatment of most osteochondrodysplasias arising from genetic defects is limited to palliation of symptoms and side effects; there is no cure. Short stature arising from normal genetic inheritance requires no treatment. The use of growth hormone to increase adult height in children who are short but otherwise normal is sometimes attempted for aesthetic or practical reasons, but remains controversial and risky.

Osteoclast Basics and Histology

Osteoclasts are specialized multinucleated giant cells that resorb bone. This is carried out primarily due to remodeling of extracellular matrix. Osteoclasts are derived from monocyte fusion and have from about 2 to 12 nuclei per cell. They are intimately associated with the surface of bone and use a structure called a *ruffled border* to bind matrix adhesion proteins and produce resorption pits called *Howship's lacunae*. The osteoclast plasma membrane forms a seal with subjacent bone, the Howship's lacunae are acidified, which solubilizes minerals in the ossified tissues, and secreted enzymes dissolve the matrix. Osteoclasts can be differentiated histologically by immunohistochemical stains for tartrate-resistant acid phosphatase.

Cytokine Regulation of Osteoclasts

Numerous cytokines have been shown to regulate osteoclast formation and function; therapies that target these cytokine actions could be used in the future to reduce the effects of inflammatory diseases on bone.

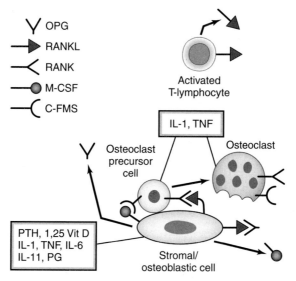

Fig. 163-1 Osteoclast formation. Osteoclasts form from osteoclast precursor cells, which are derived from hematopoietic lineage cells. These express C-FMS (the receptor for M-CSF) and RANK and attach to stromal/osteoblastic cells, which express M-CSF (both membrane-bound and soluble), membrane-bound RANKL, and OPG under the influence of stimulators of resorption (PTH, 1,25-Vit D, IL-1, TNF, IL-6, IL-11, or PGs). If stromal or osteoblastic cells produce more RANKL than OPG, osteoclasts are formed and activated, which increases bone resorption. If stromal or osteoblastic cells produce more OPG than RANKL, OPG binds the available RANKL and new osteoclast formation is prevented. During states of inflammation, T lymphocytes are activated and produce both membrane-bound and soluble RANKL, which can, in turn, stimulate osteoclast-mediated bone resorption. It has also been shown that IL-1 and TNF can augment the effects of RANKL and M-CSF on osteoclast formation and bone resorption by directly stimulating osteoclast precursor cells and mature osteoclasts. *IL*, Interleukin; *M-CSF*, macrophage colony-stimulating factor; *OPG*, osteoprotegerin; *PG*, prostaglandin; *PTH*, parathyroid hormone; RANK, receptor activator of nuclear factor kB; RANKL; RANK ligand; *TNF*, tumor necrosis factor; *1,25 Vit D*, 1,25-dihydroxyvitamin D. *(From Kronenberg HM, et al: Williams Textbook of Endocrinology, 11th ed. Philadelphia, Saunders, 2008.)*

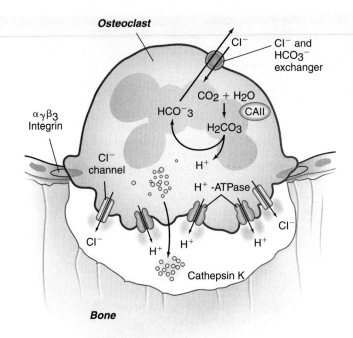

Fig. 163-2 Functional elements of the fully differentiated osteoclast. Osteoclasts attach to bone via podosomes containing $\alpha v \beta 3$ integrin. Protons are generated through the actions of carbonic anhydrase II (CA II), which is transported into the resorption space by the vacuolar-type H^+-ATPase "proton pump." A chloride channel coupled to the proton pump facilitates charge neutrality across the membrane while passive exchange of chloride for bicarbonate in the basolateral membrane removes excess bicarbonate. Cathepsin K is an important enzyme for the removal of the organic components of bone in the acid environment of the resorption space. *(Redrawn from Tolar J, Teitelbaum SL, Orchard PJ. Osteopetrosis. N Engl J Med 2004; 351:2839-2849. From Kronenberg HM, et al: Williams Textbook of Endocrinology, 11th ed. Philadelphia, Saunders, 2008.)*

RANKL, RANK, OPG

Receptor activator of nuclear factor kappa-B ligand (RANKL) is a tumor necrosis factor (TNF) superfamily member that has potent activity as a stimulator of both the formation of osteoclasts from precursor cells and bone-resorbing activity of mature osteoclasts. Marrow stromal and osteoblastic cells produce RANKL, and regulation of its mRNA has been shown to correlate with activation of osteoclastogenesis. Osteoprotegrin (ORG) is a novel cytokine secreted TNF receptor superfamily member and a potent inhibitor of osteoclast formation because of its ability to act as a decoy receptor for RANKL. In murine studies, it has been shown that a lack of OPG resulted in osteoporosis and increased numbers of osteoclasts, while the overexpression of OPG caused osteopetrosis and decreased numbers of osteoclast. The receptor for RANKL is RANK. Like OPG, RANK is a TNF receptor superfamily member present on osteoclast precursor cells and mature osteoclasts.

M-CSF

In addition to RANKL, macrophage colony-stimulating factor (M-CSF) is critical for normal osteoclast formation. M-CSF facilitates the differentiation of osteoclasts from precursor cells and prolongs the survival of mature osteoclasts. M-CSF is a potent stimulator of RANK expression on osteoclast precursor cells.

IL-1

Interleukin-1 is the most potent peptide stimulator of in vitro bone resorption that has been identified. There are two separate interleukin gene products (IL-1 alpha and IL-1 beta), which have identical activities. Its resorption effects are due to direct stimulation of osteoclasts and stimulation of RANKL production.

TNF

TNF also represents a family of two related polypeptides (alpha and beta), which both have similar biologic activities and stimulate bone resorption. In murine models, in vivo administration of TNF-alpha was shown to increase the serum calcium of mice and stimulate new osteoclast formation and bone resorption. The activity of TNF appears to be upstream in the IL-1, M-CSF, and RANK cascade in that its activity has been shown to be stopped in IL-1, M-CSF, and RANK knockout models. TNF can stimulate osteoclastogenesis and osteolysis via activation of IL-1, M-CSF, and RANK, but it has also been shown to directly stimulate osteoclast formation independent of RANK.

IL-6

IL-6 is produced by osteoblasts and bone marrow stromal cells after stimulation by IL-1 and TNF. The function of IL-6 appears to be in the regulation of osteoclast progenitor cell differentiation into mature osteoclasts. It appears to play a role in the increased resorption of bone seen clinically in Paget's disease.

Definition: Osteochondromas (exostoses) are benign cartilage tumors that arise from the surface of either a flat or long bone that usually occur at the metaphyses. The tumor arises from aberrant foci of cartilage on the surface of the bone that acts like a typical physis. As the cartilage cap grows, a bony stalk forms and its growth parallels the growth of the patient. Once the physes are closed, the osteochondroma will also cease to grow. Multiple hereditary exostoses (MHE) is an autosomal dominant form of the disorder in which there are multiple exostoses.

Etiology: A single exostosis may be the result of "ectopic nests" of skeletal dysplasia or neoplastic mutations. Studies of MHE have demonstrated involvement of EXT tumor suppressor gene that results in defects of EXT1 and EXT2. These genes encode glycosyltransferases required for the biosynthesis of heparin sulfate, which is a component of the extracellular matrix.

Associations: Potential for cartilage cap to undergo malignant transformation into chondrosarcoma (~1% of all osteochondromas; 10% of MHE).

Incidence: One third of all benign bone tumors (most frequent). One in 10 of all bone tumors.

Age: Typically 10 to 30 years.

Clinical Findings: Palpable bony protuberance with or without tenderness. Osseous deformity that may limit range of motion, symptomatic bursa formation, vascular injury, neurologic compromise, or malignant transformation. Growth deformities are associated with MHE.

Symptoms: Often asymptomatic, although there may be pain, usually of the overlying soft tissue, which becomes irritated (i.e., pes anserine bursa). *Beware* of new-onset pain in previously asymptomatic patients because this may indicate malignant transformation.

Signs: Palpable bony protuberance with or without tenderness. Rarely, pseudoaneurysm of popliteal artery; neurologic findings consistent with spinal cord or nerve compression.

Diagnostic Studies: Radiographs demonstrate bony protuberances that maintain continuity of medullary space. The cartilage cap itself should be less than 2 cm in thickness. If the cartilage cap is larger or if cartilage type calcification (stipples and rings) greater than 2 cm from the subchondral bone is visible, then malignant change is highly probable. Magnetic resonance imaging is used to evaluate the thickness of the cartilage cap.

Pathology: The microscopic appearance is similar to the normal physeal plate. At the base of the cartilage cap, the chondrocytes are arranged in a linear fashion. Beneath the subchondral bone there is normal fatty and hematopoietic marrow. There is no nuclear atypia and the lesion does not have the lobular pattern of growth seen with chondrosarcomas.

Surgical Care: Patients usually tolerate exostoses well (even with deformity) and do not require surgery. Resection of osteochondromas may be considered for symptomatic patients and is indicated if secondary complications arise (e.g., vascular, neurologic, or malignant transformation).

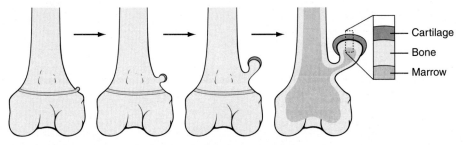

Fig. 164-1 Schematic of the development over time of an osteochondroma, beginning with an outgrowth from the epiphyseal cartilage. (*From Kumar V, et al: Robbins and Cotran Pathologic Basis of Disease, 7th ed. Philadelphia, Saunders, 2005.*)

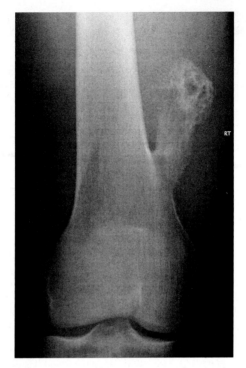

Fig. 164-2 Osteochondroma. AP radiograph showing a typical pedunculated osteochondroma of the distal femur. *(From Adam A, et al: Grainger & Allison's Diagnostic Radiology, 5th ed. Philadelphia, Churchill Livingstone, 2008.)*

Definition: An inherited disorder of the connective tissue (impaired synthesis of type 1 collagen), also known as "brittle-bone disease," in which the bones are unusually brittle and fragile. The tendency to fracture sometimes diminishes at adolescence. There are six types of varying severity, the worst being lethal at birth.

Incidence: In the United States, the prevalence of osteogenesis imperfecta (OI) is estimated to be 1 per 20,000 live births, but the mild form is underdiagnosed so the actual prevalence may be higher. Internationally, prevalences appear to be similar worldwide, although an increased rate has been observed in the southern half of Zimbabwe.

Age: The age when symptoms (i.e., fractures) begin varies widely. Patients with mild forms may not have fractures until adulthood, or they may present with fractures in infancy. Patients with severe cases present with fractures in utero.

Gender: No differences based on gender are reported.

Race: No differences based on race are reported.

Etiology: Osteogenesis is an inherited disorder. In most cases, the mode of inheritance in OI is dominant or involves a new dominant mutation regardless of the clinical form of OI observed. A recessive pattern of inheritance has been demonstrated in some families from South Africa. Some have proposed possible germ-cell mosaicism as an explanation for cases occurring in families with healthy parents that have more than one child with OI.

Pathophysiology: People with OI either have less collagen than normal or the quality is poorer than normal. Because collagen is an important protein in bone structure, this impairment causes those with the condition to have weak or fragile bones.

Signs: In severe cases, prenatal screening sonography performed during the second trimester may show bowing of long bones, fractures, limb shortening, and decreased skull echogenicity. Patients may bruise easily and have repeated fractures after mild trauma. However, these fractures heal readily. In addition, about 50% of type I OI patients have deafness by age 40 years.

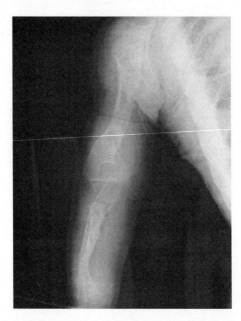

Fig. 165-1   Osteogenesis imperfecta. *(From Dormans J: Core Knowledge in Orthopaedics: Pediatric Orthopaedics. St. Louis, Mosby, 2005.)*

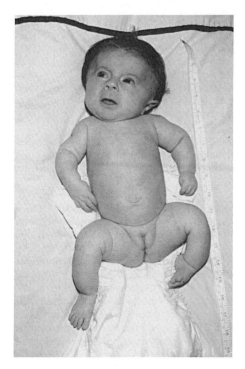

Fig. 165-2   Osteogenesis imperfecta. *(From Behrman R, et al: Nelson Textbook of Pediatrics, 17th ed. Philadelphia, Saunders, 2004.)*

Type I Symptoms: Mild (collagen is of normal quality, but not in sufficient quantity). Over a lifetime, numbers of fractures can range from 1 or 2 to 60. Bones fracture easily, especially before puberty. Bone deformity is absent or minimal. Patients are of near-normal stature, have loose joints and muscle weakness, have a tendency toward spinal curvature, and have a triangular face. Patients usually have blue, purple, or gray tinted sclera; protrusion of the eyes, brittle teeth, and hearing loss beginning in their early 20s or 30s. Types IA and IB are distinguished by the absence or presence of dentinogenesis imperfecta.

Type II Symptoms: Extremely severe (collagen is not of sufficient quality or quantity). Frequently lethal at or shortly after birth. Causes of death include respiratory failure, extreme fragility of the ribs, pulmonary hypoplasia, and malformations or hemorrhages of the central nervous system. All patients have in utero fractures, which may involve the skull, long bones, and/or vertebrae. Patients may have broad/thin and short/longer long bones with/without broad/ thin beaded ribs. In addition, patients may have small stature, limb shortening, progressive deformities, blue sclera, and a small nose and/or micrognathia.

Type III Symptoms: Severe (collagen is sufficient in quantity but not of high quality). Patients may have symptoms already mentioned in types I and II. Other findings may include vertigo, basilar invagination, hypercalcuria, constipation, and hernias; respiratory complications secondary to kyphoscoliosis are common. Type III is distinguished among the other classifications as being the "progressive deforming" type, wherein a neonate presents with mild symptoms at birth and develops the aforementioned symptoms throughout life. Lifespan may be normal, albeit with severe physical handicapping.

Type IV Symptoms: Not clearly defined. Type IV is between types I and III in severity. Fractures usually begin in infancy, but in utero fractures may occur. The long bones are bowed and bone deformity is mild to moderate. Patients may have short stature, spinal curvature, barrel-shaped rib cage, brittle teeth, a triangular face, and early loss of hearing. Sclera are white or near-white. Types IVA and IVB are distinguished by the absence/presence of dentinogenesis imperfecta.

Types V and VI: Patients are clinically within the type IV group, but have a distinct pattern to their bone. There are no data regarding mutations in the type I collagen genes.

Type V Symptoms: Clinically similar to type IV. The bone has a "meshlike" appearance when viewed under the microscope. Type V is further characterized by the V triad, consisting of (1) radio-opaque band adjacent to growth plates, (2) hypertrophic calluses at fracture sites, and (3) calcification of the radioulnar interosseous membrane.

As per Drs. Francis Glorieux and Frank Rauch and Leanne Ward, the Shriners OI type V leads to calcification of the membrane between the radius and ulna, making it difficult to turn the wrist. Another symptom is abnormally large amounts of repair tissue (hyperplasic callus) at the sites of fractures.

Type VI Symptoms: People with this type of OI are moderately to severely affected. The alkaline phosphatase (an enzyme linked to bone formation) activity level is slightly elevated in OI type VI, and this can be determined by a blood test. Because the clinical features are so similar to other moderate forms of OI, a bone biopsy is the only method by which OI type VI can be diagnosed with certainty. The bone from people with this form has a distinctive "fish scale" appearance when viewed under the microscope.

Medical Treatment: Because OI is a genetic condition, it has no cure. Treatments are aimed at increasing overall bone strength to prevent fracture and maintain mobility.

Cyclic administration of intravenous pamidronate reduces the incidence of fracture and increases bone mineral density while reducing pain and increasing energy levels. Doses vary from 4.5 to 9 mg/kg/day depending on the protocol used.

Surgical Treatment: This aims to correct and prevent the deformity resulting from multiple fractures. Surgical interventions include intramedullary rod placement, surgery to manage basilar impression, and correction of scoliosis.

Metal rods can be surgically inserted along the long bones to improve strength; however, this can have the side effect of reduced joint mobility, although not always. In patients with bowed long bones, intramedullary rod placement may improve weight bearing and thus enable the child to walk at an earlier age than he or she might otherwise.

Definition: Osteoid osteoma is a benign bone-forming lesion that occurs most often in the long bones of the lower extremities. They are very small tumors that do not grow larger than half an inch in diameter. They usually emerge sometime during the teenage years or early adulthood. Osteoid osteoma accounts for approximately 10% of benign bone tumors.

Etiology: Unknown; tumoral origin considered to be most likely, some authors postulate viral, immunologic, or inflammatory origin.

Associations: No known associations.

Incidence: The proximal femur is the most common location, followed by the tibia, posterior elements of the spine, and the humerus. Osteoid osteoma is found in the diaphysis or the metaphysis of the proximal end of the bone more often than the distal end.

Age and Gender: The tumor occurs most frequently in the second decade and affects males twice as often as females.

Clinical Findings: Osteoid osteoma has a distinct clinical picture of dull pain that is worse at night and disappears within 20 to 30 minutes of treatment with nonsteroidal anti-inflammatory medication.

Symptoms: Local symptoms can include an increase in skin temperature, increased sweating, and tenderness.

Signs: The signs and symptoms of osteoid osteoma may resemble other medical conditions or problems. Occasionally, children with undiagnosed osteoid osteomas have been thought to have a psychological or psychiatric condition.

Diagnostic Studies: The classic radiologic presentation of an osteoid osteoma is a radiolucent nidus surrounded by a dramatic reactive sclerosis in the cortex of the bone. The lesion can occur only in the cortex, in both the cortex and medulla, or only the medulla. The reactive sclerosis may be present or absent. The four diagnostic features include (1) a sharp, round, or oval lesion that is (2) less than 2 cm in diameter, (3) has a homogeneous dense center, and (4) a 1- to 2-mm peripheral radiolucent zone. Computed tomography is the preferred method of evaluation, especially if the lesion is in the spine or obscured by reactive sclerosis. Magnetic resonance imaging scans are less useful, in that they will show extensive edema, which may be mistaken for a marrow-replacing neoplasm

Pathology: On gross examination, osteoid osteoma is a brownish red, mottled, gritty lesion that is distinct from the surrounding bone. It can be present in the cortex or medullary canal. Osteoclasts are present. The nidus is surrounded by sclerotic bone with thickened trabeculae.

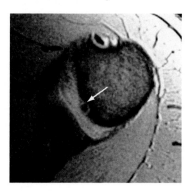

Fig. 166-1 Osteoid osteoma of the proximal humerus. MRI features. Axial T2-weighted gradient-echo MRI shows the nidus in a medial subperiosteal location (*arrow*). (*From Adam A, et al: Grainger & Allison's Diagnostic Radiology, 5th ed. Philadelphia, Churchill Livingstone, 2008.*)

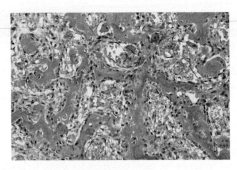

Fig. 166-2 Osteoid osteoma composed of haphazardly interconnecting trabeculae of woven bone that are rimmed by prominent osteoblasts. The intertrabecular spaces are filled by vascular loose connective tissue. *(From Kumar V, et al: Robbins and Cotran Pathologic Basis of Disease, 7th ed. Philadelphia, Saunders, 2005.)*

Microscopically, the nidus consists of a combination of osteoid and woven bone surrounded by osteoblasts. The oval-shaped nidus is well vascularized and clearly separate from the reactive woven or lamellar bone.

Surgical Care: Osteoid osteoma will resolve without treatment in an average of 33 months. If the patient does not wish to endure the pain and prolonged use of nonsteroidal anti-inflammatory medications, surgical removal or percutaneous ablation of the nucleus is indicated. Surgical fixation frequently involves resection from the long bone and posterior fusion of the spine, if the posterior elements are afflicted.

Definition: Osteomyelitis is an acute or chronic inflammatory process of the bone and its structures secondary to infection with pyogenic organisms. Bacterial causes are the most common and may arise from a variety of sources. Depending on the duration, there are both subacute and chronic forms of the disease. The bacterial pathogen varies depending on the patient's age and the mechanism of infection.

Etiology: Osteomyelitis may be the result of hematogenous spread, direct inoculation, trauma, surgical procedures (postoperative infections after open reduction and internal fixation of fractures), or contiguous spread from adjacent infections. In the adult patient, the tibia is the most common site of osteomyelitis. Hematogenous osteomyelitis is uncommon in adults but may occur in intravenous drug abusers. The most common pathogen is *Staphylococcus aureus*; however, a variety of organisms may be involved depending on the clinical setting.

Associations: Sickle cell disease often predisposes to osteomyelitis caused by the bacteria *Salmonella*. In addition, open trauma has been shown to be a significant risk factor for osteomyelitis. Chronic draining sinuses may be complicated by malignant transformation and development of squamous cell carcinoma (Marjolin's ulcer) in approximately 1% of patients.

Incidence: The incidence of osteomyelitis is 2 in 10,000 people.

Age and Gender: In general, osteomyelitis has a bimodal age distribution. Male-to-female ratio is approximately 2:1. Spinal osteomyelitis is more common in persons older than 45 years than in younger persons.

Clinical Findings: Osteomyelitis may manifest with a combination of clinical findings, including pain, erythema, warmth, fluctuance, tenderness to palpation, and draining sinuses.

Signs and Symptoms: Abrupt onset of high temperature (present in only 50% of neonates with osteomyelitis), fatigue, irritability, malaise, restriction of movement (pseudoparalysis of limb in neonates), local edema, erythema, and tenderness.

Diagnostic Studies: Radiographic changes usually reflect the destructive process of osteomyelitis, but lag at least 2 weeks behind the process of infection. Computed tomography can also help identify areas of necrotic bone. One disadvantage of this study is the scatter phenomenon, which occurs when metal is present in or near the area of bone infection and results in a substantial loss of image resolution. Magnetic resonance imaging has been recognized as a useful modality for diagnosing the presence and scope of musculoskeletal infection. Bone scans are also helpful in identifying infected bone.

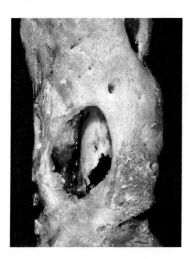

Fig. 167-1 Resected femur in a patient with draining osteomyelitis. The drainage tract in the subperiosteal shell of viable new bone (involucrum) reveals the inner native necrotic cortex (sequestrum). *(From Kumar V, et al: Robbins and Cotran Pathologic Basis of Disease, 7th ed. Philadelphia, Saunders, 2005.)*

347

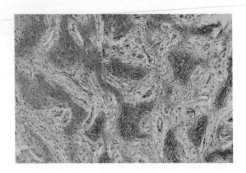

Fig. 167-2 Tissue from the central mandible is minimally inflamed and has a fibro-osseous appearance. *(From Regezi JA, et al: Oral Pathology: Clinical Pathologic Correlations, 5th ed. Philadelphia, Saunders, 2008.)*

Pathology: Culture should be obtained from the affected area and sent for appropriate stains, culture, sensitivity, microscopic evaluation, cell count, and differential. Cultures should be obtained without the presence of antibiotics.

Medical Treatment: Whereas immunocompromised patients may be afflicted by less common organisms such as fungi and mycobacteria, the most common gram-negative organism is *Pseudomonas aeruginosa*, and the most common anaerobe is *Peptostreptococcus* species. Antibiotic treatment should be tailored to specific flora.

Surgical Treatment: The cornerstone of treating osteomyelitis is adequate débridement of necrotic bone, soft tissue, and sinus tracts followed by skeletal stabilization and eradication of the infection. This treatment can then be followed by reconstruction including tissue transfer, bone grafting, or distraction osteogenesis as needed.

Definition: A genetically inherited disorder characterized by excessive bony density and medullary canal occlusion resulting from a failure of bony resorption. First described by German radiologist Albers-Schönberg in 1904.

Etiology: Failure of the osteoclasts to reabsorb bone is the primary cause of osteopetrosis, whereas numerous genetic and molecular defects are posited to affect osteoclastic function.

Incidence: No epidemiologic studies have been conducted; estimated 1 in 100,000 to 500,000; however, true incidence is unknown and as many as 50% of adult types may go undiagnosed.

Associations: Renal tubular acidosis and calcification due to carbonic anhydrase isoenzyme II deficiency. Severe anemia, bleeding, infection.

Age and Gender: Infantile (usually results in mortality by the first decade) and adult onset (described as type I and type II).

Symptoms: Bone pain, pathologic fracture in 40%; however, it is estimated that one half of all patients are asymptomatic.

Signs: Growth retardation, bony defects, and sequelae such as stiffness and neuropathies. Extramedullary hematopoiesis, pancytopenia, and recurrent infections occur with this disorder.

Subtypes: (See Table 168-1)

Pathology: A disorder characterized by a failure of bone to be reabsorbed.

Studies: Serum calcium, parathyroid hormone (elevated), acid phosphatase (increased), creatinine kinase (elevated). Radiologic studies are diagnostic, illustrating osteosclerosis, skull thickening, or possibly osteomyelitis.

Medical Care: Calcitriol (stimulate osteoclasts), erythropoietin (anemia), corticosteroids (bone resorption and anemia), gamma interferon (infection).

Surgical Care: Bone marrow transplantation is the only curative treatment for this disease but the procedure carries inherent risks. Other surgical interventions are warranted to correct for deformity and degenerative joint disease.

Complications: Severe anemia secondary to bone marrow failure as well as bleeding, risk of infection, and growth retardation.

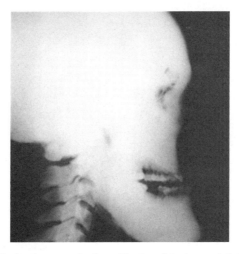

Fig. 168-1 Osteopetrosis showing generalized opacification of the jaws and skull. *(From Regezi JA, et al: Oral Pathology: Clinical Pathologic Correlations, 5th ed. Philadelphia, Saunders, 2008.)*

349

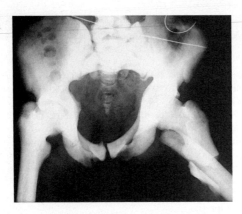

Fig. 168-2 Osteopetrosis. In this disease, also called "marble bone" disease, an abnormality in osteoclast function occurs. As a result, the bones become very dense or white, but they are almost chalklike and fracture easily. The patient broke his femur by just falling out of bed. Differential diagnosis of uniformly increased bony density would include fluorosis and myelofibrosis. *(From Mettler FA, Jr: Essentials of Radiology, 2nd ed. Philadelphia, Saunders, 2005.)*

Table 168-1. SUBTYPES OF OSTEOPETROSIS

Characteristics	Adult (Benign)	Infantile (Severe)	Intermediate
Inheritance	Autosomal dominant	Autosomal recessive	Autosomal recessive
Bone marrow failure	None	Severe	None
Prognosis	Good	Poor	Poor
Diagnosis	Often diagnosed incidentally	Usually diagnosed before age 1 year	

Definition: Osteoporosis is characterized by low bone mass and the structural deterioration of bone tissue, leading to an increased susceptibility to fractures of the hip, spine, and wrist.

Etiology: *Primary osteoporosis* can be divided into three types based on a unique etiology.

Type 1: Postmenopausal osteoporosis is characterized by the disproportionate loss of trabecular bone secondary to estrogen depletion. It is associated with fractures at sites rich in cancellous bone such as the vertebral body and distal radius.

Type 2: Age-associated osteoporosis affects all skeletal sites with both cortical and cancellous bone such as the proximal femur.

Type 3: Idiopathic osteoporosis affects premenopausal women as well as middle-age and young men.

Secondary osteoporosis can be caused by an identifiable agent such as glucocorticoids, or by a disease such as hyperthyroidism, myeloma, and even alcoholism.

Associations: Although there is an association of low body weight and bone mass, low body weight may be an independent risk factor.

Incidence: Twenty-eight million Americans are afflicted with osteoporosis, 80% of whom are women.

Age and Gender: Based on the World Health Organization (WHO) criteria, approximately one third of women older than age 65 years have osteoporosis, while rates for Hispanic and African American women are lower.

Clinical Findings: Patients with decreased bone density usually have no specific abnormal physical findings. Those with vertebral compression fractures will have kyphosis, protruding abdomen, and height loss. Back tenderness is usually only present after an acute fracture. Gait speed and grip strength are often reduced in patients who have or are about to have a hip or distal radius fracture.

Symptoms: Progressive loss of height, pain due to the compression of the spinal nerve, curvature of the spine (kyphosis), digestive, and breathing problems can occur due to the severe curvature of the spine, which starts to reduce the space under the rib cage, and incontinence, which can occur as the internal organs become pressed on the bladder.

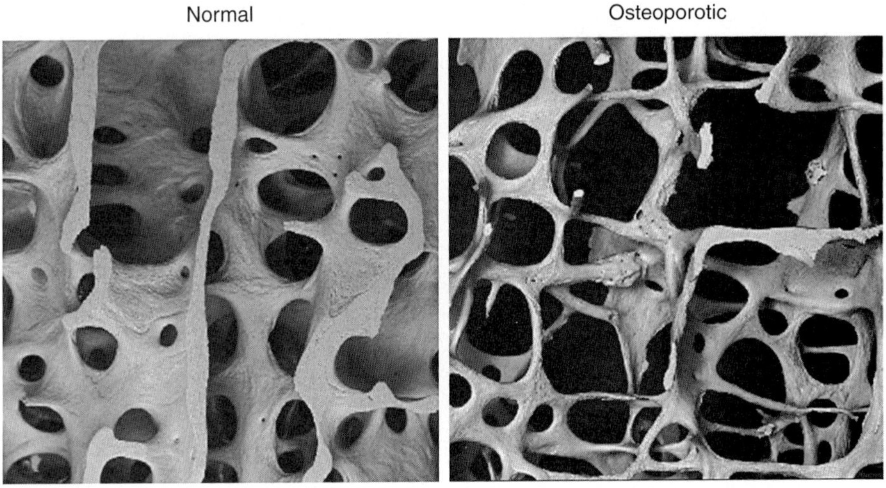

Normal   Osteoporotic

Fig. 169-1 Scanning electron micrographs of a normal vertebra from a 31-year-old man and an osteoporotic vertebra from an 89-year-old woman showing extensive loss of trabecular bone architecture with conversion of plates to rods and a microfracture. *(From Boyd A: Morphologic detail of aging bone in human vertebrae. Endocrine 17:5–14, 2002.)*

351

Signs: There are very few physical warning signs for osteoporosis until the disease has established itself.

Diagnostic Studies: The most commonly used method is dual-energy x-ray absorptiometry (DEXA). This measures the bone density of the hip and spine within a few percent. Urine and blood tests measure various markers of bone resorption (e.g., urinary N-telopeptide crosslinks and pyridinoline) and bone formation (e.g., serum osteocalcin and bone-specific alkaline phosphatase).

Pathology: Histologically, osteoporotic bone is lamellar in character and without osteoid seams, resorption cavities, or osteoblastic and osteoclastic activity.

Medical Treatment: Gonadal hormone replacement, calcitonin, selective estrogen-receptor modulators, and bisphosphonates are pharmacologic agents typically used; however, they predominately reduce bone resorption with little effect on bone remodeling.

Surgical Treatment: The vast majority of compression fractures may be treated nonoperatively with the use of analgesics, orthotic devices, and rest. Recently, kyphoplasty and vertebroplasty have been offered to reduce the pain associated with vertebral compression fractures. In rare cases, unstable fractures do occur in the axial spine requiring surgical fixation, especially when neurologic compromise exists. The major problem in treating these unstable fractures is gaining adequate purchase for implants. The majority of long bone fractures in the elderly are treated by early surgical stabilization with a goal of achieving early weight-bearing status for the lower extremity and rapid restoration of functional capacity in the upper extremity.

Definition: Osteosarcoma is a highly malignant tumor of the bone, which is characterized by the production of neoplastic osteoid (bone tissue).

Etiology: The etiology of osteosarcoma remains obscure; however, several etiologic agents have been associated with the disease. Some agents shown to induce osteosarcomas are radiation, chemicals including beryllium, and viruses. Many osteosarcomas are also found to contain a mutation in the retinoblastoma gene. Additionally, osteosarcoma is described in an osteoblastic, fibroblastic, and chondroblastic forms.

Associations: There is an increased incidence of osteosarcoma in patients with Paget's disease, electrical burns, and trauma and in some hereditary syndromes such as Rothmund-Thomson syndrome, Bloom syndrome, and Li-Fraumeni syndrome.

Incidence: It is the most common primary malignant bone tumor, with an annual incidence reported of 4.6 per million in whites and 5.2 per million in African Americans.

Age: The peak incidence of osteosarcoma is in the second decade of life.

Gender: Osteosarcoma is more common in males than females (1.5:1).

Symptoms: Pain related to strain is the most common symptom and is seen in 85% of patients with osteosarcoma. Unrelenting pain that increases with rest or at night is often considered a symptom of malignant bone tumors but is only seen in 21% of patients with osteosarcoma.

Signs: Palpable painful bone mass or limping in children are common presenting signs of the disease.

Location: Fifty percent of cases arise in the distal femur or the proximal tibia.

Studies: X-ray findings show a destructive lesion predominately osteoblastic with or without an osteolytic component. Poorly defined margins and periosteal reaction are common:

Codman's Triangle: Triangular area of bone seen on roentgenography produced by periosteal elevation.

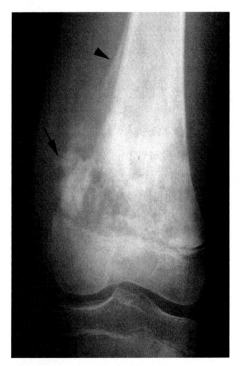

Fig. 170-1 Conventional central osteosarcoma. AP radiograph of the distal femur showing a classic osteosarcoma with mixed lytic and sclerotic areas, tumor bone formation in the extraosseous mass (*arrow*), and a proximal Codman's triangle (*arrowhead*). (*From Adam A, et al: Grainger & Allison's Diagnostic Radiology, 5th ed. Philadelphia, Churchill Livingstone, 2008.*)

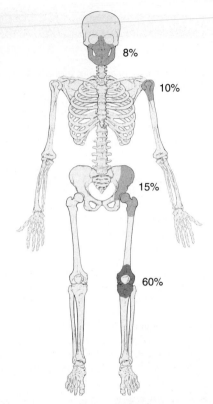

Fig. 170-2   Major sites of origin of osteosarcomas. The numbers are approximate percentages. *(From Kumar V, et al: Robbins and Cotran Pathologic Basis of Disease, 7th ed. Philadelphia, Saunders, 2005.)*

Sun Burst: Reactive ossification of bone spicules perpendicular to long bones. Computed tomography, magnetic resonance imaging, and radionuclide bone scan with Tc 99-methylene diphosphonate are recommended.

Pathology: Histologic examination shows malignant osteoblasts, osteoid, and poorly organized neoplastic bone.

Staging: Histologic grade of the tumor (low grade versus high grade), the anatomic location of the tumor (intracompartmental versus extracompartmental), and the absence or presence of metastatic disease. The staging system is typically depicted as follows:

I-A: Low-grade tumor, intracompartmental
I-B: Low-grade tumor, extracompartmental
II-A: High-grade tumor, intracompartmental
II-B: High-grade tumor, extracompartmental
III: Any tumor with evidence of metastasis

Treatment: Two surgical interventions are performed; biopsy and resection. Surgical extirpation with wide margins and adjuvant chemotherapy are recommended. Limb salvage surgery versus amputation appears to have similar outcomes.

Prognosis: Surgery and adjuvant chemotherapy have shown greater than 60% 5-year survival rates in nonmetastatic osteosarcoma.

Definition:
- Inconsistently present accessory bone posterior to talus, usually asymmetrical
- Round, oval, or triangular; variable size
- Nonunited portion of lateral tubercle
- Arises from separate ossification center posterior to lateral tubercle of posterior talar process

Incidence: Reported to be 1.7% to 7% (Chao, 2004), 2.5% to 14% (wheelessonline.com), or up to 50% of normal feet (Koval, 2002).

Etiology: Forced plantar flexion → impingement of os trigonum vs. posterior tibial plafond. Most commonly seen in ballet (Marotta, 1992); also seen in soccer, running, and other sports.

Acute/Trauma: Fracture; disruption of cartilaginous synchondrosis between talus and os trigonum.

Chronic: Repetitive ossicle impingement.

Metatarsocuneiform Involvement: Os trigonum-talus, may also involve flexor hallucis longus (FHL) tenosynovitis, ankle osteochondritis, subtalar joint disease, and fracture

Age: Related to etiology.

Gender: Related to etiology.

Race: Related to etiology.

Signs and Symptoms:
- Painful plantar flexion, symptoms reproduced with forceful passive plantar flexion
- Associated FHL or posterior tibial tendinitis (posteromedial tenderness) or avulsion fracture

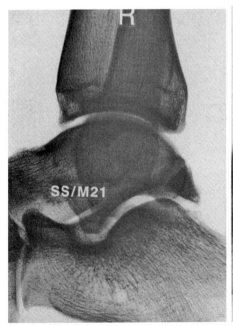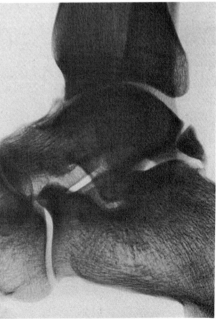

Fig. 171-1 Post-traumatic syndrome of the os trigonum of the right ankle. Plain lateral x-rays (*left*) reveal an undisrupted os trigonum. Additional posteromedial impingement view (PIM) with the foot in 25-degree external rotation in the same patient shows that the os trigonum is disrupted. (*From Porter DA, Schon LC: Baxter's The Foot and Ankle in Sport, 2nd ed. Philadelphia, CV Mosby, 2007.*)

Imaging: Lateral hindfoot x-rays of forced plantar flexion may demonstrate posterior impingement. Magnetic resonance imaging may show bone marrow edema within os trigonum and surrounding fluid.

Treatment:

Conservative: Restricted activity, immobilization, nonsteroidal anti-inflammatory drugs, local steroid injection.

Surgical:

- Excision often improves motion and eliminates pain.
- Posterolateral approach is safer than medial approach; subtalar arthroscopy bears similar results (Abramowitz, 2003).
- Surgery is performed at level of ankle joint, directly posterior to peroneal tendons.
- Consider lateral approach for isolated posterior impingement.
- Identify sural nerve and FHL tunnel to avoid injury and complications.
- Appropriate excision and decompression allow plantar flexion without impingement.

Definition: A disorder of increased bony turnover resulting from enhanced osteoclastic resorption. First described in 1876 by Sir James Paget.

Etiology: Unknown. Leading theories include slow virus, dog distemper virus, and exposure to arsenic. Additionally, human leukocyte antigen (HLA) on chromosome 6 and the gene on chromosome arm 18q may play important roles.

Incidence: Common (1 in 500 persons in the United States). Very common in Anglo-Saxons (Europe, North America, Australia, New Zealand), while rare in Asia, Africa, and Scandinavia.

Age: Most common in older adults, with the majority of cases in persons older than age 60 years. Fewer cases in persons in the 30- to 40-year age range. Rare in patients younger than 25 years.

Gender: Male-to-female ratio 3:2.

Signs and Symptoms: Mostly asymptomatic or discovered incidentally; however, minority of patients experience various symptoms such as bone pain, thickening of the skull, hearing loss, and joint pain with warmth. Bowing and severe deformity can occur (osteitis deformans).

Clinical Findings: Bony deformity (monostotic, 33%; polyostotic, 67%). High output cardiac failure, deafness, fractures, and occasional malignancy. Abnormal mechanical axis may play a role in causing joint overload or impingement. Rarely (1 in 1000) may present with malignancy related pain. Fracture not uncommon.

Staging: Three stages are osteoclastic, osteoblastic, and osteosclerotic distribution. Most cases are polyostotic, while fewer are monostotic.

Micropathology: Bone has trabecular appearance with wide canaliculi.

Medical Treatment: None if asymptomatic. Bisphosphonates, calcitonin, and analgesics are currently used to treat symptoms.

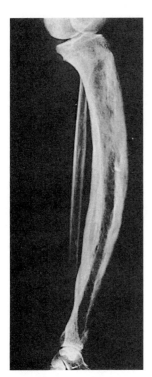

Fig. 172-1 Paget's disease of the tibia. Note the bowing and the marked irregularity of the anterior cortex and the flame-shaped lytic lesion of the posterior cortex. *(Courtesy of Dr. Ethel S. Siris. From Kronenberg HM, et al: Williams Textbook of Endocrinology, 11th ed. Philadelphia, Saunders, 2008.)*

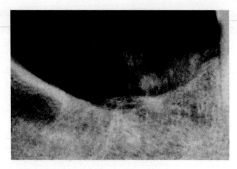

Fig. 172-2 Paget's disease with fibrotic marrow and numerous osteoblasts and osteoclasts. *(From Regezi JA, et al: Oral Pathology: Clinical Pathologic Correlations, 5th ed. Philadelphia, Saunders, 2008.)*

Surgical Treatment: Total joint arthroplasty for those with degenerative joint disease; osteotomy for severe deformity (fracture healing slightly retarded). Excision and adjuvant treatment of malignancy.

Studies: Alkaline phosphatase (increased), urinary hydroxyproline (increased), x-rays. Discrete areas of osteolysis are an early feature as well as osteoporosis circumscripta. In the vascular stage, areas of porosis shaped like a candle flame are seen in the cortex (arrow or flame sign). Also, raised urinary hydroxyproline and alkaline phosphatase are indicators.

Sequelae: Malignancy (Paget's osteosarcoma) most common. The histologic findings differ from classic osteosarcoma. Fibrosarcoma and chondrosarcoma can result in 1% to 6% of cases.

Complications: Metabolic complications such as hypercalciuria and hypercalcemia (both rare) can be seen in patients with severe involvement who are immobilized. High-output cardiac failure has also been described. Hyperparathyroidism, if present, is usually coincidental.

Definition: A low-grade osteosarcoma occurring on the surface of metaphyses of long bones. Classically described on the posterior aspect of the distal femur, as well as the proximal tibia and humerus and arises from the osteoblastic layer of the periosteum. Originally described in 1951 by Geschickter and Copel.

Incidence: Between 3% and 4% of primary bone malignancies.

Age and Gender: Suggested that gender distribution is greater in females than in males, with the peak incidence at 30 to 50 years.

Clinical Findings: Often painless or manifests with pain, swelling, and a palpable mass that may have been present for weeks or months.

Radiologic Findings: No cortical erosion, discrete lesion with mottled calcification. Often a dense, heavily ossified, broad-based mass that appears to encircle the metaphysis is visible.

Differential: Trauma, myositis ossificans, osteochondroma. Differentiate from periosteal osteosarcoma, which tends to be diaphyseal. There is a sunburst sign radiologically and cortical erosion histologically of intermediate grade. Prognosis differs between classic and parosteal osteosarcoma.

Staging: Stage 1A (low-grade) is the most common presentation. Medullary invasion does not signify a poor prognosis. Parosteal osteosarcoma may on occasion (10%), typically after multiple recurrences, dedifferentiate into a stage IIB (high-grade) sarcoma with features of malignant fibrous histiocytoma or conventional high-grade osteosarcoma. Dedifferentiated parosteal osteosarcoma has a high metastatic potential.

Studies: Computed tomography, magnetic resonance imaging (after biopsy), and ultrasonography.

Pathology: Slightly atypical spindle cells that in one in six cases have regions of high-grade sarcoma. Frequently cartilaginous component is present. Parosteal osteosarcomas are typically densely ossified tumors arising from a broad base on the adjacent bone. Unlike osteochondromas, parosteal osteosarcomas involve no continuation of the medullary cavity into the tumor. Dedifferentiation signifies poor prognosis.

Medical Care: Chemotherapy or irradiation is not necessary for the majority without marked atypia and clear margins.

Surgical Care: Wide surgical resection is often curative, with about 80% to 95% long-term survival with local surgical control; however, recurrence should be considered.

Complications: The survival rates are excellent at 5 to 10 years, at 80% to 90%. Intramedullary back growth has previously been reported to imply a worse prognosis.

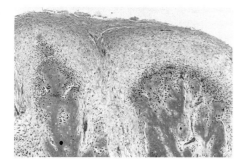

Fig. 173-1 Parosteal osteosarcoma of the left maxilla. Biopsy specimen shows a pale peripheral myxoid zone overlying a cellular zone and tumor osteoid. *(From Regezi JA, et al: Oral Pathology: Clinical Pathologic Correlations, 5th ed. Philadelphia, Saunders, 2008.)*

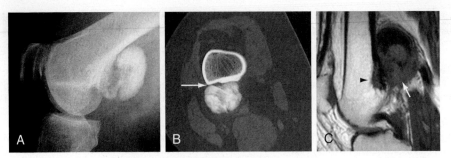

Fig. 173-2 Parosteal osteosarcoma. **A,** Lateral radiograph of the knee showing a dense, lobulated mass of bone arising from the posterior distal femur. **B,** Axial CT shows a lucent line (*arrow*) separating the lesion from the underlying cortex. **C,** Sagittal T1-weighted spin-echo MR image shows the low SI mass with central intermediate SI (*arrow*) indicating a region of dedifferentiation to high-grade tumor. Note also the intramedullary extension (*arrowhead*). (*From Adam A, et al: Grainger & Allison's Diagnostic Radiology, 5th ed. Philadelphia, Churchill Livingstone, 2008.*)

Definition: Lateral displacement of the patella from the patellofemoral groove is the most common dislocation. Superior, medial, and intra-articular dislocations have been described. They all typically spontaneously reduce.

Etiology: Dislocations can occur from a direct blow (10%) to the medial patella or more commonly from an indirect injury. Indirect dislocations usually occur with a combination of strong quadriceps contraction while the knee is in a flexed and valgus position and the femur is rotated internally with an externally rotated tibia. Risk factors include shallow patellofemoral groove, patella alta, excessive Q angle, or generalized ligamentous laxity. Football, basketball, baseball, gymnastics, and cheerleading are activities that are most commonly associated.

Age: 16 to 20 years old, rarely older than 30.

Gender: Females are associated with higher incidence. Twenty-four percent of patients have a positive family history.

Symptoms: Anterior knee pain, swelling, and ecchymosis, often accompanied by a history of the knee "giving out," which may present grossly dislocated. If the patella is still dislocated, then the patient will present with the knee flexed and a prominent medial femoral condyle.

Clinical Findings: Hemarthrosis may track superomedially; apprehension test should be performed with a lateral displacement of the patella with the knee 30 degrees flexed to produce reflex quadriceps activation; superomedial tenderness (medial retinaculum); superolateral tenderness (lateral femoral osteochondral fracture).

Diagnostic Studies: Aspiration of knee is indicated. Hemarthrosis implies traumatic mechanism and presence of fat droplets associated with osteochondral (OCD) fracture; serosanguinous fluid may indicate articular cartilage lesion. Radiographs help rule out fracture. Magnetic resonance imaging can be used for determination of detailed osseous alignment of the patella, evaluation of soft tissues (i.e., medial patellar femoral ligament [MPFL]), and diagnosis of OCD lesions.

Treatment: Reduction of acute dislocations is accomplished by gently extending the knee, avoiding forceful medial patella pressure. Aspiration of tense hemarthrosis will aid diagnosis and provide pain relief. Management of acute dislocations is controversial. Surgical treatment should initially be considered in young, athletic patients, especially those requiring surgery for OCD lesions. Surgical repair is the accepted treatment for recurrent dislocations.

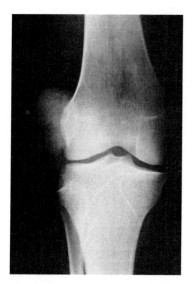

Fig. 174-1   Anteroposterior radiograph of the knee of an adolescent girl who sustained a patellar dislocation. Note that the patella is laterally displaced. *(Courtesy of Dr. Neil E. Green. From Green NE, Swiontkowski MF: Skeletal Trauma in Children, 3rd ed. Philadelphia, Saunders, 2003.)*

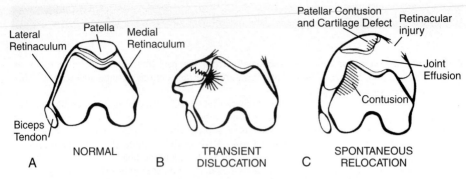

Fig. 174-2 Transient patellar dislocation. **A,** Normal relationship of the patella and retinacula in extension. **B,** Transient lateral patellar dislocation results in disruption of the medial retinaculum. Contractile force of the vastus medialis causes the medial facet of the patella to strike the lateral femoral condyle. The patella usually reduces back into the intercondylar notch spontaneously with knee extension. **C,** The resultant MR findings are delineated: disruption of the medial patellar retinaculum, patellar and femoral contusions, and joint effusion. *(Reprinted with permission from Kirsch MD, et al: Transient lateral patellar dislocation: Diagnosis with MR imaging. Am J Roentgenol 161:109-113, 1993.)*

Nonoperative: Knee immobilizer and rehabilitation focusing on quadriceps strengthening, especially the vastus medialis obliquus (VMO).

Operative: Repair of MPFL, lateral retinacular release if patellar tilt, and repair of any significant malalignment. OCD lesions should be addressed arthroscopically. Surgery should be followed with similar rehabilitation to nonoperative patients.

Complications: Risk of recurrent dislocation following nonoperative treatment is reported between 15% and 44%. Risk is as high as 60% for patients younger than 14 years and decreases with age. Following surgical repair, the re-dislocation rate is less than 10%.

Definition: The patella functions to improve the lever arm of the extensor mechanism. Joint contact forces are greater than 3 times body weight during stair climbing and greater than 7½ times body weight while squatting with maximum tensile forces at 45 to 60 degrees of flexion. Fractures and extensor mechanism disruptions can result in serious consequences.

Incidence: Patellar fractures represent nearly 1% of all skeletal fractures.

Age: Patellar fractures affect both children and adults equally. Females are more likely than males to have patellar dislocation. Patellar tendon ruptures usually occur in younger patients (younger than 40 years), whereas quadriceps tendon ruptures usually occur in older patients (older than 40 years). Patellar dislocations usually occur in patients in their mid-20s.

Pathology: Patellar fractures include transverse, vertical, marginal, and osteochondral classifications. Typically, these fractures follow direct trauma, resulting in a comminuted fracture pattern. Fractures caused by indirect trauma usually result in displaced, transverse fractures. Patellar tendon ruptures most commonly occur at the proximal insertion.

Signs and Symptoms: Patients with patellar fracture present with persistent patellar tenderness and pain or a joint effusion with a history of a direct or indirect injury. Extensor mechanism disruptions are most often unilateral, but can be bilateral in patients with underlying systemic diseases (diabetes mellitus, rheumatoid arthritis, systemic lupus erythematosus) or who are on systemic steroids.

Diagnostic Studies: Radiography, magnetic resonance imaging, and computed tomography. Anteroposterior radiographs may obscure findings of patellar fractures, whereas lateral views may be useful in evaluating comminution and separation of fracture fragments.

Treatment:

Nonoperative: For fractures with less than 2-mm step-off and less than 3-mm diastasis without an extensor lag. Long leg cylinder cast or knee immobilizer for 4 to 6 weeks with weight bearing as tolerated is recommended. Nonoperative treatment has a limited role in the care of patellar tendon ruptures

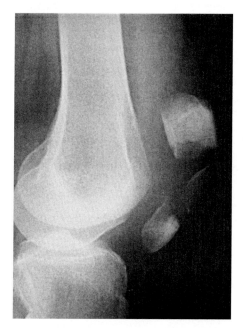

Fig. 175-1 Displaced transverse fracture of the patella. Lateral radiograph. *(From Browner BD: Skeletal Trauma: Basic Science, Management, and Reconstruction, 3rd ed. Philadelphia, Saunders, 2003.)*

363

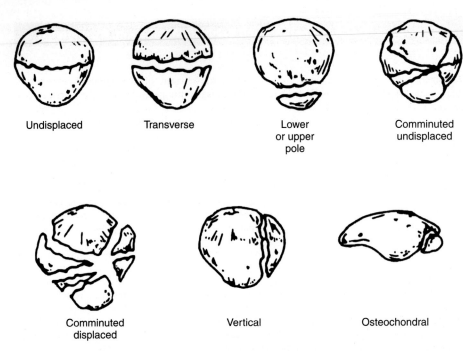

Undisplaced   Transverse   Lower
                                          or upper
                                          pole

Comminuted
undisplaced

Comminuted   Vertical   Osteochondral
displaced

Fig. 175-2   Classification of patellar fractures. *(From Wiss DA, Watson JT, Johnson EE: Fractures of the knee. In Rockwood CA Jr, Green DP, Bucholz RW, et al, eds: Rockwood and Green's Fractures in Adults, 4th ed, Philadelphia, Lippincott-Raven, 1996.)*

Operative: For displaced fractures with an extensor lag. Tension band, lag screws, cannulated lag screws with tension band through the screws (strongest construct), or partial patellectomy is indicated. A partial patellectomy or re-approximate patellar tendon at the level of the joint to avoid articular surface step-off is also performed as a surgical treatment. Surgical treatment followed with No. 5 nonabsorbable sutures using a Bunnell or Krackow technique passed through drill holes in the patella (usually three holes: medial, lateral, and central) is recommended. In general, repair of tendons involves suturing the torn tendon through bone tunnels within the patella or tibial tubercle.

Complications: Knee stiffness, quadriceps weakness/atrophy, and re-rupture.

Nonoperative: Early range of motion with patellar support bracing. Two thirds have good results; 26% have residual instability.

Operative: Repair of medial patellar femoral ligament (usually avulsed from its femoral attachment).

Long-term Treatment: Lateral release, vastus medialis obliquus advancement or reefing, tibial tubercle transfer (i.e., Fulkerson).

Definition: Patellofemoral syndrome is among the most common causes of knee pain complaints, particularly among adolescent and young adult patients. In particular, younger females are especially vulnerable to this diagnosis. Oftentimes, the patellofemoral joint itself is often the source of the pain. This pain can be caused by such disorders as chondromalacia patella, patellofemoral arthralgia, and lateral patellofemoral compression syndrome.

Common Causes: Many injuries and anatomic issues can predispose patients to patellofemoral misalignment, leading to the diagnosis of patellofemoral syndrome. Some of the predisposing conditions can include imbalance of quadriceps strength, patella alta, recurrent patellar subluxation, direct trauma to the patella, and meniscal injuries.

Symptoms: Patients frequently complain of anterior knee pain, especially associated with climbing up and down stairs, or with rising from a seated position. They also frequently have difficulty localizing the source of their complaint, but normally they complain of pain around the patella, beneath, or within the patella. Patellofemoral syndrome can also have complaints of crepitus, joint locking, or sensations of joint instability. None of these complaints is usually elicited on examination.

Physical Examination: Physical examination is not as useful as history in establishing the diagnosis. A common examination finding is reproduction of symptoms when the knee is held in slight flexion and gentle pressure against the patella is applied as the patient contracts the quadriceps muscles. In some cases, with the knee extended and the quadriceps relaxed, the typical pain may be reproduced by digital pressure under the medial or lateral border of the patella, with side-to-side movement of the patella itself.

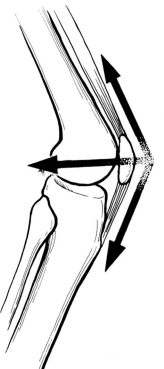

Fig. 176-1   Patellofemoral resultant force increases with knee flexion due to position and muscle actions. *(From DeLee DJ, Drez D: Orthopaedic Sports Medicine, 2nd ed. Philadelphia, Saunders, 2003.)*

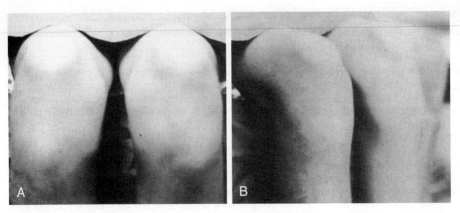

Fig. 176-2 A and B, Patella alta in a 14-year-old boy who had grown 6 inches over the previous 6 months. *(From DeLee DJ, Drez D: Orthopaedic Sports Medicine, 2nd ed. Philadelphia, Saunders, 2003.)*

Treatment: Therapy includes strengthening of the quadriceps and avoidance of aggravating actions. Physical therapy is helpful in educating the patient about home exercises. Many patients learn that the most effective therapy is bicycling. Most cases resolve either on their own or with formal therapy. Conservative treatment is the rule, with physical therapy and nonsteroidal anti-inflammatory drugs being the mainstay.

Definition: Differences between the lengths of the upper and/or lower legs.

Incidence: True incidence is unknown; however; it is suggested that the majority of individuals have at least a small degree of discrepancy.

Etiology: Etiology includes congenital disorders (developmental dysplasia of the hip, dysplasias, anisomelia, proximal femoral focal deficiency, hemihypertrophy), trauma (physeal injury, malunion), infection, neuromuscular disorders (polio, cerebral palsy), and tumors.

Age: Diagnosed during infancy or later in childhood, depending on the cause.

Gender: Leg-length discrepancy due to trauma and trauma-related conditions is observed more commonly in males than in females. However, the incidence of congenital conditions corresponds to the gender predilection of the underlying condition.

Race: No predilection.

Signs and Symptoms: Associated with a limp when the discrepancy is greater than 2 cm. Other clinical findings relate to the specific disorder causing the length discrepancy. May observe scoliosis, contractures, and pelvic obliquity. Patients with spasticity or weakness have less ability to compensate. The severity of symptoms may be linked to the degree of discrepancy between the lengths of the lower extremities.

Diagnostic Studies: Accurate measurement of leg lengths and skeletal age are critical. Moseley straight-line graph is used to determine final discrepancy at maturity. Clinically, leg lengths can be measured by placing blocks under the foot until the iliac crests are level (less accurate). X-ray evaluation with orthoroentgenogram (overlapping radiographs of entire bilateral lower extremities) may be a more precise method. Gruelich and Pyle use anteroposterior x-ray studies of the hand and wrist to determine bone age.

Classification: Moseley suggested a graphic method that facilitates the recording and interpretation of data in cases of leg-length discrepancy. This graph provides a mechanism for predicting future growth that automatically takes into account the child's growth percentile and the degree of growth inhibition in a short leg.

Treatment: Dependent on the amount of inequality. Goals are equal leg length, level pelvis, and providing an appropriate mechanical axis for weight bearing. A discrepancy of less than 2 cm is usually acceptable. A 2- to 5-cm difference can be treated with a shoe lift, epiphysiodesis of long leg, or resection osteotomy once skeletal maturity has been reached. Leg shortening is associated with increased incidence of physeal arrest. At greater than 5 to 15 cm, lengthening of the short limb is recommended. Lengthening does not affect the rate of growth; timing is less critical. Lengthening up to 1 mm/day is advised. The Ilizarov method of lengthening (distraction osteogenesis) is favored.

Sequelae: Back pain, gait disturbances, compensatory scoliosis, degenerative arthrosis of lumbar spine and sacroiliac articulations, foot calluses, equinus contracture of the ankle, long leg, degenerative hip, and patellofemoral arthrosis are possible sequelae.

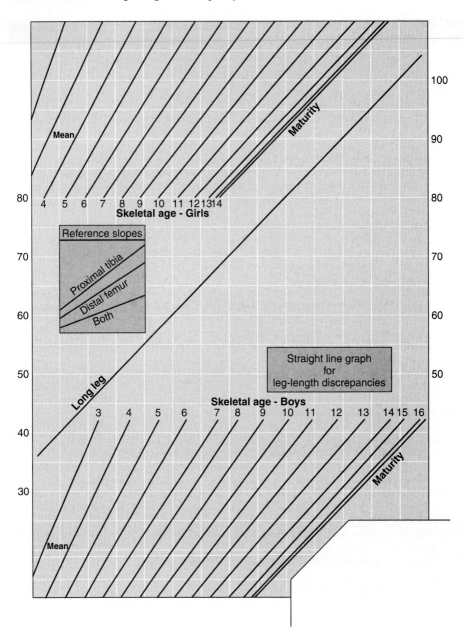

Fig. 177-1 Moseley straight-line graph. *(From Moseley CF: Straight-line graph for leg-length discrepancies. J Bone Joint Surg [Am] 59:174-179, 1977.)*

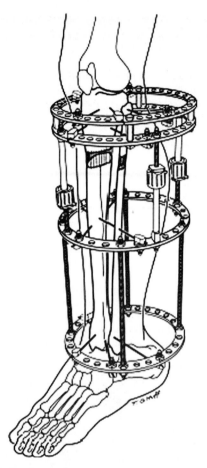

Fig. 177-2 Ilizarov method of leg lengthening. *(From Canale ST: Campbell's Operative Orthopaedics, 10th ed. St. Louis, Mosby, 2003, pp. 1043-1059.)*

Definition: Genu varum (bow legs) is improper growth of the tibia in the leg, causing the knees to appear to "bow" out from the body. The tibia may bow anteriorly, posteriorly, or laterally. Genu valgum ("knock knees"), on the other hand, is when a child's legs curve inward abnormally so that the distance between the knees seems smaller than expected.

Incidence: Knock knees are less common than bow legs. Lateral bowing of the tibia is extremely common; as long as it is bilateral, it is developmentally normal and settles spontaneously by age 4. Anterior bowing is always significant, whereas posterior bowing is rare.

Age: Bow legs are typical in infants to age 12 to 14 months, and may be normal to age 2. Knock knees are typical in children ages 3 to 7 years.

Etiology and Pathophysiology: In older children, bow legs can be caused by many different problems, including abnormal bone growth in the legs, leg injury, infection, severe vitamin D deficiency, and other problems of the bone or cartilage. Some other causes of tibial bowing are congenital absence of the fibula, neurofibromatosis type 1, and osteogenesis imperfecta.

Signs and Symptoms: Both bow legs and knock knees are usually noticed by parents and can be checked for using the tests described below. Either bow legs or knock knees, if not treated, can cause osteoarthritis in the knees later in life.

Diagnostic Studies: Diagnosis of bow legs or knock knees is best accomplished through physical examination. In addition, x-ray studies may be done when needed to obtain more information about the knee joint. Less often, a patient may need a magnetic resonance imaging scan or other tests to check the cartilage in the knees. In addition to the torsional profile test for bow legs and knock knees, angulation should be quantified by measuring the intercondylar or

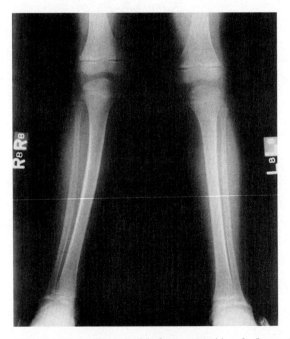

Fig. 178-1 Anteroposterior standing radiograph of the lower extremities of a 5-year-old boy who sustained a nondisplaced fracture of the right proximal tibial metaphysis 15 months previously. The fracture healed uneventfully. The valgus deformity occurred shortly after cast removal. In terms of the mechanical axis, the right knee has a 22° valgus alignment versus 5° on the left. *(From Browner BD, et al: Skeletal Trauma in Children, 3rd ed. Philadelphia, Saunders, 2003.)*

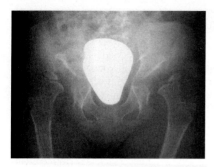

Fig. 178-2 Mucopolysaccharidosis Type IV. Radiographs showing absent odontoid peg. *(From Adam A, et al: Grainger & Allison's Diagnostic Radiology, 5th ed. Philadelphia, Churchill Livingstone, 2008.)*

intermalleolar distance. Intercondylar distance measures the degree of genu varum and is the distance between the medial femoral condyles when the lower extremities are positioned with the medial malleoli touching. The intermalleolar measurement quantifies genu valgum and is the distance between the medial malleoli with the medial femoral condyles touching. Intermalleolar and intercondylar have the disadvantage of being relative measurements that are affected by the child's size. Measuring the femoral tibial angle with a goniometer is a more accurate way to quantify angulation. Reasons for concern in bow legs and knock knees are excessive knee angle, knee angles that are not equal on each side, knee angle associated with pain or other complaint, bow legs after age 3 years, and knock knees greater than 15 degrees. If physiologic genu varum or genu valgum persists beyond 7 to 8 years of age, orthopedic referral is indicated. Pathologic conditions should be referred for appropriate management.

Treatment: Treatment is usually conservative. Special shoes, cast, or braces are rarely beneficial and have no proven efficacy. Surgery is reserved for older children with a deformity of 3 to 4 standard deviations from normal. Surgery is performed only on asymmetrical limbs or those with debilitating torsional abnormalities. Most bow legs are symmetrical and stable, and spontaneously resolve. Bracing has shown benefit to age 34. Surgery is most often indicated for those with an abnormality of the growth plate, a condition known as *Blount's disease.*

Osteotomy is usually indicated for treatment of symptomatic dysplasia in young, active patients who have mild or no arthritis. There are generally three basic categories in procedures correcting acetabular pathomorphology, which include (1) reshaping, (2) reorientation, (3) augmentation.

Reshaping Procedures: Reshaping procedures essentially describe trimming of an excessive acetabular rim, which causes pincer type femoroacetabular impingement (FAI). The surgical procedure comprises reducing overcoverage by excising the bony prominence at the rim. The torn and degenerative area of the labrum is excised and the remainder of the labrum is reattached to the rim using a suture anchor. Femoral osteoplasty (bumpectomy), if necessary, is performed. The hip is then reduced and checked for impingement-free range of motion. The midterm results of this procedure have been reported as encouraging, with significant improvement of pain and function.

Reorientation Procedures: This is an osteotomy around the acetabulum to achieve an improved position over the femoral head. For developmental dysplasia, reorientation osteotomies are preferred because they change the orientation of the acetabular articular surface, thereby correcting the anterolateral deficiency. In majority of dysplastic hips, there is sufficient articular surface in the posteroinferior quadrant to allow reorientation. The periacetabular (Ganz) osteotomy is most widely used procedure because it allows large potential correction that is obtainable in all planes with a single approach. Additionally, it has potential for medial translation of the hip joint center, thus reducing the lever arm of the hip and joint loading. It also does not alter the shape of the true pelvis or jeopardize stability of the pelvis. The surgical procedure comprises five steps: (1) incomplete ischial osteotomy, (2) complete pubic osteotomy, (3) chevron supra-acetabular osteotomy, (4) retroacetabular osteotomy, (5) completion of whole osteotomy by controlled fracture of the original incompletely osteotomized ischium. Most challenging part of this procedure is performing the actual fragment correction accurately. The reported long-term results of Ganz osteotomy have demonstrated good or excellent clinical outcome in more than 80% of patients with early stage arthrosis. Other reorientation procedures, including rotational acetabular osteotomy and juxta-articular triple osteotomy, have also been performed with the same purpose.

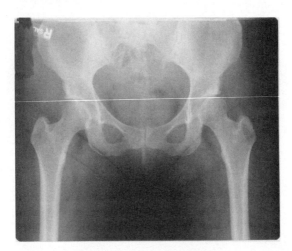

Fig. 179-1   Patient with developmental dysplasia of left hip. Note undercoverage of femoral head.

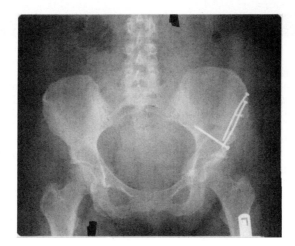

Fig. 179-2   Same patient following periacetabular osteotomy.

Augmentation Procedures: The purpose of the augmentation procedures, such as the Chiari osteotomy, dome, and shelf procedure is to reduce joint load forces by augmenting the main weight-bearing area of the joint. These are indicated in cases with very short and relatively normally oriented acetabulum or occasionally with a more advanced subluxation. The Chiari osteotomy is one of the most widely used salvage procedures (iliac osteotomy from sciatic notch to just proximal to the joint, followed by medial displacement of the acetabulum). With weight bearing, the capsule undergoes metaplastic transformation to fibrous cartilage. However, the labrum remains within the main weight-bearing area and is subjected to chronic shear stress and might cause pain. Even though this augmentation procedure can provide reliable pain relief for some years, it is currently regarded as a salvage procedure. Because the indications for total hip arthroplasty have expanded to young adults with promising results, the overall frequency of this procedure continues to decrease and is now rarely performed.

Peripheral Nervous System
Comprises less than 0.1% of all nerve tissue. The somatic peripheral nervous system (PNS) is defined by the presence of Schwann cells. This includes the primary roots, dorsal root ganglia, mixed spinal nerves, plexuses, nerve trunks, autonomic nervous system, and cranial nerves III through XII. Peripheral nerve trunks are composed of one, few, or many fascicles of axons with surrounding epineurium, blood vessels, and connective tissues. Conduction is provided by gaps between Schwann cells or nodes of Ranvier. Each Schwann cell encircles its axon segment with a myelin sheath. The three main types of peripheral nerve fibers are shown in Table 180-1.

Peripheral Neuropathy: Peripheral nerve lesions that are not due to trauma. Pathology is rather mainly from metabolic disturbances or vascular disease. The two main kinds of peripheral neuropathy are axonal and demyelinating neuropathies.

Axonal Neuropathy (AN): Involve axonal degeneration. Characterized by decreased sensory and motor amplitudes, which results in responses that cannot be elicited at all stimulation points. There is only mild slowing of conduction velocity and latency as they are measured from unaffected axons. Fibrillations can occur with severe motor nerve involvement. Diabetes and alcohol abuse are the most common causes of AN.

Demyelinating Neuropathy (DN): Characterized by blocking or slowing of conduction velocity and latency by greater than 40%. When conduction is slowed along different fibers to different degrees, sensory and motor amplitudes decrease. Clinically, these abnormalities manifest as muscle weakness, fasciculations, cramps, and paresthesias. Guillain-Barré syndrome, lead exposure, compression, and uremia are the most common causes.

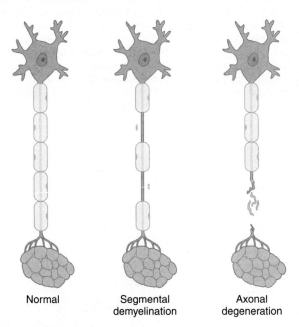

Normal   Segmental   Axonal
demyelination   degeneration

Fig. 180-1 Types of peripheral nerve damage. *(From Frontera WR: Essentials of Physical Medicine and Rehabilitation, 2nd ed. Philadelphia, Saunders, 2008.)*

Table 180-1. MAIN TYPES OF PERIPHERAL NERVE FIBERS

Type	Diameter	Myelination	Speed	Examples
A	10 to 20 μM	Heavy	Fast	Touch
B	<3 μM	Intermediate	Medium	Autonomic nervous system
C	<1.3 μM	None	Slow	Pain

Table 180-2. NERVE CONDUCTION STUDIES OF PERIPHERAL NEUROPATHY

Disorder	Action Potential		Conduction Velocity	F-Wave Latency
	Amplitude	Duration		
Axonal neuropathy	Decreased	Normal	>70%	Mild increase
Demyelinating neuropathy	Decreased	Increased	<50%	Increased

Definition: A disorder, in which the common peroneal nerve is damaged, manifested by a loss of movement and/or sensation in the foot and leg.

Etiology: Trauma is the most common cause of a localized injury to a single nerve. Direct trauma or injury to the knee, fracture of the fibula, tight-fitting casts or immobilizers of the lower leg, pressure to the lateral aspect of the knee from positions during sleep or coma, and injury to the knee during surgery or dislocation.

Associations: More common in emaciated bedridden patients and in thin persons who habitually cross their legs or from wearing high tight-fitting boots. A minor association exists with some polyneuropathies such as diabetic neuropathy, polyarteritis nodosa, and Charcot-Marie-Tooth disease.

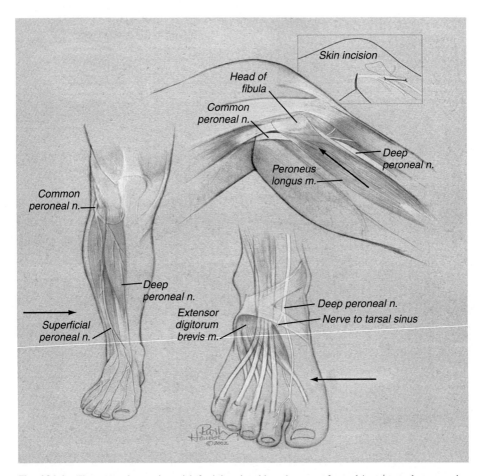

Fig. 181-1   The peroneal nerve is at risk for injury in athletes because of stretch/traction and compression of the common peroneal nerve at the fibular neck, the superficial peroneal nerve as it exits the fascia in the distal third of the leg, and the deep peroneal nerve as it crosses the dorsum of the ankle and the foot. For the deep peroneal nerve, the most common site of entrapment is beneath the extensor hallucis longus tendon. These three sites are noted by arrows. *(From Porter DA, Schon LC: Baxter's The Foot and Ankle in Sport, 2nd ed. Philadelphia, Mosby, 2007.)*

Incidence: Overall incidence is rare, with most noted after total knee arthroplasty or traumatic dislocation of the knee. Incidence of peroneal nerve palsy after total knee arthroplasty varies from 0% to 9.5% in the literature. Injury to peroneal nerve following traumatic knee dislocation has a reported incidence varying between 25% and 40%.

Age and Gender: Men and women equally affected with an age range anywhere from 20 to 80 years.

Clinical Findings: Loss of sensation, numbness, tingling over portions of the L4, L5, S1, and S2 dermatomes (especially dorsum of the foot). Loss of motor function of the tibialis anterior, extensor hallucis longus, extensor digitorum longus, peroneus longus, peroneus brevis, peroneus tertius muscles.

Symptoms and Signs: Foot drop, "slapping" gait, and weakness of ankles or feet; also a decreased sensation to dorsum of foot.

Diagnostic Studies: Physical examination; finding Tinel's sign over the fibular neck may help localize the site of nerve compression. Electromyography is used to objectively document conduction block; however, it is more commonly used in follow-up within 1 month of injury to document extent of injury.

Pathology: Peroneal nerve palsy is primarily caused by direct compression of the nerve or by direct trauma/traction injury during knee dislocations or total knee arthroplasty. The common peroneal nerve enters the popliteal space and winds lateral to the fibular head and has a fixed attachment in the region of the neck of the fibula. At this level, the nerve is superficial and susceptible to direct compression or trauma. The nerve proximal to this fixed location is also vulnerable to a traction injury when the knee is subjected to varus and hyperextension forces.

Surgical Care: Conservative treatment is the first line of therapy to prevent further injury: knee and hip flexed to 20 to 45 degrees, and constrictive dressings removed. If there is no neurologic improvement after 2 to 3 months, operative decompression is indicated. If the nerve is not disrupted, external neurolysis of the nerve at the level of the fibular head is often performed. If the nerve is completely ruptured, nerve repair is desirable, although not always technically feasible. Nerve grafting may have a role in repair; however, prognosis remains poor in these cases.

Definition: Abnormally high arched foot, forefoot in plantar flexion relative to hindfoot. Associated deformities include varus hindfoot, plantar flexed first metatarsal, and claw toes.

Etiology:

Neuromuscular: Charcot-Marie-Tooth (CMT) and polio are most common. Others include amyotrophic lateral sclerosis, Huntington's disease, Friedreich's ataxia, cerebral palsy. Also occurs in adults with stroke and closed head injury.

Traumatic: Deep posterior compartment syndrome. Severe scarring after burn, crush injury, and venous stasis can pull foot into cavoarus. Talar neck fracture malunion can leave the distal portion of the talar neck shortened, dorsally and medially translated, resulting in fixed varus. Injury to the deep branch of peroneal nerve or L5 nerve root.

Idiopathic: Imbalance of extrinsic-intrinsic muscles.

Symptoms: Variable, depending on degree of deformity. Pain in overstressed parts of the foot.

CMT: Overload of the lateral border, first metatarsal head as well as lateral metatarsal heads. Can manifest with stress fractures, most common in fifth metatarsal, and lateral ankle instability.

Diagnostic Studies:

- Coleman block test—flexible versus fixed hindfoot deformity: 1-inch wooden block under patient's hindfoot and lateral forefoot, with first metatarsal head off the block. Flexible deformity will evert into valgus when the plantarflexed first metatarsal is not bearing weight.
- Standing lateral x-ray study—assessment of ankle joint position, calcaneal pitch, midfoot and forefoot position and their contribution to the deformity
- Anteroposterior x-ray study—metatarsus adductus component or other deformities
- Calcaneal axial view
- Magnetic resonance imaging
- Electromyography
- Neuromuscular workup

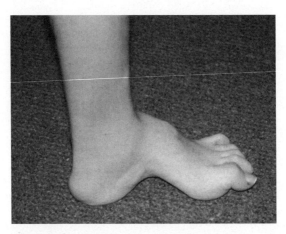

Fig. 182-1 Clinical picture demonstrating pes cavus. *(From Kliegman RM, et al: Nelson Textbook of Pediatrics, 18th ed. Philadelphia, Saunders, 2007.)*

Treatment:

Nonoperative: Shoe modification, orthotics, brace

Surgical: Dependent upon etiology; correct spinal pathology; reconstruction including plantar fascia release, selected tendon transfers to improve muscle balance, Achilles tendon lengthening for equines contracture, wedge of calcaneus to correct heel varus, dorsal wedge osteotomy of first metatarsal, claw toe realignment

Complications: If left untreated, the condition is often progressive, especially in the child, leading to poor function and pain.

Definition: Pigmented villonodular synovitis (PVNS), first described by Jaffe and colleagues in 1941, is a rare inflammatory granulomatous condition. This disorder can be considered as a benign tumor of the synovium located at the lining of joints, bursae, and tendon sheaths anywhere. Regardless of its benign histologic characteristics, it sometimes displays an aggressive invasion to the adjacent bone and cartilage if left untreated.

Etiology: Unknown. Genetic predisposition, chronic inflammation and even vascular trauma have been postulated. Trisomy 7 and 5 have been strongly linked as a predisposing factor to PVNS.

Associations: Abnormalities in the short arm of chromosome 1 are linked with hemorrhage because the locus for coagulation factors III and V is located there. Some studies have shown that patients with PVNS have this chromosomal defect. Also, alterations on the regulatory pathways at cell division, such as the p53 pathway and the RB pathway, have been associated with PVNS.

Incidence: Reported as 1 to 2 cases per million in the United States.

Age: Young adults with a bimodal presentation in the third and fourth decades.

Gender: No preference.

Signs and Symptoms: The diagnosis is not usually reached clinically, because the symptoms are similar to those of osteoarthritis and rheumatoid arthritis, taking an average delay of 4.4 years from the beginning of symptoms. The knee is the joint most affected in 66% to 80% of the cases. Other joints include hip, ankle, shoulder, elbow, wrist, foot, spine (especially cervical spine), and temporomandibular joint. Even the retroperitoneal mass, femoral triangle, and gluteal region have been reported.

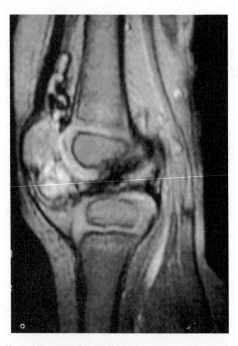

Fig. 183-1   Pigmented villonodular synovitis. This child was unusual in that he was only 3 years of age at the time of diagnosis. Sagittal T1 MRI illustrating a mixed signal mass with areas of low hemosiderin and high signal (hemorrhage). *(From Adam A, et al: Grainger & Allison's Diagnostic Radiology, 5th ed. Philadelphia, Churchill Livingstone, 2008.)*

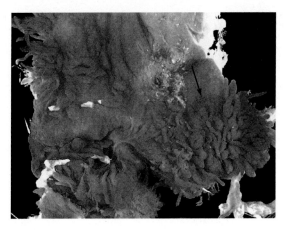

Fig. 183-2   Excised synovium with fronds and nodules typical of pigmented villonodular synovitis (PVNS) (*arrow*). (*From Kumar V, et al: Robbins and Cotran Pathologic Basis of Disease, 7th ed. Philadelphia, Saunders.*)

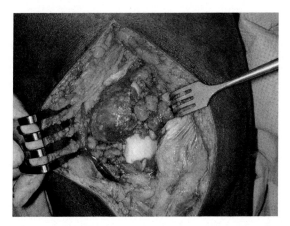

Fig. 183-3   Intraoperative photograph of pigmented villonodular synovitis. (*From Canale ST, Beaty JH [eds]: Campbell's Operative Orthopaedics, 11th ed. Philadelphia, Mosby, 2007.*)

Diagnostic Studies: Aspiration will render hemarthrosis in more than 60% of patients, but usually is still normal for standard laboratory testing, which increases the delay in the diagnosis. It is often difficult to differentiate from trauma, hemophilia, giant cell tumors of tendon sheaths (GCTTS), and other sarcomas. X-ray study occasionally shows a periarticular mass with no other changes initially. Ultrasound has failed to yield specific images for this pathology. Magnetic resonance imaging, especially T2-weighted images, helps when there is a heavy deposition of hemosiderin inside the nodules.

Macropathology: The joint appears swollen, with increased and edematous synovial tissue with a characteristic brownish discoloration due to hemosiderin deposits. Subchondral resorption and cyst formation are seen in advanced PVNS.

Micropathology: There are mainly two types of presentation, a diffuse type that is mostly villous in character and a localized type that is predominantly nodular. Histologic findings typically show large amounts of mononuclear cells with hemosiderin deposition, multinucleated giant cell, and occasionally intranuclear inclusions. Chronic inflammation increases the chance

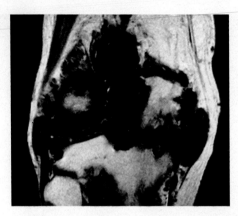

Fig. 183-4 Pigmented villonodular synovitis (PVNS). Coronal T1-weighted MR image showing dark synovial masses due to haemosiderin deposition against a background of degenerative joint disease. *(From Adam A, et al: Grainger & Allison's Diagnostic Radiology, 5th ed. Philadelphia, Churchill Livingstone, 2008.)*

of intra-articular bleeding, thus the predisposed PVNS tissue will have more iron available, which in turn probably stimulates the mononuclear cells and fibroblasts, creating a vicious cycle.

Treatment: Resection of the synovium by means of arthroscopy is useful; open arthrotomy is advisable, requiring in most cases adjuvant treatment with radiotherapy. Extensive bone destruction can necessitate joint reconstruction. Cryosurgery directed to the synovium layers avoiding the cartilage has been reported also as curative, with no recurrence. Tumor necrosis factor alpha (TNF-α) blockade for resistant or refractory PVNS has been reported with good results at long-term follow-up.

Complications: Recurrence is higher when simple synovectomy is used and especially in the diffuse type. Contamination of the portals used in an arthroscopy on patients with PVNS leading to spreading of the pathology into subcutaneous tissue has been described.

Sequelae: Joint destruction and subsequent limitation. Malignant transformation is associated with trisomy 5 and 7.

Definition: Fracture through growth plate.

Incidence: 15% to 30% of all childhood fractures.

Etiology: Growth plate = weakest area of growing bone.

Age-Appropriate Responses to FOOSA (Fall onto out-stretched arm) Injury:

- Infant—greenstick fracture
- Adolescent—physeal fracture
- Young adults—joint fracture and dislocation
- Older adults—metaphyseal fracture

Classification Salter-Harris (S-H) Types I-IX: Types I-V (SALTR 5 separation, above, lower, through, reduction: 1963 Robert Salter and W. Robert Harris of Toronto).

- Type I—transverse fracture through hypertrophic zone/physis; increased physeal width and point tenderness at the epiphyseal plate
- Type II (most common)—through physis and metaphysis; epiphysis *not* involved; variably sized triangular bone fragment of metaphysis (Thurstan Holland fragment)
- Type III—through the hypertrophic layer of the physis, extends to split the epiphysis, damages the reproductive physeal layer; Tillaux fracture = S-H type III ankle fracture prone to disability

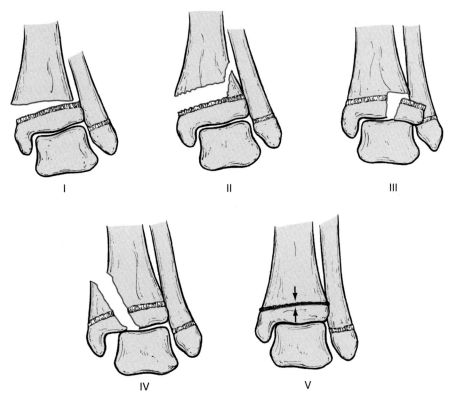

Fig. 184-1 Salter-Harris classification of physeal injury. I, pure separation through the physis; II, metaphyseal spike; III, separation through the physis and vertically through the epiphysis; IV, fracture through the metaphysis, through the physis, and vertically through the epiphysis; V, pure compression injury. *(From Browner BD, et al: Skeletal Trauma in Children, 3rd ed. Philadelphia, Saunders, 2003.)*

- Type IV—passes through epiphysis, physis, and metaphysis; intra-articular Thurstan Holland sign
- Type V—compression/crush injury with no associated epiphyseal or metaphyseal fracture; initial diagnosis may be difficult and is often made retrospectively; typically axial load injury, poor prognosis
- Type VI—injury to perichondral structures
- Type VII—isolated injury/epiphyseal plate
- Type VIII—isolated injury/metaphysis; potential injury related to endochondral ossification
- Type IX—periosteal injury; may interfere with membranous growth

Age: Adolescents to 16F (11 to 13 most common) and 18M (14 to 16 most common); physeal fracture occurs before physis closes; ligaments 2 to 5 times stronger vs. growth plates.

Gender: Male preponderance 2:1.

Race: No preponderance.

Associations: Approximately 50% wrist.

Imaging: Anteroposterior radiographs.

Treatment: reduction, any mild deformity left after growth plate fracture almost always remodels

Contraindications:

Absolute: When risks of sedation or general anesthesia outweigh the potential benefits of reduction.

Relative: SH I/II fracture with clinically insignificant displacement; great displacement fracture with delayed presentation.

Complications: Growth acceleration, premature closure (rare); 2% significant functional disturbance.

Definition: Intra-articular fracture of the tibial plafond. Pilon fractures are also referred to as a *plafond fracture* or a *high-energy fracture.*

Etiology: Although it represents a small percentage of lower extremity fractures, pilon fractures most commonly result from a traumatic axial loading force with or without a rotational force, such as from a fall or motor vehicle accident. This was described by Destot in 1911 based on the talus likened to a pestle (French *pilon*).

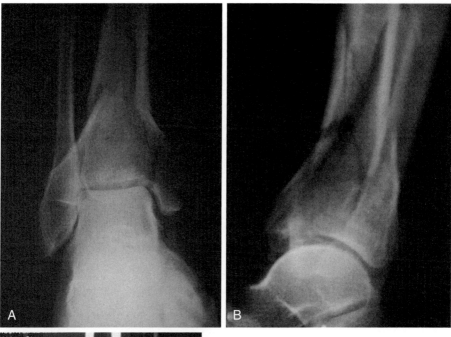

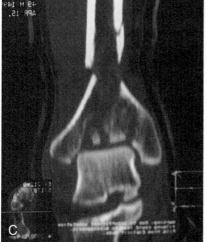

Fig. 185-1   This type C3 pilon fracture was sustained by a 40-year-old man who fell off his bicycle at high speed. **A, B,** Anteroposterior and lateral radiographs reveal a displaced pilon fracture with comminution extending well into the diaphysis. **C,** A computed tomographic scan (coronal reconstruction) shows articular comminution, displacement, and impaction. *(From Browner BD: Skeletal Trauma: Basic Science, Management, and Reconstruction, 3rd ed. Philadelphia, Saunders, 2003.)*

Incidence: 5% to 7% of all tibial fractures; less than 1% of all lower extremity fractures.

Gender: No preponderance.

Symptoms: Inability to bear weight is a cardinal sign, in addition to swelling, gross deformity of the ankle, fracture blisters, and crepitus motion.

Classification: Ruedi-Allgower Classification.

• Type I—nondisplaced
• Type II—significant displacement without comminution
• Type III—impacted and comminuted.

Examination: Neurologic examination assessing motor and sensory skills, as well as a vascular examination assessing tibial and dorsalis pedis pulses should be administered.

Studies: Anteroposterior and lateral radiographs of the foot, ankle, tibia, and knee, as well as the contralateral side should be obtained. Computed tomography should be considered an essential study and can often identify fracture lines and fragments missed on x-ray study.

Treatment: The overriding goals are restoration of the articular surface and range of motion, stable fixation of the metaphysis to the diaphysis, and preventing complications. Immobilization such as casting and splinting are indicated for type I fractures. Open reduction and internal fixation versus a limited open reduction and external fixation should be considered for types II and III fractures. Additionally, the use of intramedullary nailing may be indicated. Consideration should be made for delayed reconstruction aimed at tissue recovery after swelling has resolved.

Complications: The most common complication is post-traumatic osteoarthritis, followed by complications in wound/soft tissue healing with excessive swelling. Compartment syndrome may also manifest after such fractures.

Definition: Most common cause of inferior (plantar) heel pain in both the athletic and nonathletic populations.

Etiology: Most cases are the result of a biomechanical fault that causes abnormal pronation. A tight Achilles tendon or a pes planus or pes cavus deformity can increase the loading of the plantar fascia during normal standing activities and may be associated with plantar fasciitis.

Associations: Conditions that cause a pronation deformity, which increases tension on the plantar fascia, are associated with plantar fasciitis. They include tibia vara, ankle equinus, rearfoot valgus, and limb length inequality.

Incidence: Plantar fasciitis comprises approximately 15% of all foot complaints in the United States.

Age and Gender: More common in middle-age women and young male runners. Obesity is present in 90% of affected females and 40% of affected males.

Clinical Findings: Positive findings may include flat foot, highly arched foot, or excessively pronated foot. Gait alteration may reveal a supinated foot to redistribute the load laterally. Other findings may include tenderness of the heel with dorsiflexion of the foot or great toe that resolves with plantar flexion of the foot, which relaxes the plantar fascia. Also, mild edema and small granulomas palpable along the medial fascial origin may be appreciated.

Symptoms: Classically described as heel pain on taking the first steps in the morning, with symptoms lessening as walking continues. Pain is usually insidious, with no history of trauma. Another highly characteristic feature is the location of pain, usually at the origin of the medial plantar fascia from the medial tubercle of the calcaneus.

Signs: Mild swelling of the feet and pain with dorsiflexion of the foot or great toe. Direct palpation of the medial calcaneal tubercle often causes severe pain.

Diagnostic Studies: The diagnosis of plantar fasciitis is still based mainly on history and clinical presentation. Heel and ankle radiographs are useful to exclude fractures and may identify heel spurs.

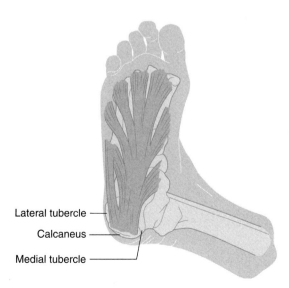

Lateral tubercle

Calcaneus

Medial tubercle

Fig. 186-1   Plantar view of origin and insertion of plantar fascia. *(From Frontera WR: Essentials of Physical Medicine and Rehabilitation, 2nd ed. Philadelphia, Saunders)*

Pathology: Specimens of inflamed fascia obtained during surgery reveal collagen necrosis, angiofibroblastic hyperplasia, chondroid metaplasia, and matrix calcification. These changes are consistent with a chronic degenerative/reparative process secondary to repetitive stress.

Treatment: Plantar fasciitis is best treated initially with rest, orthotics, stretching, and nonsteroidal anti-inflammatory drugs (NSAIDs). Treatment several times per day consisting of ice massage, heel cord stretching, posterior tibial and peroneal strengthening, heel cushioning, and NSAIDs have been shown to be therapeutic. In cases with symptoms lasting more than 6 weeks, casting may be required for absolute rest. Release of the fascia, either open or endoscopic, has been shown to be effective.

Definition: Bites from insects, arachnids, arthropods, reptiles and diseased animals can all be considered toxic to the recipient. Although many bites typically manifest as pruritic erythematous papules, some insects serve as disease vectors and their bites pose a more serious health risk. Certain species of snake and arachnid contain significant toxins in their venom that are released during a bite.

Incidence: Insect bites and stings are common across the United States. In the Mid-Atlantic region, mosquitoes, biting flies, and ticks account for most bites. In arid areas, such as California and much of the desert Southwest, crawling arthropods are the primary cause of bites and stings. Incidences of poison bites from reptiles also occur in the southwestern and southeastern United States, but they are rare.

Age: Poison bites can occur at any age.

Gender: Distribution between genders is equal.

Etiology and Pathophysiology: Most snake venom from poisonous snakes is composed of neurotoxins. Enzyme concentrations vary among species, thereby causing dissimilar envenomations. Most lesions indicative of insect bites are the result of the victim's immune response. Serious toxicity related to insect bites results not from the bite itself, but from the transmission of disease through bacterial or viral infection on contact with an infected insect.

Associations: Insects and their related diseases:

Fleas: Plague.

Lice: Lice infestation.

Mosquitoes: Arborviral encephalitides (viral diseases causing brain inflammation and encephalitis, including eastern equine encephalitis, Japanese encephalitis, La Crosse encephalitis, St. Louis encephalitis, West Nile virus, western encephalitis), dengue fever, malaria, rift valley fever, and yellow fever.

Ticks: Babesiosis, Crimean Congo hemorrhagic fever, Ehrlichiosis, Lyme disease, Rocky Mountain spotted fever, tick typhus, tularemia.

Arachnid bites can result in tissue loss and necrosis, whereas poisonous snake bites can induce neurotoxic effects and cardiac and respiratory failure.

Signs and Symptoms: Most commonly, poison bites manifest as intensely pruritic erythematous papules grouped in areas where the bites occur. Vesicular and bulbous reactions are common, and large pseudolymphomatous nodules may occur. In the case of poisonous snake and arachnid bites, tissue necrosis surrounding the bite may appear. Exposure to certain toxins induced during a bite or sting, especially if the victim is hypersensitive, may result in anaphylactic shock.

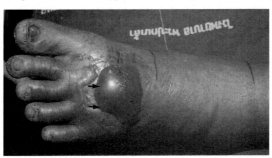

Fig. 187-1   Characteristic local necrotic lesion produced by bites of African spitting cobras and Asian cobras. In this case, the patient was bitten by a monocellate Thai cobra (*Naja kaouthia:* family Elapidae) near Chantaburi, eastern Thailand. Two days after the bite, there was a darkened anesthetic area at the site of the bite (fang marks indicated by arrows) surrounded by blisters. There was an odor of putrefaction. *(From Auerbach PS: Wilderness Medicine, 5th ed. Philadelphia, Mosby, 2007.)*

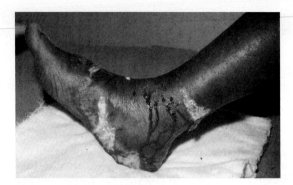

Fig. 187-2 Profuse and persistent bleeding from incisions, performed as an ill-advised first aid method after a bite by a saw-scaled viper *(Echis ocellatus)* near Gombe, Nigeria. On admission to the hospital 20 hours after the bite, the hematocrit was only 15%. *(From Auerbach PS: Wilderness Medicine, 5th ed. Philadelphia, Mosby, 2007.)*

Diagnostic Studies: Serologic tests can help in the diagnosis of diseases borne by insects and arthropods.

Macropathology: Poisonous bites can occur anywhere on the body but are most commonly seen on extremities.

Treatment: Typically, bites are managed with topical antipruritics and corticosteroids. In the case of tick bites, ticks must be carefully removed with forceps to ensure complete removal of the tick body. Many envenomations are minimal and can be treated conservatively by copious ingestion of fluids and careful monitoring for more serious symptoms. Physicians should be vigilant in monitoring vital signs after envenomations. For severe envenomations as a result of poisonous snake or spider bites, where the patient is at risk for acute complications, antivenom is recommended. However, it is important to administer the appropriate antivenom, which can only be determined if the biting species is known.

Definition: A linear polymer of the simple ethylene molecule synthesized as a fine white powder. Ethylene consists of covalently bound carbons and pendant hydrogens.

History: High-density polyethylene (HDPE) was introduced as a bearing surface in orthopedics in 1962 by Sir John Charnley from Manchester, England.

Manufacture: Polyethylene is created through polymerization of ethene. It can be produced through radical polymerization, anionic polymerization, and cationic polymerization. Powder is molded into sheets by compression molding. Electron beaming followed by annealing above the melt temperature and shaping are the next steps. Finally, the polyethylene is gas sterilized. It appears that direct molding favorably affects rate of wear but is costly. Standard, cross-linked, and Hylamer are types available to the orthopaedic surgeon.

Wear: *Tribology* is the study of lubrication and wear. All bearing surfaces result in wear to varying degrees. Wear can be divided into adhesion, abrasion, transfer, fatigue, and third body. From its inception there have always been concerns regarding the production of polyethylene debris via wear at the bearing interface. Much orthopedic research has focused on improving the performance of polyethylene and searching for alternative and more durable bearing.

Osteolysis: Resorption of bone results from the inflammatory response to polyethylene debris depending on debris size. This is the most common cause of failure of hip arthroplasty.

Reducing Wear:

Surgeon: Implant selection, alignment (impingement causes wear), and avoidance of debris, which causes 3rd body wear.

Patient: Weight reduction and reasonable activities will maximize durability of the polyethylene.

Implant Design: Conformity, especially in total knee replacement, reduces wear but increases forces at bone–prosthesis interface and may lead to loosening. Offset total hip replacement increases results by decreasing joint reaction force. Ceramic is better than cobalt chrome, yet fracture risk and expense should be considered. Proper storage prevents oxidation, and reduces failure and fatigue strength changes to the polyethylene. Thin polyethylene (<6 mm) promotes accelerated wear by delamination because of concentrated subsurface stress and fatigue wear.

Gold Standard: Simulators suggest that ceramic on molded ultra-high molecular weight polyethylene (UHMWPE) that is highly cross-linked may be the current gold standard without the potential problem of ceramic on ceramic wear, which may result in catastrophic failure. Future goals are to improve mechanical strength, decrease wear, and eliminate oxidation without remelting the polyethylene.

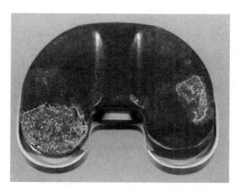

Fig. 188-1 Reinforcement of tibial polyethylene with carbon fiber often led to rapid wear and failure. *(From Canale ST, Beaty JH [eds]: Campbell's Operative Orthopaedics, 11th ed. Philadelphia, Mosby, 2007.)*

Definition: Synovial cyst located in the popliteal fossa.

Etiology: Fluid distention of the gastrocnemio-semimembranosus bursa, which is located posterior to the medial femoral condyle between the tendons of the medial head of the gastrocnemius and semimembranosus muscles. The fluid usually communicates with the joint at the posteromedial aspect of the knee capsule superior to the joint line. Arthritis is the most common condition associated with a Baker's cyst, typically osteoarthritis rather than inflammatory. Additional causes include chondromalacia patellae, chronic ligamentous or meniscal tear, chronic low-grade infection, pigmented villonodular synovitis, and persistent capsulitis. Direct trauma is the most common cause of these cysts in children.

Incidence: No racial or gender predilection has been identified. Popliteal cysts are more frequent in adults than in children.

Signs and Symptoms: The most common symptom is a mass or swelling in the popliteal fossa. Additional findings include aching, knee effusion, thrombophlebitis, clicking, buckling, and locking of the knee.

Differential Diagnosis:

Vascular: Popliteal artery aneurysm, cystic adventitial degeneration of the popliteal artery, deep vein thrombosis.

Nonvascular: Abscess, hemorrhage within a cyst, ganglion cyst, traumatic tear of gastrocnemius muscle.

Tumor: Peripheral nerve sheath tumor, myxoid liposarcoma, lipoblastoma.

Studies: The quickest, most cost effective study is an ultrasound. Baker's cysts appear as an anechoic mass with posterior acoustic enhancement. Calcified loose bodies can often be found. On computed tomography scan, a Baker's cyst appears as a fluid-containing mass but is not as sensitive as magnetic resonance imaging, which demonstrates a homogenous high signal intensity on all sequences. Addition of intra-articular gadolinium is the most vivid way to display a popliteal cyst.

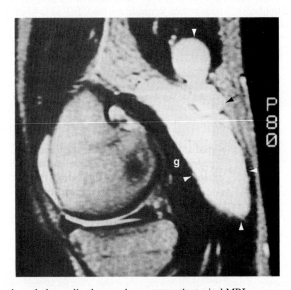

Fig. 189-1   Image through the popliteal space demonstrates the typical MRI appearance of synovial cysts. *(From DeLee D, Drez D [eds]: DeLee and Drez's Orthopaedic Sports Medicine, 2nd ed. Philadelphia, Saunders 2003.)*

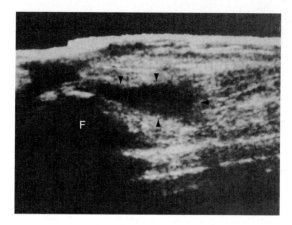

Fig. 189-2   Sonography of a popliteal cyst. Sagittal sonographic section through the popliteal space in this patient demonstrates a sonolucent fluid collection *(arrowheads)* posterior and inferior to the medial femoral condyle (F). *(From DeLee D, Drez D [eds]: DeLee and Drez's Orthopaedic Sports Medicine, 2nd ed. Philadelphia, Saunders, 2003.)*

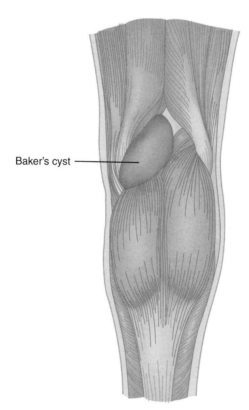

Baker's cyst

Fig. 189-3   Baker's cyst is an extension of the semimembranosus bursa posteriorly. This bursa often is connected with a joint cavity. *(From Marx J: Rosen's Emergency Medicine: Concepts and Clinical Practice, 6th ed. Philadelphia, Saunders.)*

Treatment: Initial treatment of Baker's cysts includes nonsteroidal anti-inflammatory agents, ice, and assisted weight bearing. Treatment of the underlying disorder may help resolve the cyst, including quadriceps strength training for patellofemoral syndrome. Joint replacement may be needed in cases of severe osteoarthritis. In some cases, venous sclerosant is used to prevent recurrence. The cysts tend to involute spontaneously in children. Needle aspiration of the cyst is an effective therapy and, depending on the predisposing cause of the cyst, generally results in a cure.

Surgical Treatment: Sansone and colleagues reported good clinical results in 95% of 30 patients who had arthroscopic treatment for a popliteal cyst and associated intra-articular pathology at 32-months' follow-up. If the cyst does not appear to communicate or if significant changes cannot be treated arthroscopically, an open procedure is indicated. Most cysts can be approached by a posteromedial (Henderson) incision.

Complications: The most common complication is the rupture or dissection of fluid into adjacent muscle belly, which often results in pseudothrombophlebitis syndrome mimicking symptoms of deep vein thrombosis (DVT). Incidence of cyst rupture is 3.4% to 10%. Baker's cyst may be a risk factor for DVT secondary to compression of the popliteal vein. Posterior compartment syndrome usually is caused by trauma but can also occur from a Baker's cyst. Infected cysts are rare; increased white blood cell count, fever, and elevated erythrocyte sedimentation rate help make the diagnosis.

Definition: The stretching or tearing of the posterior tibial tendon, resulting in adult acquired flatfoot deformity.

Anatomy: The tibialis posterior muscle originates at the posterior tibia and fibula. It inserts at the navicular, cuneiforms, cuboid, and bases of the second, third, and fourth metatarsals. It plantarflexes the ankle and inverts the subtalar joint.

Epidemiology: Posterior tibial tendon dysfunction (PTTD) is the primary cause of acquired flatfoot in adults. It is more common in obese, middle-age women.

Etiology: The main causes of PTTD are age-related overuse and degeneration and trauma. In cases of trauma, the common sites of rupture are proximal to the medial malleolus or at its insertion on the navicular.

Dysfunction of posterior tibial tendon may result from tenosynovitis of tendinosis. Symptoms include pain and swelling over course of tendon, and loss of tendon function results in loss of longitudinal arch

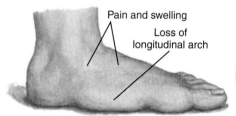

Pain and swelling

Loss of longitudinal arch

Medial view of pronated foot reveals flattened longitudinal arch

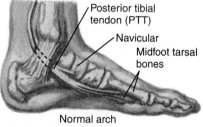

Posterior tibial tendon (PTT)

Navicular

Midfoot tarsal bones

Normal arch

Insertion of posterior tibial tendon extends beyond navicular to all midtarsal bones of foot and is the major supporting structure of midfoot

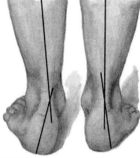

PTT dysfunction   Normal

Posterior view reveals hyperpronation in left foot. In normal foot, midlines of calcaneus and leg are aligned or deviate less than 2°.

JOHN A.CRAIG—AD

Standing. In the standing position, increased heel valgus and "too many lateral toes" may be observed on posterior view

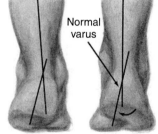

Normal varus

PTT dysfunction   Normal

Heel rise. On toe standing, normal PTT function pulls heel into varus. PTT dysfunction allows heel to remain in valgus position

Fig. 190-1 Posterior tibial dysfunction *(From Greene WB: Netter's Orthopaedics. Philadelphia, Saunders, 2006.)*

Symptoms: Early symptoms are pain and swelling at the medial foot and ankle and difficulty standing on tiptoes. Later symptoms are a flatfoot deformity due to collapse of the medial longitudinal arch and lateral pain as the fibula impinges against the calcaneus.

Physical Examination: Patients present with tenderness and swelling at the posteromedial ankle and foot. They are either unable to perform a single limb heel rise test or can do so with pain. The deformity that develops is pes planovalgus with subtalar joint eversion, hindfoot valgus, midfoot abduction, and pes planus. The fourth and fifth toes become visible while the patient is standing and facing away from the examiner, and is known as the "too many toes" sign.

Imaging: Anteroposterior radiographs show lateral subluxation of the talonavicular joint and an increased talo–first metatarsal angle. Lateral weight-bearing radiographs show an abnormal talo–first metatarsal (Meary's) angle with the talus plantarflexed, collapse of the longitudinal arch, and sag at the talonavicular, navicular-cuneiform, and metatarsal-cuneiform joints. As the disease worsens, the talonavicular, calcaneocuboid, subtalar, and tibiotalar joints develop arthritis.

Classification:

Stage I: Tendon degeneration with its normal length preserved. Patients present with medial foot and ankle pain and swelling, and mild weakness. They can perform a normal single limb heel rise, but with pain.

Stage II: Tendon is incompetent or ruptured. Patients exhibit a flexible flatfoot deformity and the "too many toes" sign. They cannot perform a single limb heel rise.

Stage III: Flatfoot deformity becomes fixed. Hindfoot and midfoot show arthritis.

Stage IV: Patients develop deltoid ligament dysfunction and/or tibiotalar degeneration.

Treatment:

Stage I: Nonoperative treatment is attempted. This involves short leg immobilization, physical therapy, and nonsteroidal anti-inflammatory drugs. If these measures are unsuccessful for 3 to 4 months, surgical synovectomy and PTT débridement, repair, and tenodesis to the flexor digitorum longus (FDL) tendon is performed.

Stage II: Nonoperative treatment can be tried but often fails. Surgical treatment involves PTT reconstruction with an FDL transfer to the navicular and a medializing calcaneal osteotomy with or without lateral column lengthening.

Stage III: Nonoperative treatment rarely helps. Surgical treatment is a triple (subtalar, talonavicular, and calcaneocuboid) arthrodesis.

Stage IV: Nonoperative treatment rarely helps. Surgical treatment is a tibiotalocalcaneal (TTC) or pantalar fusion.

Definition: Proximal femoral focal deficiency (PFFD) is a developmental disturbance in the proximal femur that results in a failure of formation or differentiation of the proximal femur and associated acetabulum.

Incidence: 1:50000 live births.

Age: PFFD is a birth defect.

Etiology and Pathophysiology: A tranquilizer, thalidomide, is the only known cause. Radiation, ischemia, chemicals, hormones, bacterial toxins, viral infections, and mechanical and thermal injuries are all suspected causes.

Clinical Presentation: PFFD manifests as a shortened, flexed, abducted, and externally rotated thigh. PFFD may be bilateral or unilateral. It often manifests with fibular aplasia/hypoplasia and lateral foot abnormalities. Contralateral limb abnormalities, unstable knee due to a cruciate deficiency, missing or small and high-riding patella, shortened tibia and fibula, and a dislocated patellofemoral joint may also be present.

Pathology: The proximal femoral growth plate has chondrocyte abnormalities.

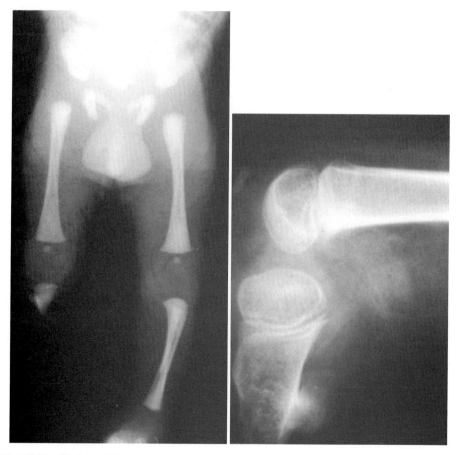

Fig. 191-1   Newborn with congenital amputation through proximal tibia. *(Courtesy of Robert N. Hensinger, MD. From Canale ST, Beaty JH [eds]: Campbell's Operative Orthopaedics, 11th ed. Philadelphia, Mosby.)*

Diagnostic Procedures: The deformity is usually noticed by inspection during clinical examination. Radiology may also be used to diagnose PFFD.

Treatment: The treatment varies with the classification. The goal in treating PFFD is to stabilize the femur and pelvis and to provide a stable basis for ambulation. Type A is typically treated by a proximal femoral osteotomy to correct the varus deformity. Type B may be treated by a proximal femoral osteotomy followed by a knee fusion and a rotationplasty, often Van Ness, for fitting of a below-knee prosthesis. Types C and D often require creative prosthetic applications.

Table 191-1. CLASSIFICATION (AITKEN)	
Type A	A gap is present between the proximal and distal femur. This gap will ossify eventually. The femur lengths are unequal and there is severe subtrochanteric varus.
Type B	Both the femoral head and acetabulum are hypoplastic and the femoral gaps will not ossify. The femoral shaft is deformed and short.
Type C	The femoral head is absent with marked dysplasia and consequent proximal migration of the shortened femur. The acetabulum is dysplastic.
Type D	The femoral head and acetabulum are absent. The femoral shaft is deformed and shortened.

Aitken GT: Proximal femoral focal deficiency. In Limb Development and Deformity: Problems of Evaluation and Rehabilitation. Springfield, Ill, Charles C Thomas, 1969.

Definition: Complete/partial split or dislocation of the radial head. The radial head is intra-articular and moves in both flexion and extension as well as with forearm rotation.

Etiology: Radial head fractures are most frequently caused by direct longitudinal loading after a trauma such as falling on an outstretched hand. The force of impact is transmitted up the hand through the wrist and forearm to the radial head, which is forced into the capitellum. Injuries that can cause elbow dislocations can also result in radial head fractures. Congenital dislocation of the radial head includes the following findings: bilateral involvement, familial occurrence, irreducible by closed means, hypoplastic capitellum, short ulna with long radius and convex radial head.

Anatomy: The radial head can be found in the lesser sigmoid notch. The radial head maintains contact with the ulna throughout forearm pronation and supination and force transmission is found at all angles, although it is greatest in full extension. The radial head also contributes to valgus stability when tested in laboratory settings. The elbow joint is constrained by the medial lateral collateral ligaments. The radioulnar joint is constrained by the annular ligament.

Frequency: The radial head is fractured in about 20% of cases of elbow trauma. Thirty-three percent of elbow fractures and dislocations include injury to the radial head and/or neck; 60% of congenital dislocations occur with malformation syndromes or connective tissue disorders.

Symptoms: Typically, isolated fractures of the radial head cause pain on the lateral side of the elbow, which is aggravated by forearm rotation. Motion may elicit crepitus around the elbow or mechanical block may be present. Swelling may be present around the elbow and any pain or swelling around the wrist should be further worked up for fracture, radioulnar dissociation, or ligamentous injury. A high suspicion for nerve injury should be suspected, particularly radial nerve palsies.

Classification: Mason classification of radial head fractures is based on degree of displacement or comminution (Table 192-1).

Diagnostic Studies: Most radial head fractures can be assessed with standard plain radiography. Two views perpendicular are required to adequately assess most fractures. For the normal elbow, a line drawn through the radial head and shaft should always line up with the capitellum, and with a supinated lateral view, lines drawn tangential to the head anteriorly and posteriorly should enclose the capitellum. If a fat pad sign is present without a noticeable fracture, radiocapitellar views may be helpful. This view is taken with the forearm in neutral rotation and x-ray tube angled 45 degrees cephalad.

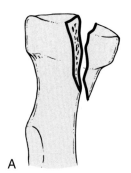 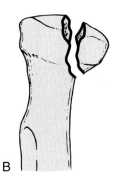 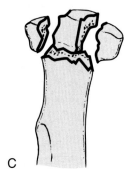

A   B   C

Fig. 192-1 Classification system of Schatzker and Tile for radial head fractures. **A,** Type I: wedge. This fracture may be displaced or nondisplaced. **B,** Type II: impaction. Part of the head and neck remains intact. The fracture is tilted and impacted, and comminution is variable. **C,** Type III: severely comminuted. No portion of the head and neck remains in continuity; comminution is severe. *(From Browner BD: Skeletal Trauma: Basic Science, Management, and Reconstruction, 3rd ed. Philadelphia, Saunders, 2003.)*

Table 192-1.	MASON CLASSIFICATION OF RADIAL HEAD FRACTURES IS BASED ON DEGREE OF DISPLACEMENT OR COMMINUTION
Type I	Nondisplaced or minimally displaced fracture of head or neck Forearm rotation is limited only by acute pain and swelling Intra-articular displacement of the fracture is less than 2 mm
Type II	Displaced fracture (greater than 2 mm) of head or neck Motion may be mechanically limited or incongruous Without severe comminution Fracture involves more than a marginal lip of the radial head
Type III	Severely comminuted fracture of the radial head and neck Not reconstructable Requires excision for movement

Treatment: Nonsurgical treatment for type I and minimally displaced type II fractures include sling immobilization and early active motion. Function typically returns after 2 to 3 months. Closed reduction treatments for type II injuries are advocated when the fracture involves less than one third of the articular surface, less than 30 degrees of angulation, and less than 3 mm of displacement. Surgical intervention is indicated for displaced, comminuted, open fractures or those that demonstrate a mechanical block to movement. Surgical treatment includes self-compressing screws (Herbert, Acutrak) and miniplates. In cases of severe comminution, excision of the radial head and possible replacement with metal or silicone replacements are available.

Complications: Radial head fractures may often be complicated by additional injuries. A Monteggia fracture is an ulna fracture in the proximal one third with associated radial head dislocation. An Essex-Lopresti fracture involves disruption of the distal radial ulnar joint, associated with a radial head fracture and tear in the interosseous ligament. This fracture is at risk for proximal migration of the radius with radial head excision.

Hans Conrad Julius Reiter (1881-1969), a German bacteriologist, treated his first patient suffering from a disease marked by urethritis, conjunctivitis, and arthritis in World War I and published reports of his discoveries in 1916. He discovered the causative organism of Weil's disease; he named and investigated *Treponema pallidum*, described symptoms of digitalis intoxication, and wrote about the use of vaccines.

Definition: Spondyloarthropathy (ankylosing spondylitis, Reiter's, psoriatic arthritis, inflammatory bowel disease)

Incidence: 3.5/100,000, estimated less than 200,000 in the United States.

Etiology: Occurs 3 weeks after initiating event, such as infection with, for example, *Chlamydia, Salmonella, Shigella, Campylobacter,* or *Yersinia*.

Pathogenesis: Incompletely known.

- 100 to 200 times more frequent in HIV-positive population; 5% to 10% prevalence
- Oligoarticular, predisposition for lower extremities, Achilles tendonitis
- Amino acid sequences shared b/t HLA-B27, *Klebsiella pneumoniae, Shigella*
- European variant includes diarrhea instead of urethritis; pathogenesis involves *Salmonella, Shigella,* and *Yersinia*

Age: Young adults, 20 to 40 years old

Gender: Male-to-female ratio 5:1

Race: White

Signs and Symptoms:

- "Can't see, pee, or climb a tree"
- Conjunctivitis early (before arthritis), mild, painless nongonococcal urethritis (NGU)/cervicitis, asymmetrical arthritis of large joints (<6 weeks, involves knees, ankles), uveitis, skin lesions (keratoderma blennorrhagicum— hard, tender lumps and scaly patches/pustules on soles and fronts of legs), balanitis circinata, sacroiliitis, spondylitis, enthesopathy, dactylitis "sausage digits" (uncommon, but specific), "lover's heel"—calcaneus.

Associations:

- MHC I, HLA-B27
- Urogenital infection in 90%; enteric infection in 50%
- Predilection for metatarsophalangeal joints and first interphalangeal joint over the distal/proximal interphalangeal joint

Diagnosis: Polymerase chain reaction, chest x-ray study.

Imaging periostitis, ill-defined erosions, bilateral asymmetrical distribution, joint space narrowing, fusiform soft tissue swelling, beaklike nonmarginal syndesmophytes, exuberant periostitis/heel

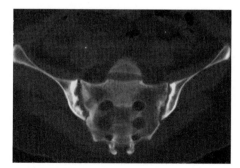

Fig. 193-1 CT scanning in reactive arthritis. An oblique axial image through the sacroiliac joints shows erosions with associated new bone formation predominating in the iliac bones. *(From Harris ED Jr: Kelley's Textbook of Rheumatology, 7th ed. Philadelphia, Saunders.)*

Treatment:
- Nonsteroidal anti-inflammatory drugs, steroids, disease-modifying antirheumatic drugs
- Consider phenylbutazone, sulfasalazine for HIV-positive patients; do *not* give MTX, as may exacerbate the immunosuppressive effects of HIV
- Antibiotics not proven to treat chronic/latent infection in mouse model
- 1g azithromycin by mouth or 100 mg doxycycline by mouth twice a day for 7 days. If pregnant: erythromycin or amoxicillin.
- Centers for Disease Control and Prevention recommends screening for chlamydial infection in women younger than 25 years old and those at high risk
- Consider workup and treatment for gonococcal joint sepsis

Prognosis: Good; 20% have chronic symptoms.

Definition: Rheumatoid arthritis is an autoimmune disease causing chronic inflammation, primarily of the joints, but also of tissues and various body organs.

Incidence: Affects more than 2 two million people in the United States each year.

Age: Most commonly symptoms begin between the ages of 40 and 60 years old.

Gender: Three times more common in women than in men.

Race: No racial preference.

Etiology and Pathophysiology: The immune system activates lymphocytes, which cause cytokines to be expressed at the affected area, causing pain and inflammation.

Associations: Caused by infection or environmental factors. The disease has also been linked to genetic inheritance.

Signs and Symptoms: Signs that suggest rheumatoid arthritis include edema, redness, and sensitivity in the affected area. Symptoms include muscle aches, joint pain, joint stiffness, lack of appetite, fatigue, and fever.

Diagnostic Studies: Diagnosis is made by reviewing the history of symptoms, examining the patient, and obtaining blood test results. X-rays are also used to confirm the presence of the disease and monitor patient progress. The disease is either inactive, when the patient may experience no symptoms, or active, when the patient is experiencing a "flare" and has the symptoms previously mentioned.

Micropathology: The synovium is inflamed due to the expression of cytokines causing the tissue to thicken and produce excess synovial fluid.

Macropathology: Edema and redness occur. Firm protuberances under the skin called *rheumatoid nodules* may occur in areas of frequent pressure, such as the fingers and elbows.

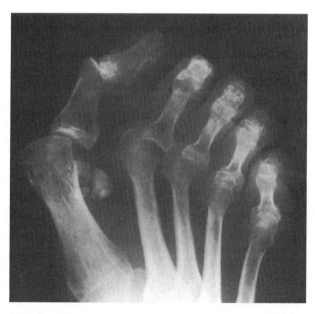

Fig. 194-1   Classic forefoot deformities of rheumatoid arthritis. *(From Resnick D, Niwayama G: Diagnosis of Bone and Joint Disorders. Philadelphia, WB Saunders, 1988.)*

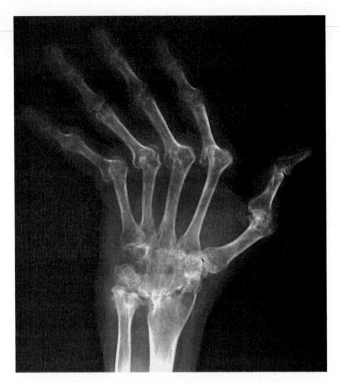

Fig. 194-2 Ulnar deviation in rheumatoid arthritis. Severe ulnar deviation is present at the metacarpopha-langeal joints with extensive erosions. Pancompartmental bony ankylosis and erosion are also seen in the wrist. *(From Harris ED Jr: Kelley's Textbook of Rheumatology, 7th ed. Philadelphia, Saunders, 2005.)*

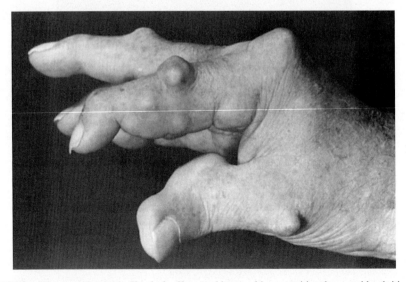

Fig. 194-3 Rheumatoid arthritis. Hand of a 60-year-old man with seropositive rheumatoid arthritis. There are fixed deformities and gross rheumatoid nodules. *(From Canoso JJ: Rheumatology in Primary Care, Philadelphia, WB Saunders, 1997.)*

Treatment: Nonsteroidal anti-inflammatory drugs and corticosteroids reduce inflammation, whereas more aggressive drugs, called disease-modifying anti-rheumatic drugs, or DMARDs, are used to prevent progressive damage to bone, cartilage, and surrounding tissues. Regular exercise is crucial in building muscle to relieve pressure on the diseased areas, and devices such as braces and canes may provide some assistance. Surgical intervention may include arthroscopic surgery or full or partial replacement surgeries in the case of a severely damaged joint.

Definition: Rickets is the inadequate calcification of osteoid into mature bone. Calcification involves the formation of hydroxyapatite crystals.

Incidence: In the United States, mild nutritional rickets still affects high-risk populations; however, severe nutritional rickets is now rare. The incidence of hypophosphatemic rickets, also known as *vitamin D–resistant rickets,* is rare and unknown.

Age: Rickets occurs during growth phase. However, when it occurs in adults, it is called *osteomalacia,* which means bone softening.

Gender: Even though vitamin D–resistant rickets causes lowered phosphate levels in both males and females, the calcification of osteoid is more prohibited in males.

Etiology and Pathophysiology: There are two major causes of rickets: nutritional deficiencies and the genetic disorder hypophosphatemia, which causes vitamin D–resistant rickets. Nutritional rickets can be caused by nutritional deficiencies in vitamin D, calcium, or phosphate, or by malabsorption of these nutrients. Vitamin D–resistant rickets is caused by phosphate loss in the proximal tubules of the kidneys. Both genetic hypophosphatemia and nutritional deficiencies of vitamin D, calcium, and phosphate prevent the formation of hydroxyapatite crystals.

Clinical Presentation: Rickets is most evident in the bowing of weight-bearing long bones, especially the femur and the tibia. The limb deformity can be genu varum or valgum. It may also cause a short stature, skeletal deformities, widened joint spaces, delayed dentition, and bone pain.

Pathology: The gross appearance of rickets is of widened and cupped metaphyses with a periosteum that appears separated from the diaphysis. Osteopenia and coarse trabeculae are observable.

Diagnostic Procedures: Radiographs of the wrist, knee, and long bones can determine the presence of rickets. Blood samples and urine samples can be used to determine the cause of rickets. Blood samples should be taken to test for levels of vitamin D, calcium, phosphate, creatinine, alkaline phosphates, parathyroid hormone, plasma bicarbonate, and magnesium. Urine samples should be tested for levels of calcium, phosphate, and creatinine. Vitamin D–resistant rickets can be diagnosed by calculating the renal tubular phosphate reabsorption.

Treatment: Nutritional rickets can be improved with supplementation, usually vitamin D supplements. Medications that enhance calcium reabsorption can be used to treat X-linked hypophosphatemic rickets. When treated early, most deformities are corrected through growth; however, an osteotomy may be needed in order to realign severely deformed bones.

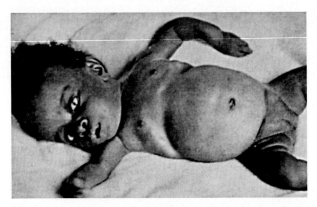

Fig. 195-1   Deformities in rickets showing curvature of the limbs, potbelly, and Harrison groove. (*From Kliegman RM, Behrman RE, Jenson HB, Stanton BF: Nelson Textbook of Pediatrics, 18th ed. Philadelphia, Saunders, 2004.*)

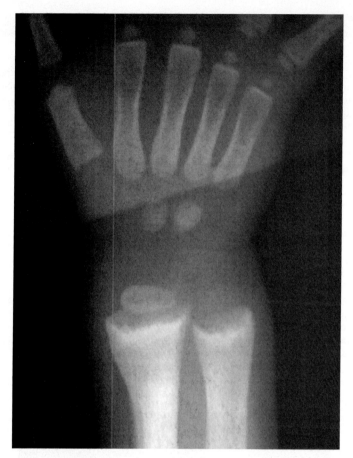

Fig. 195-2 The child with rickets has metaphyseal fraying and cupping of the distal radius and ulna. *(From Kliegman RM, Behrman RE, Jenson HB, Stanton BF: Nelson Textbook of Pediatrics, 18th ed. Philadelphia, Saunders, 2004.)*

Definition: Tears to the rotator cuff are a common cause of pain, weakness, and decreased range of motion to the shoulder joint. Ninety percent of tears result from years of repetitive, overhead activities. Acute injuries to the rotator cuff do take place, occurring during falls or while catching and throwing heavy objects. In the case of chronic tears, the mechanism of insult is impingement of the cuff tendon, leading to microtrauma. Swelling, edema, and tissue softening occur, leading to further impingement until the rotator cuff tendon tears.

Prevalence: Rotator cuff tears are more prevalent in the demographic 40 years of age and older or in athletes participating in sports with repetitive, overhead motions such as swimming, volleyball, tennis, and baseball.

Age: With the exception of certain athletic sports, rotator cuff tears are age related. Studies have shown that asymptomatic patients undergoing magnetic resonance imaging (MRI) studies have revealed partial or full thickness tears in 4% of patients younger than 40 years of age but in 54% in those older than 60 years of age.

Gender: Gender does not appear to be a predictor of rotator cuff tears. However, women 65 and older seem to have worse surgical outcomes than males of the same demographic.

Signs and Symptoms: Symptoms include nonspecific, localized, shoulder pain. Additionally, pain can occur with the arm placed above the head or at night when lying on the affected shoulder, and pain can be worsened by activity. *Note:* Subacromial bursitis and rotator cuff tendonitis can cause similar types of pain. Shoulder weakness and decreased range of motion are both positive signs for a rotator cuff tear.

Physical Examination: Findings may include maximum tenderness over the insertion of the supraspinatus tendon on the greater tubercle of the humerus. Full assessment of the cervical nerves innervating rotator cuff muscles is essential. Positive signs during specific tests may indicate a tear and suggest the need for further imaging studies.

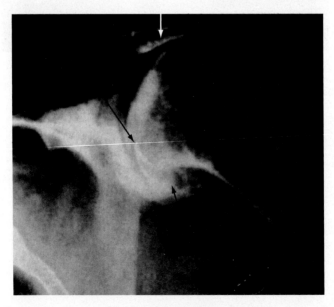

Fig. 196-1 X-ray: arrows show loss of joint space from rotator cuff arthropathy. *(From Canale ST: Campbell's Operative Orthopaedics, 10th ed. Philadelphia, Mosby, 2003.)*

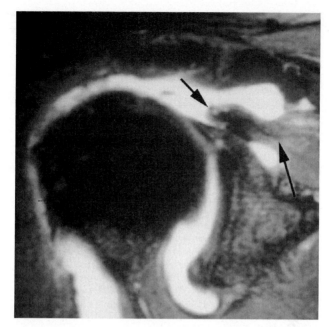

Fig. 196-2 Complete rotator cuff tear with musculotendinous retraction, magnetic resonance imaging. Oblique coronal T_2-weighted MR image demonstrates a complete tear of the supraspinatus tendon (*short arrow*), with marked retraction of the musculoskeletal junction (*long arrow*). A chronic rotator cuff tear is present in this patient with a high-riding humeral head and large joint effusion. (*From DeLee D, Drez D: DeLee and Drez's Orthopaedic Sports Medicine, 2nd ed. Philadelphia, Saunders.*)

Specific Rotator Cuff Pathology Tests:
- Neer Impingement Sign—with scapula stabilized, arm is forward flexed passively; anterior or lateral pain in the range of 90 to 140 degrees is a positive sign for tear.
- Hawkins-Kennedy Impingement Sign—with arm in 90 degrees of forward flexion, patient's arm is internally rotated; pain with internal rotation is a positive sign.
- Painful Arc Sign—arm is abducted as far as possible; positive result if patient has pain from 60 to 120 degrees.
- Cross-Body Adduction Test—with arm in 90 degrees of forward flexion, examiner adducts arm across body; pain with adduction is a positive sign.
- Drop Arm Test—patient slowly elevates arm and reverses motion; if the arm drops suddenly or pain occurs, the test is considered positive.

Diagnostic Studies: Radiographic views of the shoulder may show a narrowing of the subacromial space or a spur on the undersurface of the acromion. However, the definitive studies for diagnosing rotator cuff tear are MRI, MRI arthrogram, and ultrasound.

Classifications: Damage to the rotator cuff is classified by extent of the tear. The supraspinatus tendon is the most frequently torn. Partial tears are twice as common as full thickness tears and involve the inferior aspect of the tendon. Partial thickness tears tend to be the result of trauma; this is especially true in younger patients. Full thickness tears usually require surgical intervention.

Classification of Tears:
- Group I—partial thickness tears
- Group II—full thickness tears involving the entire supraspinatus
- Group III—full thickness tears involving more than one tendon
- Group IV—massive tears with secondary osteoarthritis

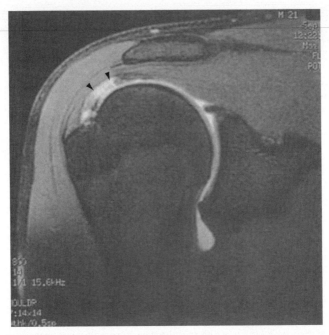

Fig. 196-3 MRI arthrogram: Professional pitcher with partial tear of the supraspinatus. *(From Harris ED Jr: Kelley's Textbook of Rheumatology, 7th ed. Philadelphia, Saunders, 2005.)*

Treatment: Initially, management of rotator cuff injury employs conservative measures. Activity modification, anti-inflammatory medication, and physical therapy are all directed at regaining normal function of the rotator cuff tendons to improve glenohumeral mechanics. Corticosteroids are injected subacromially if conservative treatment does not improve patient condition. Once conservative measures fail (attempted for at least 3 months), surgical intervention is required. An anterior acromioplasty is performed to alleviate compression of the rotator cuff. The cuff is then mobilized and the degenerated margins of the tendons are débrided. The edges are sutured into the bone at their insertion to restore function. Postoperatively, a shoulder immobilizer is worn for up to 6 weeks and rehabilitation is required to regain strength and range of motion.

Complications: Failure to repair a torn rotator cuff will result in deterioration of the shoulder joint. Complications during repair are more common with large and massive tears and are more likely to tear a second time after reattachment. Postoperatively, anterior instability and weakness with internal and external rotation can occur because of transposition of any one of the rotator cuff muscles. Stiffness from immobilization and persistent night pain may be present even after surgical repair. Eighty percent of patients undergoing surgical rotator cuff repair have complete pain relief and return to normal function.

Definition: Fracture involving the bony sacrum.

Etiology: Most commonly from a traumatic loading force. Usually from a fall or motor vehicle accident.

Incidence: Occurs in 30% of all pelvic ring fractures. Accounts for approximately 1% of all spinal fractures.

Gender: No preponderance.

Symptoms: Pain, neurologic deficit (up to 40%), trauma patients should be carefully examined for sacral root dysfunction, which is suggested by decreased perianal sensation and rectal sphincter disturbance. Decreased ankle jerk reflexes and absence of a bulbocavernosus reflex also may suggest sacral root injury.

Classification: Denis Classification:

Zone 1:
Alar—lateral to the foramina, associated with 6% neurologic injury with the L5 nerve root most common.

Zone 2:
Transforaminal—with an associated 28% risk of neurologic injury unilateral to L5, S1, and S2.

Zone 3:
Central Sacral Canal—medial to the foramina and involves the central sacral canal. Associated with 56% neurologic injury.

Diagnostic Studies: Because transverse sacral fractures may be missed on pelvic radiographs and computed tomography scans, a lateral radiograph of the sacrum is the preferred view for identifying these fractures.

Treatment: Conservative management with protected weight bearing for stable, minimally displaced fractures without neurologic injury. This includes bedrest for 2 to 3 months. Surgical decompression indicated in the presence of neurologic injury or sacral deformity and fracture fragments resulting in neural compression. Open reduction and internal fixation for fractures displaced greater than 1 cm are recommended. Sacroiliac screws—use fully threaded screws to avoid over compression, especially in zone 2 injuries. Sacral laminectomy allows for exploration of nerve roots. Posterior tension band plating and transiliac sacral bars have also been reported.

Complications: Pain and neurologic injury. Transverse sacral fractures may also develop late kyphotic deformities. Additionally, neural compression may compromise genital, bladder, anal, and rectal functions.

Definition: Most commonly fractured bone in the carpus. Diagnosis of a scaphoid (also known as the carpal "navicular") fracture is frequently delayed, which may ultimately alter the prognosis for union.

Etiology: Usually results from a fall onto the outstretched hand (FOOSH) that results in forceful dorsiflexion and impaction of the scaphoid against the dorsal rim of the radius. Contact sports such as football are also frequent causes of scaphoid injury, as are high-energy injuries associated with motor vehicle accidents.

Associations: No known correlation exists between race and scaphoid fractures. Scaphoid injuries are most commonly associated with a younger, athletic population. This injury is rarely seen in children, however, because they more often suffer injuries to the distal radius.

Incidence: In the upper extremity, the incidence of fractures of the scaphoid is second only to that of fractures of the distal radius. Fractures of the scaphoid account for 11% of hand fractures and 60% of carpal fractures.

Age and Gender: In an epidemiologic study from Norway, it was found that 82% of scaphoid fractures occurred in males, with the highest incidence occurring between the ages of 20 and 30 years.

Clinical Findings: Tenderness with palpation over the scaphoid tubercle and anatomic snuff-box and tenderness with longitudinal compression are physical findings that have been shown to have a diagnostic sensitivity of 100% during the initial evaluation of scaphoid fractures.

Symptoms: Patients often complain of radial sided wrist pain, exacerbated by wrist motion. Grip strength is often decreased.

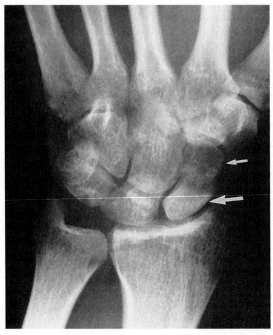

Fig. 198-1 Scaphoid or navicular fracture of the wrist of a patient who fell on his outstretched hand. A later complication shows aseptic necrosis of the proximal fragment (*large arrow*). Note that this fragment has maintained normal mineralization because the blood supply has been interrupted. In contrast, the remainder of the carpal bones demonstrate loss of calcium due to hyperemia and disuse after the fracture. (*From Mettler FA, Jr: Essentials of Radiology, 2nd ed. Philadelphia, Saunders, 2005.*)

Signs: Range of motion may be reduced and swelling around the radial and posterior aspects of the wrist is common.

Diagnostic Studies: With a suspected scaphoid injury, a scaphoid series (including a posteroanterior view with the wrist in ulnar deviation in addition to anteroposterior, lateral, and oblique views) is useful. Comparison views of the contralateral wrist may be necessary. If plain films are equivocal, a variety of other modalities including technetium bone scan, computed tomography, magnetic resonance imaging and ultrasound are useful.

Treatment: For nondisplaced fractures, a long arm thumb spica cast with the wrist in slight palmar flexion and radial deviation for 6 weeks, followed by the use of a short arm thumb spica cast until clinical and radiographic healing takes place is an acceptable treatment plan. Open reduction and internal fixation (ORIF) is indicated for displaced, angulated, or comminuted fractures. Percutaneous fixation and compression screw fixation to prevent malunion are options for ORIF. Nonunion of scaphoid fractures is influenced by delayed diagnosis, gross displacement, associated injuries of the carpus, and impaired blood supply. Nonunions may be treated by radial styloidectomy, excision of the proximal fragment, proximal row carpectomy, traditional bone grafting, and total or partial wrist arthrodesis.

Primary Scapular Winging

Neurologic Disorders
Trapezius Winging
- Due to injury of the spinal accessory nerve (CN XI) by blunt/penetrating trauma or traction
- Can be caused iatrogenically during surgical biopsy of cervical lymph nodes or radical neck dissection
- Manifests with shoulder depression, lateral scapular translation, and lateral rotation of the inferior angle of the scapula
- Patients often have trapezius wasting, inability to shrug the shoulder, weakness with forward elevation and abduction of the arm, and pain and spasm due to attempts at compensation

Treatment:
- For blunt trauma or traction, physical therapy to maintain glenohumeral motion and prevent frozen shoulder. Electromyogram (EMG) at 3 months and then serially at 6-week intervals to follow nerve recovery.
- For penetrating trauma, consider neurolysis/nerve grafting if no nerve function is found on EMG. Results are variable, but results are better if procedure is performed within 6 months of injury.
- For persistent winging, patients with debilitating symptoms for more than 1 year are unlikely to improve without surgery.
  - *Static Stabilization:* Scapulothoracic fusion (limits motion)
  - Fascial sling procedures (tend to fail)

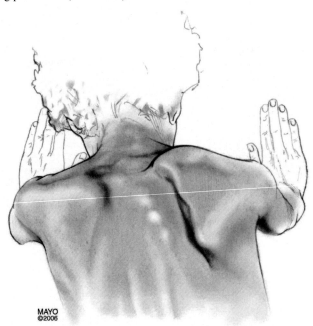

Fig. 199-1 Winging of the right scapula with forward flexion of the extended arms due to injury of the long thoracic nerve. Note the upward displacement of the scapula with prominence of the vertebral border and medial displacement of the inferior angle. *(Reprinted with permission of Mayo Foundation for Medical Education and Research. © Mayo Foundation, 2007. From Frontera WR: Essentials of Physical Medicine and Rehabilitation, 2nd ed. Philadelphia, Saunders.)*

414

- *Dynamic Stabilization:* Muscle transfers are the procedure of choice
- Eden-Lange procedure (most commonly performed)
- Lateral transfer of the scapular attachments of the levator scapulae, rhomboideus major, and rhomboideus minor, which substitute for the upper, middle, and lower thirds of the trapezius muscle

Serratus Anterior Winging
- Results from injury to the long thoracic nerve (C5-7)
- Can be caused iatrogenically during radical mastectomy, first rib resection, or axillary lymph node dissection
- Manifests with shoulder elevation, medial scapular translation, and medial rotation of the inferior angle
- Difficulty and pain with elevation of the arm above 120 degrees; attempts at arm elevation increase the degree of winging
- Severe pain may suggest Parsonage-Turner syndrome

Treatment:
- *Early:* Similar to that for trapezius winging (mostly conservative)
- *Late:* Static and dynamic, with muscle transfer procedures preferred
  - Marmor-Bechtol procedure (most commonly performed)
  - Transfer of sternocostal head of pectoralis major to inferior angle of scapula

Rhomboideus Major/Minor Winging
- Results from injury to the dorsal scapular nerve (C5)
- Much less common
- Winging usually minimal at rest; accentuated by lowering arm from elevated position (lateral winging as with trapezius)

Treatment:
- Treated with trapezius strengthening with fascial sling operations described for chronic cases
- *Osseous Causes:* Osteochondromas (most common scapular tumor) and malunion of scapular fractures
- *Muscular Causes:* Traumatic avulsions or congential absence of periscapular muscles
- *Bursal Causes:* Scapulothoracic bursa inflammation; snapping scapula

Secondary Scapular Winging

- Pain or limitation of glenohumeral motion, causing abnormal scapulothoracic mechanics
- Can be seen with contracture after obstetric palsy, deltoid fibrosis, or common conditions such as cuff tears, frozen shoulder, or impingement/tendinitis

Voluntary Scapular Winging

- Very rare
- Treat nonoperatively
- Consider underlying psychiatric issues

Definition: Scheuermann's disease is a developmental disorder that causes patients to have a stooped forward or bent-over posture as a result of excessive kyphosis of the thoracic spine.

Incidence: This condition affects between 0.5% and 8% of the general population

Age: Affects mostly teenage boys.

Gender: It is more common in males and appears in adolescents, usually toward the end of their growth spurt.

Etiology and Pathophysiology: The etiology of Scheuermann's disease is unknown, but is thought to be due to a growth abnormality of the vertebral body. The growth plate anteriorly stops growing but the posterior part of the growth plate continues to grow. This is due to a condition known as *osteochondrosis*.

Associations: Most patients with Scheuermann's also have a mild scoliosis.

Sign and Symptoms: Because Scheuermann's disease occurs during periods of bone growth, it often first appears in adolescence at the time of puberty. Parents typically bring their child in to see the doctor with a complaint of poor posture or slouching, sometimes with sporadic occurrences of fatigue and mild pain in the thoracic area of the spine. In severe cases, patients may have other symptoms, including pain, a rigid curve of the spine that gets worse when bending forward and only partially corrects itself when standing, coexistent scoliosis, chest pain, or, in rare circumstances, difficulty breathing caused by decreased lung capacity.

Diagnostic Studies: The diagnosis of Scheuermann's disease is made on the basis of a physical examination and radiographs of the spine. A physical examination is used to determine where the apex of the curve is located, where the patient is experiencing back pain, and how flexible the curve is. Currently, the most commonly accepted criteria for the radiographic diagnosis of Scheuermann's disease is the presence of at least 5 degrees of vertebral body wedging over three adjacent levels.

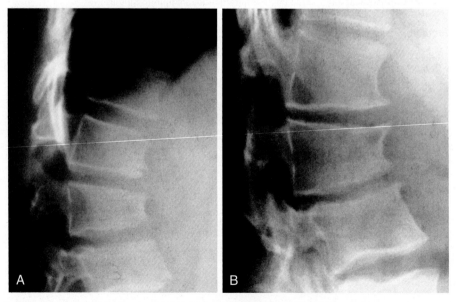

Fig. 203-1 **A,** A radiograph of a 12-year-old gymnast with nagging back pain shows thoracolumbar Scheuermann's disease. **B,** At the age of 19 years, she is pain free, but this radiograph shows permanent wedging. *(From Green NE, Swiontkowski MF: Skeletal Trauma in Children, 3rd ed. Philadelphia, Saunders, 2003.)*

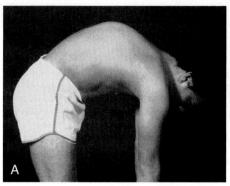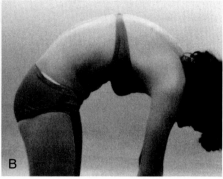

Fig. 203-2 **A,** Scheuermann kyphosis. **B,** Postural kyphosis. *(From Canale ST, Beaty JH: Campbell's Operative Orthopaedics, 11th ed. Philadelphia, Mosby, 2007.)*

Treatment: If a patient is young, has a mild curve, no back pain, and normal pulmonary function, then continued observation by a doctor is usually prescribed, with repeat clinical examinations and radiographs at regular intervals. Other forms of treatment, including bracing and surgery, are considered when there is a rapid increase in the size of the curve; worsening of the vertebral body wedging, back pain that will not improve with conservative measures, and difficulties with pulmonary function that are related to the kyphotic deformity.

Definition:
- Lateral deviation and rotational deformity of the spine. It is a three-dimensional deformity (sagittal, coronal, and rotation).
- Numerous types: idiopathic (infantile, juvenile, and adolescent), neuromuscular, and congenital.

Idiopathic Scoliosis

Infantile:
- Presentation younger than 3 years old, male predominance, left-sided thoracic curves, skull flattening (plagiocephaly), and other congenital defects (heart, kidneys)
- Progression affected by curve magnitude and apical rib-vertebral angle difference (of Mehta), with curves less than 25 degrees with rib-vertebral angle greater than 20 degrees, tending to spontaneously resolve.

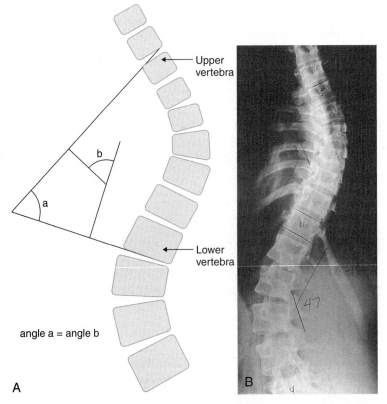

Fig. 201-1 **A,** Measurement of idiopathic scoliosis by the Cobb angle. **B,** Idiopathic adolescent scoliosis. There is a primary thoracic dextroscoliosis (convexity to the right side) measuring 52 degrees and a compensatory lumbar levoscoliosis (convexity to the left side) measuring 47 degrees. *(Reprinted with permission from Katz DS, Math KR, Groskin SA: Radiology Secrets. Philadelphia, Hanley & Belfus, 1998.)*

- Preoperative magnetic resonance imaging (MRI) scan to rule out an intraspinal anomaly (20% incidence).
- Surgical options include growing rods without fusion or combined anterior spinal fusion (ASF) and posterior spinal fusion (PSF).

Juvenile:
- Presentation between 3 and 10 years of age. High risk of progression; 70% need treatment (50% brace, 50% surgery).
- Better to delay surgery until onset of adolescent growth spurt. Need to assess skeletal maturity before fusion. If immature, options are instrumentation without fusion (growing rods) or combined ASF/PSF to prevent crankshaft phenomenon (rotational deformity of the spine after PSF due to continued anterior spinal growth around a tethered posterior fusion mass).

Adolescent:
- Most common form; patients are older than 10 years.
- Right thoracic curves are most common (apical convexity), then double-major curves (right thoracic, left lumbar). Left thoracic curves are rare and require MRI evaluation of the entire spine to rule out an intraspinal anomaly (Arnold-Chiari, syrinx, or diastematomyelia).
- Peak growth velocity is best predictor of progression. Risk factors for progression are curves greater than 20 degrees, age younger than 12 years, and skeletal immaturity (Risser stage 0-1). Curves greater than 20 degrees with Risser stage 0-1 have an almost 70% chance of progression.
- Risser sign based on the ossification of the iliac apophysis. More helpful to determine skeletal maturity in females (not as accurate in males).
- MRI of the entire spine is warranted in the following scenarios: structural abnormalities, left-sided thoracic curve, rapid progression, progression after maturity, abnormal neurologic examination, excessive kyphosis, and related syndromes.

Treatment: Observation, bracing, and surgery. Observation is warranted in curves less than 25 degrees. Curves greater than 25 degrees should be braced. Effectiveness of bracing is dose related. Curves that progress to greater than 50 degrees should be considered for surgical treatment. PSF is considered the gold standard for correction of thoracic and double major curves. ASF alone can be considered in thoracolumbar and lumbar curves because it can achieve better correction (in axial, coronal, and sagittal planes) and still save lumbar fusion levels. Combined ASF/PSF is indicated for severe deformities (>75 degrees) and crankshaft prevention (Risser stage 0, girls younger than 10 years, boys younger than 13 years or before peak growth velocity).

Fusion Levels: Almost never necessary to fuse to the pelvis. Increased incidence of low back pain with fusion to L5 and L4. Determining curve flexibility, as well as neutral (without rotation with symmetrical pedicles) and stable vertebra (most proximal vertebra that is most closely bisected by the center sacral line), helps determine fusion levels. Two classification systems exist: the King-Moe system and the Lenke system. King-Moe was developed in the era of Harrington instrumentation and defines five curve types (thoracolumbar I, thoracolumbar II, thoracic, long thoracic, and double thoracic). Lenke and colleagues developed a classification that has six curve types, with thoracic kyphosis and lumbar modifiers, allowing determination of the fusion levels based on these criteria (which take into account curve flexibility; i.e., structural versus nonstructural curves).

Complications: Neurologic insult (monitor with somatosensory evoked potentials or Stagnara's wake-up test), pseudarthrosis (1% to 2%), early wound infection (1% to 2%), implant failure. Late infection (>1 year) with solid fusion mass necessitates hardware removal.

Neuromuscular Scoliosis

- Curves are longer, involve more levels, are less likely to have compensatory curves progress more rapidly or progress after maturity, and often have a pelvic obliquity associated with them. Braces are usually less effective.

- Increased incidence of pulmonary complications.
- Initial treatment may be with wheelchair modifications, then fusion when curves are greater than 50 degrees (the exception is in patients with muscular dystrophies who are fused early, at 25 to 30 degrees before pulmonary/cardiac function declines).

Congenital Scoliosis

- Due to developmental defect of mesenchymal cells during fourth through sixth embryologic weeks.
- *Three Types:* Failure of formation, failure of segmentation, or mixed type.
- *Worst Prognosis (Most Rapid Progression):* Unilateral unsegmented bar with contralateral fully segmented hemivertebrae (surgery on presentation). Partially segmented, incarcerated or non-segmented hemivertebrae are treated with observation; the partially segmented may require excision. Unilateral unsegmented bar or fully segmented hemivertebrae usually require fusion.
- PSF is the gold standard for treatment; bracing is ineffective in controlling curve progression.
- *Associated Anomalies:* Cardiac (10%), genitourinary (25%), dysraphism (25%).
- Renal ultrasound rules out kidney abnormality.

Definition: Infection in the joint space.

Etiology: Most septic arthritides are monomicrobial infections, but polymicrobial infections may be seen in patients with direct inoculation of the joint space. The most common bacterial isolates in native joints include gram-positive cocci, primarily with *Staphylococcus aureus* (60%). Other isolates include *Neisseria gonorrhoeae* (in sexually active young adults), streptococci, and gram-negative cocci. Other organisms less commonly isolated include mycobacteria and fungi. Gram-negative bacilli are often present in neonates, older adults, and patients with immune deficiency disorders.

Incidence: The incidence is 2 to 10 per 100,000 in the general population and 30 to 70 per 100,000 in patients with rheumatoid arthritis.

Age and Gender: In gonococcal arthritis, women are approximately 3 times as likely as men to develop this disease. No racial predisposition is recognized.

Symptoms and Signs: Patients usually present with acute onset of fever, pain, distention and redness of the affected joint. Range of motion is markedly limited. In *N. gonorrhoeae* infection, patients may have a rash over the trunk and extensor surfaces of distal extremities, pharyngitis, and ureteritis.

Pathophysiology: Bacteria may enter the joint hematogenously (the most common route), from the osteomyelitis of the adjacent bone, or directly through skin after trauma. The knee accounts for 40% to 50% of septic arthritis. In infants and young children, the hip is involved more than the knee. Synovial membrane hyperplasia develops in 5 to 7 days, and the release of cytokines leads to hydrolysis of proteoglycans and collagen, cartilage destruction, and eventually bone loss.

Differential Diagnosis: Viral arthritis, gout, pseudogout, Lyme disease, reactive arthritis, and other rheumatic diseases.

Diagnostic Studies: Synovial fluid changes include more than 100,000 white blood cells (WBCs)/mm^3, polymorphonuclear leukocytes greater than 75%, low glucose concentration, and often positive culture (85% to 95% of nongonococcal arthritis cases and approximately 25% in gonococcal arthritis cases). Plain radiography is often normal. Soft tissue swelling, widening of the joint space, and in later stages, bony erosion and joint space narrowing are the findings.

Treatment: After obtaining a synovial and blood sample, intravenous antibiotics should be started. Most patients respond to oxacillin or nafcillin in combination with intravenous ceftriaxone, cefotaxime, or ceftizoxime. In cases of methicillin-resistant *S. aureus* infection, IV vancomycin would be the drug of choice.

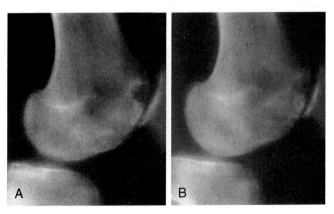

Fig. 202-1 Tomogram of right knee of a patient who has *Staphylococcus aureus* septic arthritis and periarticular osteomyelitis. Note the mixed sclerosis and lytic changes suggestive of osteomyelitis. *(From Cohen J, Powderly WG: Infectious Diseases, 2nd ed. Philadelphia, Mosby, 2004.)*

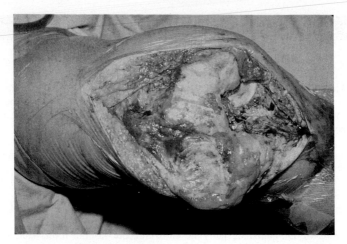

Fig. 202-2 Intraoperative photograph of right knee of a patient who has *Staphylococcus aureus* septic arthritis. Note the damaged joint and dark brown, boggy and hyperemic synovium. *(From Cohen J, Powderly WG: Infectious Diseases, 2nd ed. Philadelphia, Mosby, 2004.)*

Definition: Evaluation of intra-articular or extra-articular shoulder structures or pathology via an arthroscope.

Incidence: The most common procedure, repair of rotator cuff tear, 230,000 a year in the United States. Shoulder pain is the third most common musculoskeletal pain (low back, cervical).

Etiology of Rotator Cuff Pathology:

Anterosuperior Impingement Syndrome: Impingement of the cuff beneath coracoacromial arch is a common cause of shoulder pain. Neer—1972 paper on impingement syndrome. Impingement against anterior one third of the acromion. Traction spurs cause repeated impingement of the cuff, particularly the supraspinatus. Biglianni described three shapes of acromion: type 1, flat; type 2, curved; type 3, hooked. Neer described three progressive stages of impingement: stage 1, edema and hemorrhage, excessive overhead use (younger than 25); stage 2, fibrosis and tendonitis, mechanical inflammation (25- to 40-year-old age group); stage 3, bone spurs with incomplete or complete tears found almost exclusively in patients older than 40.

Intrinsic Hypothesis: Progressive age-related degeneration of the tendon. In 1934, Codman introduced the idea that most tears begin at the articular surface. Codman zone: poor vascularization offered as reason for the tendency of this area to tear.

Age: Most common age group for rotator cuff tear is older than 40 years. Average onset is at 55 years. Twenty-one percent of patients have shoulder symptoms at ages older than 70.

Gender: Historically thought to have a male predominance, but study data conflict—most cite an equal distribution between males and females.

Race: No predilection.

Signs and Symptoms for Rotator Cuff Repair:

Neer Impingement Test: Shoulder flexed passively with internal rotation.

Hawkins Test: Flexed to 90 degrees with internal rotation.

Jobe Test: The shoulder is placed at 90 degrees of abduction and 30 degrees of flexion in the plane of the scapula. Elevation is resisted. Test is 86% sensitive and 50% specific.

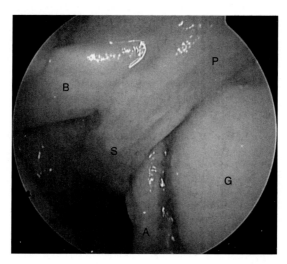

Fig. 203-1   Arthroscopic image from a posterior viewing portal. The biceps tendon (B), superior glenohumeral ligament (S), and the labrum, both anterior and posterior, are intimately related. A, anterior labrum; G, glenoid surface; P, posterior labrum. *(From Miller MD, Cole BJ: Textbook of Arthroscopy, Philadelphia, Saunders, 2004.)*

Other Tests: Infraspinatus test, teres minor test, belly press test, and lift-off test (subscapularis). Magnetic resonance imaging is the most sensitive and specific test that can be offered (90% to 95% sensitive and specific).

Procedure: Portals are placed posterior (2 cm distal and medial to posterolateral border of acromion—for viewing), anterior (lateral and inferior to coracoid process), and lateral (1 to 2 cm distal to lateral acromial edge). Other portals include Neviaser (supraspinatus) portal for anterior glenoid visualization, Port of Wilmington (anterolateral) portal, and posterolateral portals for labral or superior labrum from anterior to posterior (SLAP), and anterior inferior (5-o'clock portal) for Bankart repair or stabilization procedures (also posteroinferior 7-o'clock portal).

Definition: Pain in the subacromial space when the humerus is elevated or internally rotated.

Incidence: As the most common shoulder ailment, there is a relatively high incidence, although more so in overhead athletes or laborers. Specifics are unavailable.

Age: Varies according to Neer stages as follows: stage 1 (inflammation) before 25 years; stage 2 (rotator cuff fibrosis and tendonitis) between ages 25 and 40; stage 3 (frank tear) older than 40 years.

Gender: No correlation.

Etiology and Pathophysiology: A rigid coracoacromial arch impinges the rotator cuff tendons under the acromion, eventually leading to degeneration and tearing of the rotator cuff tendon. The supraspinatus outlet may be impinged with coracoacromial ligament thickening and acromioclavicular joint osteophytes. Non–outlet impingement results from loss of normal humeral head depression from either a large rotator cuff tear or an innervation problem (C5/6 neural lesion or suprascapular mononeuropathy). The origin of pain is unclear, but because the highest concentration of pain fibers is in the bursa, followed by the rotator cuff and biceps tendon, these are likely sources.

Associations: A hooked type 3 acromion is associated, although no causation has been proved.

Signs and Symptoms: The most common symptom is a gradual increase in shoulder pain with overhead activities, although the onset is sudden and sharp in quality in the event of a rotator cuff tear. Pain is most often in the lateral superior anterior shoulder, occasionally referred to as *deltoid*. Often present, a positive impingement sign is pain with forward flexing of the arm to 90 degrees and forcefully internally rotating the shoulder. The subacromial space can be injected once with 10 to 15 mL of 1% xylocaine and the provocative positioning repeated to assess the origin of the pain and predict the response to surgery.

Diagnostic Studies: Shoulder radiographs in two planes are recommended. An anteroposterior (AP) radiograph with the arm in internal rotation or a Grashey view of the glenohumeral joint is useful to detect a Hill-Sachs lesion or evaluate the articular cartilage, respectively. Additionally, an axillary view demonstrates the proximal humeral anatomy in addition to the glenoid rim, acromion, and coracoid shown by a regular scapular outlet view. A 30-degree caudal tilt AP view detects anterior proliferation of acromion relative to the clavicle. Magnetic resonance imaging (MRI) is the gold standard.

Macropathology: Critical hypovascular zones have been shown in both the supraspinatus and infraspinatus tendons, along with inflammation, fibrosis, and/or frank tearing of the rotator cuff. In addition, subacromial bursal effusion/hypertrophy, glenoid labral tear, coracoacromial ligament hypertrophy, and inferior acromioclavicular joint osteophytes may be seen.

Micropathology: Repetitive microtrauma causes inflammation and edema within the tendon.

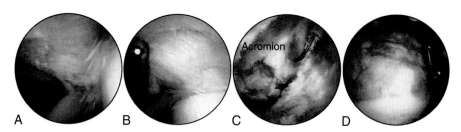

Fig. 204-1   Stages of impingement. **A** and **B,** Stage II. Supraspinatus tendon insertion extends in anteroposterior dimension from biceps to bare area. Medially, it inserts adjacent to the articular surface and fans out laterally approximately 7 mm onto tuberosity. **C,** Débridement and acromioplasty. **D,** Stage III, with massive complete rotator cuff tear. *(From Canale ST, Beaty JH: Campbell's Operative Orthopaedics, 11th ed. Philadelphia, Mosby, 2007.)*

Treatment: Initial management includes physical therapy, nonsteroidal anti-inflammatory drugs, and corticosteroid injection, although the clinical efficacy of the latter has been shown in only two of eight randomized control trials. With failure of initial management or complete cuff rupture on MRI, arthroscopic subacromial decompression with coracoacromial ligament release and resection of the subacromial bursa or, alternatively, open acromioplasty, may provide pain relief. Releasing the coracoacromial ligament may worsen superior migration with massive rotator cuff tear. Acromioplasty may not benefit in throwing athletes.

Incidence: Shoulder stability has been classified in various ways, including direction (anterior, posterior), degree (dislocation, subluxation), etiology (traumatic, atraumatic, overuse), and timing (acute, recurrent, fixed). Posterior dislocations and posterior glenohumeral joint instabilities are rare (approximately 2% to 4%). Anterior dislocations are usually the result of direct or indirect trauma, with the arm forced into abduction and external rotation. This is by far the most frequent type of shoulder dislocation and represents more than 90% of injuries. Of single acute dislocations, 40% become recurrent as a result of associated damage of the surrounding ligamentous and capsular structures that stabilize the joint.

Age: Initial dislocations have been recognized as occurring at two age peaks: at 10 to 30 years of age and at 50 to 70 years of age.

Gender: No preponderance exists for either gender.

Geography: No reported regions of greater preponderance.

Symptoms and Signs: Generalized painful or sore shoulder, worsened with activity or certain arm positions. Less common symptoms perceived by the patient are dislocation factors, subluxation, or functional symptoms such as catching or locking. Nocturnal pain is variable.

Macropathology: Several contribute to shoulder stability and compromises in one or multiple may cause instability; balance, concavity compression, superior stability, adhesion-cohesion glenohumeral suction cup, limited joint volume, and capsuloligamentous constraints.

Sequelae: The sequelae are well seen on magnetic resonance imaging (MRI) and include tears of the labrum, glenohumeral ligaments, capsule, tendons, and muscles.

Studies: X-rays, MR arthrogram, MRI, and computed tomography scan.

Medical Treatment: Treatment consists of a period of shoulder immobilization with subsequent physical therapy aimed to improve range of motion. Rehabilitation should include the scapula, serratus anterior, and then rhomboids, followed by the deltoids, and finally strengthening of the rotator cuff.

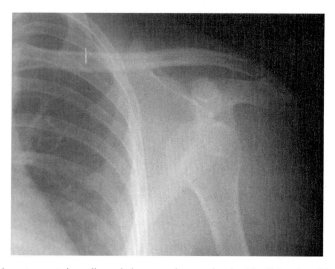

Fig. 205-1 An anteroposterior radiograph demonstrating anterior shoulder dislocation. *(From Cole BJ, Sekiya JK: Surgical Techniques of the Shoulder, Elbow, and Knee in Sports Medicine. Philadelphia, Saunders, 2008.)*

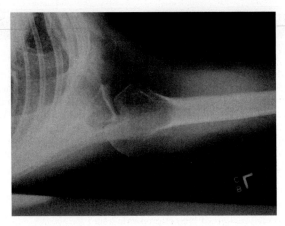

Fig. 205-2 Axillary radiograph revealing a locked posterior shoulder dislocation. *(From Miller MD, Cole BJ: Textbook of Arthroscopy. Philadelphia, Saunders, 2004.)*

Surgical Treatment: Historically, surgical repairs for posterior instability have had mixed results with failure rates as high as 50%. In general, surgical intervention is associated with a 50% to 95% success rate. Due to differences regarding classification and terminology, studies have combined groups of patients with trauma, multidirectional laxity, unidirectional or multidirectional instability, voluntary subluxation, and positional instability.

Prognosis: The recurrence of posterior capsular shift procedures is higher than the rate of repair for anterior instability. The recurrence of multidirectional instability following surgery is about 10%.

Definition: A SLAP (superior labral anterior to posterior) lesion is the detachment of the superior glenoid labrum, which serves as the insertion of the long head of the biceps. The functional importance of the long head of the biceps at the glenoid joint is its role in anterior stability and humeral head depression.

Etiology: The most common mechanisms are traction and compression. Traction includes sudden pulls inferiorly (losing hold of a heavy object), anteriorly (water skiing), or upward (grab overhead object to keep from falling). Repetitive overhead motion, such as pitching also constitutes traction. Compression injuries occur when falling on an outstretched arm or from direct blows. SLAPs may accompany rotator cuff pathology and/or anterior instability.

Incidence: Mileski and Snyder reported the results of more than 140 patients treated operatively for superior labral lesions. They noted a 6% incidence of SLAP lesions in persons undergoing shoulder arthroscopy for all diagnoses. Type I lesions have been reported to account for 9.5% to 21% of all cases; type II, 41% to 55%; type III, 6% to 33%; and type IV, 3% to 15%.

Histology: Histologic examinations reveal that the labrum consists of densely packed collagen bundles and fibrochondrocytes.

Symptoms: The two most common symptoms are pain, especially with overhead activities, and mechanical symptoms of catching, locking, popping, and grinding. Decreased range of motion, pain with activities of daily living, and loss of strength are also reported. It is difficult to distinguish a SLAP lesion from impingement syndrome on the basis of physical findings.

Clinical Findings: No physical finding is specific for SLAP lesions. Compression-rotation test (pain with internal-external rotation of humerus with patient in lateral position and arm in 90 degrees abduction) and biceps tension test (pain with resisted flexion with elbow extended and forearm supinated) may be positive. Neer and Hawkins can be positive as well even without rotator cuff pathology.

Diagnostic Studies: Magnetic resonance imaging is useful in detecting SLAP lesions and other concomitant humeral-glenoid pathology; however, diagnostic arthroscopy remains the definitive diagnostic method.

Classification and Treatment: There are four basic types of SLAP lesions:

Type I: Fraying of edge of superior labrum with firmly attached labrum and biceps anchor. Treatment consists of simple débridement.

Type II: The labrum and biceps anchor are detached from the superior glenoid and arch away from the glenoid neck. Treatment consists of fixation and stabilization of the biceps anchor to the superior glenoid.

Type III: Bucket handle tear of the superior labrum with the remaining labrum and biceps anchor still attached. Treatment is simple débridement.

Type IV: Bucket handle tear of the superior labrum with extension into the biceps tendon. Treatment should consist of suture repair of the complex or resection if less than 30% of the tendon body is involved.

Each patient also needs a thorough evaluation of glenohumeral stability under anesthesia and any concomitant instability must be addressed at the time of labral repair/débridement. Postoperative sling is used with gentle hand, wrist, elbow, and pendulum exercises prescribed. Active biceps strengthening is begun slowly at 3 to 5 weeks with 3 to 5 pounds. No stressful biceps activity is advised for 3 months.

Complications: Reported complications include adhesive capsulitis, possibly from reattachment of Buford complex (cordlike middle glenohumeral ligament that attaches at the base of biceps tendon), instability, and need for removal of hardware.

429

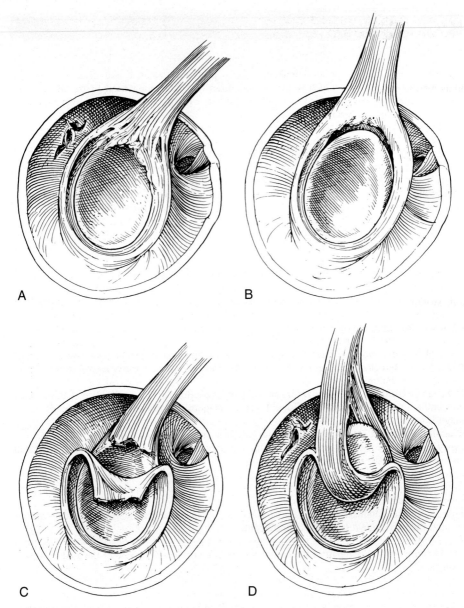

Fig. 206-1   The original Snyder classification of SLAP lesions. Type I has degenerative superior labrum tearing but attached biceps (**A**). Type II has detachment of the superior labrum/biceps tendon complex from the superior glenoid (**B**). Type II has a bucket handle tear of a meniscoid superior labrum but attached biceps (**C**). Type IV has tearing of the superior labrum up into the biceps tendon (**D**). Variable amounts of the biceps are left attached. *(From Snyder SJ, Karzel RP, Del Pizzo W, et al: SLAP lesions of the shoulder. Arthroscopy 6:274-279, 1990.)*

Definition: The most common hip disorder in the adolescent. Characterized by variable degrees of posterior slippage of the proximal femoral epiphysis.

Etiology: Several suggested etiologies including local trauma, mechanical factors including obesity, inflammatory conditions, endocrine disorders, and genetic factors. Associated with deficiency of insulin growth factors.

Incidence and Epidemiology: Approximately 11 cases in 100,000 children. Approximately 4 times higher incidence in blacks and 2.5 times higher incidence in Hispanic than in white children. More frequent in obesity. Left sided twice as common as right sided; bilateral occurrence, 25% to 40%.

Age: Rarely younger than 9 years in girls or younger than 11 in boys; most begin before puberty.

Gender: Slight male predominance. Boys, approximately 13/100,000; girls, approximately 8/100,000.

Symptoms: Variable depending on type of slip. Common complaints of pain in groin, medial thigh, or knee with limited hip motion (especially internal rotation).

Clinical Findings: Variable shortening of affected extremity, possibly fixed in external rotation. Antalgic limp. Most are chronic; more than half are mild slips.

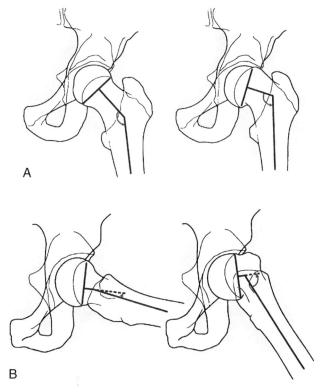

Fig. 207-1 Extracapsular base-of-neck osteotomy: measurement of head-shaft angles on radiograph. **A,** Normal anteroposterior angle compared with slipped capital femoral epiphysis (SCFE). **B,** Normal lateral angle compared with SCFE. *(From Abraham E, Garst J, Barmada R: Treatment of moderate to severe slipped capital femoral epiphysis with extracapsular base-of-neck osteotomy, J Pediatr Orthop 13:294, 1993.)*

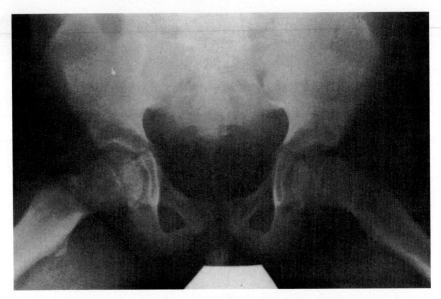

Fig. 207-2   Left slipped capital femoral epiphysis (SCFE) in an athlete who had left groin pain for several weeks. The frog-leg lateral position provides the most sensitive radiographic image for detecting SCFE. *(From DeLee D, Drez D [eds]: DeLee and Drez's Orthopaedic Sports Medicine, 2nd ed. Philadelphia, Saunders, 2003.)*

Acute: Sudden, symptoms less than 2 weeks; displacement without evidence of bone healing or remodeling.

Chronic: Gradual, symptoms more than 2 weeks; some signs of healing and remodeling along posterior and medial femoral neck on x-ray study.

Acute or Chronic: Symptoms more than 1 month with recent exacerbation.

Preslip: X-ray finding of irregularity, widening, indistinctness of physis.

Mild (Grade I): Neck displaced less than one third of the diameter of the femoral head or head-shaft angle is deviated from normal by 30 degrees or less on either projection.

Moderate (Grade II): Neck displaced between one third and one half of the diameter of the femoral head or head shaft is deviated 30 to 60 degrees

Severe (Grade III): Neck displaced more than one half of the diameter of the head or deviation of greater than 60 degrees.

Diagnostic Studies: Anteroposterior x-ray study of pelvis often is only attainable view. Lateral may help with extent of posterior displacement. Frog-leg view is useful for subtle slip, but should be avoided in acute slip. When there is clinical suspicion but negative x-ray findings, computed tomography can help with early or mild slip.

Treatment Goals: Prevent additional slipping, stimulate early physeal closure, avoid avascular necrosis, chondrolysis, osteoarthritis.

Accepted Treatment: In situ single screw fixation under fluoroscopy, multiple screws and pins and bone peg epiphysiodesis, prophylactic pinning of contralateral slip. Most treatments avoid reduction by open or closed technique.

Complications: Avascular necrosis, chondrolysis, osteoarthritis. Persistent pin penetration is most serious complication, which can lead to joint sepsis, localized acetabular erosion, synovitis, postoperative hip pain, chondrolysis, late degenerative osteoarthritis.

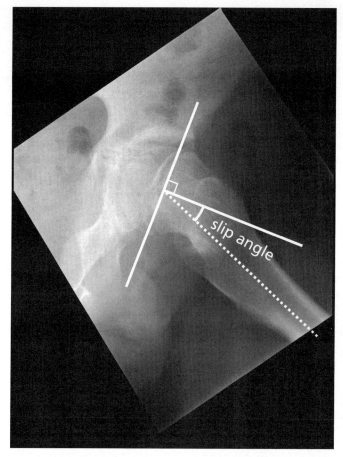

Fig. 207-3 Slipped capital femoral eppiphysis. Frog lateral, illustrating measurement of slip angle. *(From Adam A, et al: Grainger & Allison's Diagnostic Radiology, 5th ed. Philadelphia, Churchill Livingstone, 2008.*

Embryonic Time Course

Week 2-3: Embryo is bilaminar.
- Ectoderm (primarily responsible for the neural elements) and the endoderm
- Caudal end, also known as *primitive streak*
  - Cluster of cells that invaginates between the two layers
  - Forms a third layer—mesoderm

Week 3-5: Ectodermal induction—forming the neural plate.

Neural plate subsequently curls, forming the neural tube.

Neural tube begins to close centrally and continues to each end.
- Guided by the notochord
  - Derived from the primitive knob
  - Parallels the mesodermal plate
    Elongates cranially first, then adds caudally
- Failure of Closure:
  - Cranially—anencephaly
  - Caudally—spina bifida

Neural Crest Cells—a population of ectodermal cells.
- Run parallel to the closed neural tube
- Forms the peripheral nervous system

Somites—formed from the medial aspect of the mesoderm.
- Differentiates into three layers
  - Dermatome—forms skin
  - Myotome—forms muscle
  - Sclerotome—forms the skeleton
    Responsible for forming the neural arch, vertebral body, and costal process by end of fourth week

Week 6-8: Segmentation.

Each vertebra forms from each adjacent sclerotomes.

Notochord begins to degenerate between the vertebrae.
- Persists to form the nucleus pulposus

Chondrification begins here.

Week 32 Birth: Vertebral body fusion.

The two sclerotomes fuse to form a centrum.

Failure—hemivertebrae.

Year 1: The two halves of the neural arch fuse.

Year 3-6: The neural arch fuses to the centrum of the vertebral body.

Puberty: Secondary ossification centers appear.

Upper and lower body; tip of the transverse processes and spinous process.
- Longitudinal growth—via superior and inferior apophysis
- Horizontal growth—via periosteal apposition

Year 25: Ossification, which begins in the embryonic period, ends.

Definition: Narrowing of the spinal canal or neural foramina anywhere along the spine, producing neural element compression, root ischemia, and a variable syndrome of back and leg pain.

Classification: Cervical or thoracic stenosis, which can lead to myelopathy, versus lumbar stenosis, which can be divided into *central canal stenosis* with compression of the thecal sac or *lateral stenosis* with individual nerve root compression in the lateral recess or the intervertebral foramen.

Etiology and Age Distribution: Most stenosis results from acquired degenerative changes (spondylosis), although congenital stenosis places patients at earlier risk to develop symptoms from degenerative narrowing of the spinal canal. Men are slightly more affected, and most frequently in the fifth to seventh decades.

Cervical and Thoracic Stenosis: Refers to age-related changes including disk degeneration and narrowing, and spur formation with facet and ligamentum flavum hypertrophy. Cervical spondylotic myelopathy is the most common cause of spinal cord dysfunction in patients older than 55 years. Decreased motion and compression with spurs at C5-7 lead to instability and compression due to anterolisthesis and retrolisthesis at C3-5. Contributing disorders are

SPINAL STENOSIS/CLAUDICATION

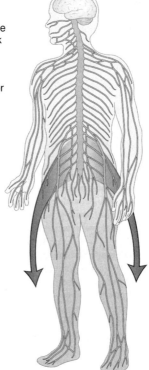

- Dull to severe pain in the buttocks and lower back triggered by walking, especially downhill

- Pain radiates into one or both legs (60%)

- Numbness, weakness, paresthesiae of lower extremities

- Relief when sitting, leaning forward, or resting

Fig. 209-1 Spinal stenosis syndromes. *(From Kronenberg HL, et al: Williams Textbook of Endocrinology, 11th ed. Philadelphia, Saunders.)*

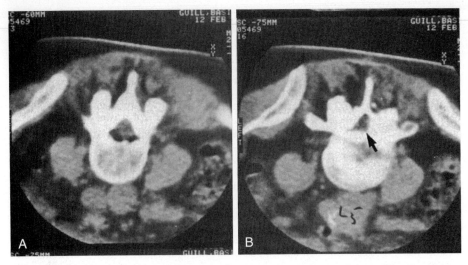

Fig. 209-2 Normal (**A**) and abnormal (**B**) CT scans of the lumbar spine. Marked narrowing *(arrow)* is present in **B** because of hypertrophic spurring. *(From Mercier R: Practical Orthopedics, 5th ed. St. Louis, Mosby, 2000, p 129.)*

rheumatoid arthritis, ankylosing spondylitis, and ossification of the posterior longitudinal ligament. Thoracic stenosis is rare, and often associated with disk bulging or herniation, posterior element hypertrophy, and occasionally ligamentum flavum calcification.

Lumbar Stenosis: Most commonly at L4-5 and L5-S1. Central canal narrowing is frequently due to anterior disk bulges/herniation, facet hypertrophy from lateral disk bulges/herniation, and flavum hypertrophy with epidermal lipomatosus from posterior disk bulges/herniation. Ischemic nerve roots elicit pain when walking, the hallmark of neurogenic claudication. Pain is relieved by leaning forward (shopping cart) or sitting. Flexing forward relieves pressure by stretching the protruding ligamentum flavum, reducing the overriding laminae and facets, and enlarging the foramina. Extensor hallucis longus weakness is the most common (L5).

Incidence: Degenerative changes of the cervical spine leading to some form of cervical stenosis are present in 95% of asymptomatic patients older than 65 years (C5-7 most common). Myelopathy develops in 20% of such patients. Lumbar spinal stenosis affects 1 per 1000 people older than 65 years.

Signs and Symptoms: Cervical myelopathy with loss of dexterity and muscle weakness, also in the proximal lower extremities. Some upper extremity reflexes may be decreased or absent. Lumbar stenosis results in back and leg pain, pseudoclaudication (see above), and giving way with numbness and weakness in the legs.

Clinical Findings: Cervical myelopathy due to stenosis. Pathologic reflexes with myelopathy: Hoffman's, clonus, up-going toes on Babinski with increased lower extremity reflexes. At increased risk for (central cord) spinal cord injury due to minor trauma, with at least one third of patients experiencing worsening myelopathy with stepwise degeneration if left untreated. Lumbar stenosis exhibits decreased reflexes, general weakness, and incidental bowel or bladder abnormalities with numbness.

Medical Treatment: Aimed at symptomatic relief. Rest and bracing with analgesics, nonsteroidal anti-inflammatory drugs, and antispasmodics can help. Epidural steroids have shown minimal effect. Temporary relief of back pain and muscle spasms can be obtained from physical therapy with strengthening.

Surgical Treatment: For significant myelopathy, radiculopathy, and/or neurogenic claudication. Posterior cervical decompression is preferred from multilevel disease, and fusion is mandatory after laminectomy. Disk herniation and spur formation are best addressed from the anterior perspective. Single or multilevel laminectomy with foraminotomy is the treatment of choice for lumbar stenosis. Partial or complete facetectomies or a diskectomy might also be necessary. Postoperative instability after a wide decompression requires fusion.

Studies: Plain radiographs can reveal a congenitally small canal, as well as degenerative spondylolisthesis. Computed tomography/myelogram provides excellent information in both axial and sagittal planes. Bony anatomy is also shown. Magnetic resonance imaging more specifically reveals compressive anatomic structures like ligaments, facet capsules, and disk fragments.

Sequelae: Conservative measures can only provide temporary relief; surgical decompression is indicated when signs and symptoms correlate with radiographic studies. Individualized treatment plans should be made to determine the need for fusion post decompression. Generally, patients have significant increases in walking distance and substantial reduction in pain and numbness postoperatively. It is one of the most satisfied patient populations after decompressive (and fusion) surgery in the spine subspecialty.

Definition: Forward slippage of one vertebral body on the one below it (anterolisthesis vs. retrolisthesis, slipping posteriorly).

Classification: Six types as listed in Table 210-1.

Severity Staging of the Slip: Based on the relative distance of forward migration over the vertebral body below: I = 0% to 25%, II = 25% to 50%, III = 50% to 75%, IV = 75% to 100%, V > 100% (spondyloptosis). Sacral inclination (kyphosis angle of posterior sacrum compared with straight vertical line) and slip angle (degree-differences in parallel lines to superior and inferior endplates of the vertebral bodies above and below the slip, respectively) have both a prognostic and cosmetic impact.

Etiology and Age Distribution: See Table 210-1.

Incidence: Depending on the type, approximately 5% of general population. Remarkably common in Inuits (>50% of white boys with hyperextension activities are prone to a pars fracture [type II], whereas degenerative spondylolisthesis [type III] is more common in African American women older than 40 years).

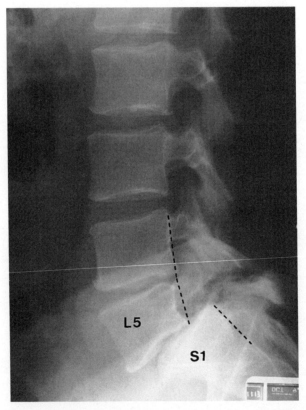

Fig. 210-1 Spondylolysis with resulting grade 2 spondylolisthesis. Discontinuity of the posterior elements of L5 has allowed L5 to slip forward on S1. The degree of slippage is ascertained by looking at the relation between the posterior portions of the vertebral bodies. *(From Mettler FA, Jr: Essentials of Radiology, 2nd ed. Philadelphia, Saunders, 2005.)*

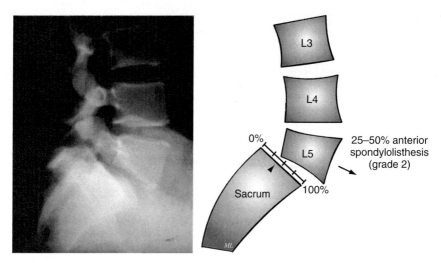

Fig. 210-2 Lateral plain radiograph and schematic diagram of grade 2 anterior spondylolisthesis of L5 on S1. Grading is based on the percentage of slippage with 0% to 25%, 25% to 50%, 50% to 75%, and greater than 75% corresponding to grades 1 to 4, respectively. *(From Marx JA: Rosen's Emergency Medicine: Concepts and Clinical Practice, 6th ed. Philadelphia, Saunders.)*

Table 210-1. TYPES OF SPONDYLOLISTHESIS

Class	Type	Age	Pathology/Etiology
I	Dysplastic	Child	Congenital defect in superior facet on S1
II	Isthmic	5 to 45 years	Elongation or fracture of the pars interarticularis (usually L5-S1)
III	Degenerative	>50 years	Facet arthrosis leading to subluxation (usually L4-5 (orientation of facets commonly in the sagittal plane))
IV	Traumatic	Teens	Acute fracture through any element other than pars (pedicle-watershed area)
V	Pathologic	Any	Incompetence of posterior elements
VI	Postsurgical	20 to 40 years	Excessive decompression/bony resection of pars interarticularis or facet joints

Signs and Symptoms: Frequently back pain (due to instability) and hamstring tightness, as well as characteristic posture (heart-shaped buttocks). Often "pelvic waddle" gait pattern with occasional radiculopathy. Isthmic type (L5-S1 most common) has exiting L5 symptoms. Degenerative type (most often L4-5) has L5 symptoms due to compression on the traversing root in the lateral recess from compression against the posterior L5 body by the hypertrophied L4 inferior facet joint.

Clinical Findings: Bandlike back pain with radiculopathy. Back pain risk is higher in cases of slips greater than 25% and L3-4 or L4-5 involvement. Cauda equina syndrome with bowel/bladder dysfunction can occur if slip acutely progresses. Spina bifida occulta occurs frequently, as does compensatory thoracic hyperkyphosis. High-grade slips usually manifest with neurologic symptoms.

Medical Treatment: None if asymptomatic. Nonsteroidal anti-inflammatory drugs for increased pain; postural exercises and trunk strengthening. Adults with grade I slip may return to all activities (including contact sports) once they become asymptomatic. Even grade II asymptomatic patients should be advised not to play football or do gymnastics. Bracing with cessation of exercise for 12 weeks can allow healing of acute pars fracture in young athletes (leg extension if L5-S1).

Surgical Treatment: For painful, low-grade slip: fusion in situ with pedicle screws after failing proper nonoperative management. This is also the treatment choice for progressive listhesis. In cases of pars defect at L4 or cranial, lag-screw fixation or wiring has been reported. Slips greater than 50% in children require prophylactic fusion.

Studies: Low-grade slips may require computed tomography scan for diagnosis of pars defect. Lateral flexion-extension views show instability at the involved level and magnetic resonance imaging may be helpful to determine cauda or root compression.

Sequelae: Risk factors for progression are high-grade slip; young age at presentation and female gender; slip angle greater than 10 degrees; sacral inclination greater than 30 degrees; dome-shaped promontorium. If posterior arch is intact (usually grade I), cauda equina can occur if slip suddenly progresses. Generally, patients perform well after stabilizing surgery.

Complications: Sudden increase in slip can cause acute neural compromise; dural tear can occur during surgery; hardware failure can occur after stabilization if (need for) anterior column support was not identified or not properly performed.

Definition: Statistics is the science and practice of developing knowledge through the use of data expressed in quantitative form.

Study Population: The group of patients to which survey results are to apply.

Data: Data can be classified into either attribute (qualitative or categorical) or numerical (quantitative) types.

Variables: A characteristic of interest that is possessed by each item in the study.

Continuous Variable: A variable that can assume any one of the countless numbers of values along a line interval. Examples include age, distance, and temperature.

Discrete Variable: A numerical variable that takes only a finite number of real values (e.g., X can equal only 1, 3, 5, and 1000).

Normal Distribution: Often called the *bell curve* or *bell-shaped curve*. Most of the scores in this graph accumulate around the middle. The mean, median, and mode are all equal, and the scores at either end of the distribution occur less often.

Mean: The arithmetic average of a set of numbers.

Median: The median is the middle value that has exactly half of the data above it and half below it.

Mode: The observation that occurs most frequently in a data set.

Type of Study: The purpose of most statistical tests is to determine whether the obtained results provide a reason to reject the hypothesis and whether the results are merely a product of chance factors. Different types of studies have been designed to test the hypothesis.

Prospective Study: A study that looks forward in time. An example is studying the results of a surgery in a group of patients.

Retrospective Study: A study that looks backward in time. Studying the cause of illness in a group of patients diagnosed with gastroenteritis is an example.

Cross-Sectional Study: A research design wherein subjects are assessed at a single time in their lives. This type of study is typically used to find incidence and prevalence.

Case-Control Study: Researchers select cases, a group of patients with a specific outcome (e.g., diagnosed with lung cancer), and controls, a second group without that outcome and study them to find a cause.

Cohort Study: Patients are selected on the basis of an exposure variable (exposed and not exposed) and follow them to determine how this exposure will affect them.

Experimental Study: A study in which the investigator specifies the exposure category for each individual (clinical trial) or community (community trial), then follows the individuals or community to detect the effects of the exposure.

Hypothesis Testing: The goal is to identify sufficient statistical evidence to reject a presumed null hypothesis in favor of an alternative hypothesis.

• *Null hypothesis (hypothesis 0)*—assumes that the means of the two study groups are the same
• *Alternate hypothesis (hypothesis 1)*—assumes that the means of the two study groups are significantly different and rejects the null hypothesis

Study Power: The probability of correctly rejecting the null hypothesis where it is false.

Sample Size: The researchers should calculate how large the patient population group should be in order to provide adequate power to the study.

Type I Error: A true null hypothesis is incorrectly rejected. The probability of making a type I error is determined by the significance level chosen, which is usually as $\alpha < 0.05$.

Type II Error: A true alternative hypothesis is incorrectly rejected. The smaller the sample, the more likely one is to commit a type II error.

Table 211-1. FORMULAS FOR SOME OF THE VALUES USED IN STATISTICS

Value	Formula
Mean	$M = \Sigma x / N$ (N: number of subjects)
Standard deviation	$S = \sqrt{(\Sigma x^2 / N)}$ (x: deviation of score from mean)
Standard error of the mean	$SE_m = s / \sqrt{N}$ (s: standard deviation, N: number of subjects)
Variance (σ^2)	$\sigma^2 = \Sigma (x_i - \mu)^2 / N$ (μ: population mean, x_i: value)
Z-test	$Z = (m - \mu) / SE_m$ (m: sample mean; μ: population mean)
Chi-square	$X^2 = \Sigma (O - E)^2 / E$ (O: observed outcome; E: expected outcome)

Definition: The sternoclavicular joint (SC) connects the clavicle to the sternum. This attachment is the only bony joint linking the bones of the arm and shoulder to the main part of the skeleton. The SC joint participates in all movements of the upper extremity. On every side, structural supports, such as the dense fibrous capsule and ligaments, reinforce the joint, making dislocations uncommon events and relatively minor.

Age: Incidence is increased in young adult males, because this population is engaged more often in activities associated with SC injury, such as motor vehicle crashes and contact sports.

Gender: Overall incidence is higher in males than in females because of the activities (e.g., motor vehicle crash, contact sports) associated with the injury. However, recurrent atraumatic anterior subluxation of the SC joint (usually associated with overall joint laxity) occurs more frequently in young girls.

Etiology: SC injury is usually the result of high-energy force sustained during a motor vehicle accident (50%) or during contact sports activity (20%). Falls and other types of accidents cause the remainder.

Pathophysiology: Only through the application of significant force do the ligaments supporting the SC joint become completely disrupted, enabling dislocation of the joint. Whether the SC joint subluxes or dislocates depends on the extent of the damage to the supporting ligaments and capsule. Simple sprains predominate among SC injuries and are graded into three types. A first-degree injury constitutes an incomplete tear of the sternoclavicular and costoclavicular ligaments. With a second-degree lesion, the clavicle subluxes from its manubrial attachment, signifying a complete breach of the sternoclavicular ligament but only a partial tear of the costoclavicular ligament. With a third-degree wound, complete rupture of the sternoclavicular and costoclavicular ligaments permits the clavicle to completely dislocate from the manubrium.

Mechanism: A substantial direct or indirect force to the shoulder region can cause a traumatic dislocation of the SC joint. Anterior dislocations of the SC joint are much more common (by a 9:1 ratio), usually resulting from an indirect mechanism such as a blow to the anterior shoulder that rotates the shoulder backward and transmits the stress to the joint. Traumatic contact driving the shoulder forward can cause posterior dislocations of the SC joint, but direct impact to the superior sternal or medial clavicle also can ensue.

Classification: SC instability can be classified according to degree (subluxation or dislocation), direction (anterior or posterior), etiology (traumatic or atraumatic), and chronicity (acute, chronic, recurrent, congenital, or developmental).

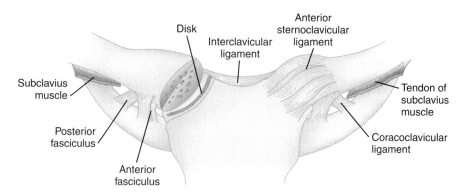

Fig. 212-1   Ligaments and the interarticular disk of the sternoclavicular joint. *(Redrawn from DePalma AF: Surgery of the Shoulder, 3rd ed. Philadelphia, JB Lippincott, 1983. In Marx JA: Rosen's Emergency Medicine: Concepts and Clinical Practice, 6th ed. Philadelphia, Saunders.)*

Signs and Symptoms:

Sprains: Mild sprains cause pain, but the joint is still stable. In moderate sprains, the joint becomes unstable.

Dislocation: This causes severe pain that gets worse with any arm movements. In anterior dislocation, the end of the clavicle juts out near the sternum. This causes a hard bump in the middle of the chest. Posterior dislocations can cause difficulty breathing, shortness of breath, or a feeling of choking.

Ligament Injury: In rare cases, patients have a stable joint but a painful clicking, grating, or popping feeling. This indicates an injury to the intra-articular disk ligament. This type of injury causes pain and problems moving the SC joint.

Degenerative Arthritis: Injury to a joint can result in the development of osteoarthritis, which tends to get worse with age, eventually causing pain and stiffness.

Diagnostic Studies: Radiographic evaluation involves standard chest radiographs as well as the serendipity view, which involves a 40-degree cephalic-tilt radiograph showing both medial joints. Normal clavicles should appear in the same horizontal plane, whereas anterior and posterior dislocations appear above and below the plane, respectively. In most cases, an MRI scan or CT scan is required to confirm the diagnosis.

Nonsurgical Treatment:

Sprains: Patients with a moderate sprain may wear a figure-eight strap wrapped around both shoulders to support the SC joint, for 4 to 6 weeks.

Anterior Dislocation: This can be treated by letting it heal where it is or by performing a closed reduction. Closed reduction involves pulling, pushing, and moving the clavicle until it pops back into place. A figure-eight strap is used afterward for 6 weeks.

Posterior Dislocation: This is treated by closed reduction. The arm is pulled out and then brought back into place. Sometimes the clavicle is grabbed and pulled out from behind the sternum. If this doesn't work, a special kind of clip is used to pull out the clavicle. A figure-eight strap is used afterward for 6 weeks.

Surgical Treatment:

Resection Arthroplasty: The most common procedure for SC joint osteoarthritis is resection arthroplasty, which involves removing the surface of the clavicle next to the sternum. This keeps the arthritic bone surfaces from rubbing on one another. The remaining end of the clavicle eventually attaches to the rib with scar tissue. This stops the end of the clavicle from moving around when moving the arm.

Graft Method: The surgeon will try to keep from disturbing the ligaments around the SC joint. But if the ligaments are damaged and loose, a tendon graft may be used to tighten the connection between the end of the clavicle and the first rib. Surgeons use a piece of tendon taken from the wrist or a piece of fascia taken from the thigh. These are referred to as tendon grafts or fascia grafts. The graft is then sewn through the end of clavicle and connected to the first rib.

Observational Designs

Case Series: Retrospective, descriptive account of a group of patients with interesting characteristics or a series of patients who have undergone an intervention (one patient = case report).
Pros: Easy to construct, generate hypotheses
Cons: Anecdotal, no hypothesis testing, weak generalization
Cross-sectional Surveys: Determine the prevalence, identify associations, treatment patterns
Pros: Cheap, simple, ethically safe
Cons: No causality established, recall bias, confounding
Case-Control Studies: Investigator identifies patients with an outcome of interest and patients without the outcome and then compares in regard to possible risk factors. Determins the odds of an outcome.
Pros: Quick, cheap, only way to study rare disorders or long lag to outcome, few subjects
Cons: Confounders, recall bias, difficult to control, selection bias
Cohort Studies: Involves identification of two groups (cohorts) of patients, one that did receive the exposure of interest and one that did not, and following these cohorts forward for the outcome of interest.
Determines relative risk
Pros: Ethically safe, events over time, eligibility criteria, standard outcomes, matched subjects, easier and cheaper than RCT
Cons: Confounding, difficult blinding, no randomization

Experimental Designs

Randomized Controlled Trial (RCT): A group of patients is randomized into an experimental group and a control group. These groups are followed up for the variables/outcomes of interest.
Pros: Randomization, easy blinding, unbiased distribution of confounders
Cons: Ethics, volunteer bias, expensive in time and money

Gold standard of clinical evidence provides valid information by minimizing effects of bias and confounding.
Bias: Nonrandom systematic error in the design or conduct of a study, although usually not intentional. It can enter at all levels of the study, from patient selection, through study performance, to outcome determination. For example:
- Selection bias—dissimilar groups are compared
- Nonresponder bias—the follow-up rate is low
- Interviewer bias—when the investigator determines the outcome

RCTs confront bias through prospective planning, randomization, and blinding.
Confounder: A variable that has independent associations with both the independent variable and the dependent variable, thus distorting their relationship. Common confounders in clinical research: gender, age, socioeconomic status, and comorbidities.

RCTs confront confounding with a priori randomization, assuring equal distribution. Also, matching can be used to assure homologous study groups. Multivariate statistical analysis can also control for confounding post hoc.

Problems with RCTs in Surgery:
- History—techniques established before research protocols
- Time—long period of recruitment vs. rapidly changing techniques/technology

445

- Logistics—recruiting large sample size for sufficient power involves many centers and surgeons
- Learning curves—complex procedures improve with the number of cases
- Quality control
- Definition—how do you define an acceptable level of variation within a procedure?
- Blinding—procedure performance affected by surgeon expectations
- Ethics—for two treatments to be compared, there must be equipoise (uncertainty with respect to preferred treatment modality)

Definition: A fracture of the distal humerus proximal to the condyles.

Incidence: Relatively rare; about 3% of all fractures in adults.

Eitology: Typically a result of a high-energy trauma or significant fall. An axial load on the elbow, with the olecranon acting as a wedge splitting the medial and lateral columns of the distal humerus, causes these fractures. The fracture pattern produced seems to be related to the degree of elbow flexion as well as the direction and magnitude of the force applied.

Age: Most common in the first decade of life (peak 5 to 8 years of age).

Gender: Boys more than girls.

Race: No predilection.

Signs and Symptoms: A painful swollen elbow, perhaps gross deformity. The elbow may appear angulated and the upper extremity shortened. Open wounds have been associated with as many as 30% of these fractures.

Classifications: Predominantly an extension mechanism (90% to 99% of reported cases); flexion accounts for 1% to 10% of cases. Displacement (distal fragment) occurs medially in 75% and laterally in 25% of cases.

Gartland Classification: Type I—nondisplaced; type II—displaced with intact posterior hinge; type III—completely displaced. Other classifications include the AO-ASIF and that proposed by Mehne and Matta.

Associations: Neurologic injury is associated in 7% to 15% of cases with the anterior interosseus nerve (AIN) being the most common (check thumb interphalangeal/index distal interphalangeal flexion) injury. Posteromedial displacement: radial > median > ulnar. Posterolateral displacement: median > radial > ulnar. Flexion angulation: ulnar nerve most common, usually a neuropraxia. Vascular injuries: Brachial artery may be injured in type III fractures (10% to 20%) and the patient will have an absent radial pulse on presentation. Preoperative arteriograms are contraindicated (because they delay treatment and do not alter the treatment plan). May observe patient with serial examinations if the hand is well perfused despite an absent radial pulse.

Diagnostic Studies: Fracture line occurs near the olecranon. Anteroposterior, lateral, and sometimes oblique views are needed to assess fracture. The anterior humeral line and Baumann's angle (average 72 degrees, normal 64 to 82 degrees, formed by an angle between the capitellar physis and the long axis of the humerus) should be evaluated.

Treatment: Type I—posterior splint for 3 to 5 days followed by a long arm cast for 3 weeks. Type II—treat with splint, followed by cast in flexion, must recheck alignment in 5 to 7 days and if there is displacement then closed reduction and percutaneous pinning (CRPP). Some perform CRPP acutely in type II fractures. Type III—CRPP. The deformity should *not* be exaggerated, so as to avoid injuring the brachial artery. Longitudinal traction/countertraction, varus-valgus angulation, and rotation are corrected and the distal fragment is pushed forward while the forearm is pronated. The goal of CRPP is to construct stability via cross pinning with two equal lateral divergent pins, two parallel lateral pins, or two pins crossing at or near the fracture site.

Complications: Nerve (iatrogenic 1% to 5%) or vascular injury, compartment syndrome (<1%), stiffness, cubitus varus, gunstock deformity associated with tardy ulnar nerve palsy, and failed closed reductions are possible complications. Additionally, ulnar nerve injury is possible with a medial pin.

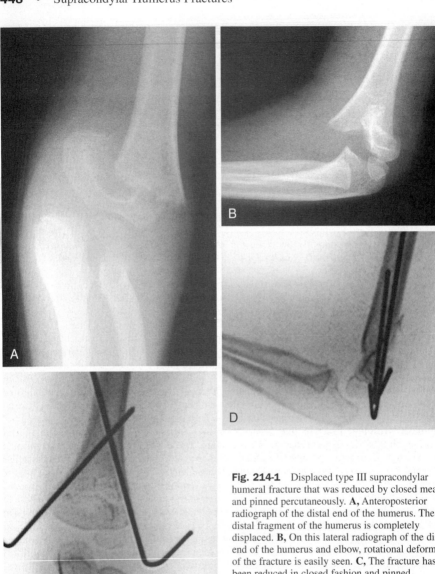

Fig. 214-1 Displaced type III supracondylar humeral fracture that was reduced by closed means and pinned percutaneously. **A,** Anteroposterior radiograph of the distal end of the humerus. The distal fragment of the humerus is completely displaced. **B,** On this lateral radiograph of the distal end of the humerus and elbow, rotational deformity of the fracture is easily seen. **C,** The fracture has been reduced in closed fashion and pinned percutaneously. This anteroposterior radiograph shows that the fracture has been reduced and pinned with medial and lateral pins. Note that the medial pin begins high on the medial epicondyle to avoid the ulnar nerve. **D,** Reduction of the fracture is complete, as seen on this lateral radiograph. *(From Green NE, Swiotkowski MF: Skeletal Trauma in Children, 3rd ed. Philadelphia, Saunders.)*

Anatomy:
- Motor nerve arising from the *upper trunk* of the brachial plexus (*C5-6,* occasional contribution from C4)
- Passes in close proximity to the posterior clavicle border to reach the suprascapular notch
- *Suprascapular Notch:* First point of potential nerve compression
- Nerve passes through the notch *beneath* the transverse scapular ligament (suprascapular artery and vein pass superior)
- Nerve generally found *3 cm* medial to supraglenoid tubercle at this point
- Distal to notch, nerve bifurcates into motor branches to *supraspinatus* and *infraspinatus*

Compression here causes weakness of both muscles.
- Cutaneous branch to lateral deltoid axillary nerve distribution in 15% of population
- Descends toward lateral margin of scapular spine
- *Spinoglenoid notch* second point of potential nerve compression
- Formed by lateral margin of the projection of the scapular spine from the body of the scapula
- Nerve generally lies *2.1 cm* medial to posterior glenoid rim at this point
- Nerve traverses some form of fibro-osseous canal present in up to 80% of patients at this notch
- Distal to notch, nerve continues inferiorly to *infraspinatus*

Compression here causes weakness of infraspinatus only.
- Compression by a *ganglion cyst* is more common here

Clinical Presentation:
- More common in patients with history of repetitive shoulder use (e.g., tennis, swimming, weight lifting, volleyball)
- Dull ache over lateral and posterior shoulder ± weakness

Suprascapular: Symptoms are usually more severe.
- Weakness of both *external rotation* (infraspinatus) and *abduction* (supraspinatus)
- Wasting of supraspinatus and infraspinatus

Spinoglenoid: Isolated wasting of infraspinatus.
- Weakness of *external rotation,* although this may be absent due to compensation by posterior deltoid and teres minor
- May be painless
- Cross body adduction and internal rotation may increase pain (must distinguish from acromio-clavicular joint pathology)

Diagnostic Studies:

Electromyography/Nerve Conduction Velocity Study: Demonstrate motor loss in one or both muscles depending on compression level

Magnetic Resonance Imaging: Optimal study for evaluating possible sites of compression. Shows space-occupying lesions (e.g., ganglion cysts) as well as muscular atrophic changes.

Treatment:
- Initial treatment is nonoperative unless there is evidence of a space-occupying lesion
- Most cases resolve completely, although this may take greater than a year
- Physical therapy emphasizing preservation of shoulder motion and strengthening of cuff, deltoid, and periscapular musculature
- Operative treatment indicated for patients with no improvement after 6 months of nonoperative management
- Suprascapular notch: Compression at the release transverse scapular ligament via superior trapezius-splitting approach
- Spinoglenoid notch: Compression at the open (posterior approach) or arthroscopic decompression (arthroscopy recommended by some authors when cyst is present due to the high incidence of associated labral pathology amenable to repair via scope)

449

Approaches (3 Classic)

Anterior Approach of Henry (to the Radius): Preferred for open reduction and internal fixation (ORIF) of the proximal and distal thirds, and for conditions of the volar forearm.

Dorsal Approach of Thompson (to the Radius): Preferred for ORIF of the middle (and proximal) third, posterior interosseous nerve (PIN) decompression, and conditions of the dorsum of the forearm.

Approach to the Ulna:

- All surgery in the proximal third of the radius is complicated by the PIN, which winds spirally around the bone close to, if not in contact with, its periosteum.
- With respect to the three classic approaches: in almost every case, only part of the approach is necessary.

Anterior Approach of Henry

- *Patient Position:* Supine, arm abducted and supinated, with tourniquet
- *Landmarks:* Biceps tendon, brachioradials (BR), radial styloid
- *Incision:* Gentle curved line from the flexor crease at the volar elbow just lateral to the biceps tendon down to the radial styloid.
- *Internervous Plane:* Proximally, pronator teres (PT) and BR; distally, extensor carpi radialis longus (ECRL) and BR

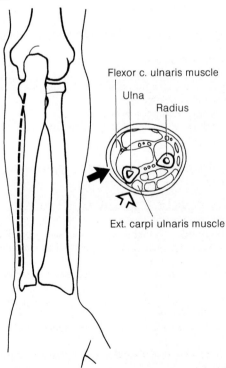

Flexor c. ulnaris muscle

Ulna

Radius

Ext. carpi ulnaris muscle

Fig. 216-1 Approach to the ulna. The skin incision is made just lateral to the subcutaneous border of the ulna. The ulna is exposed longitudinally between the flexor carpi ulnaris and extensor carpi ulnaris. *(From Schatzker J, Tile M: The Rationale of Operative Fracture Care. Berlin, Springer-Verlag, 1987.)*

450

Fig. 216-2   Incisions used in forearm in severe Volkmann contracture. **A,** Extensive opening of fascia of dorsum of forearm in dorsal compartment syndromes. **B,** Incision used for anterior forearm compartment syndromes in which skin and underlying fascia are released completely throughout. *(From Canale ST, Beaty JH [eds]: Campbell's Operative Orthopaedics, 11th ed. Philadelphia, Mosby, 2007.)*

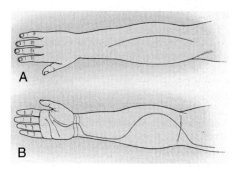

- *Superficial Dissection:* Develop the internervous plane (work from distal to proximal) by identifying the medial border of the BR, and the ECRL. Identify the superficial radial nerve and the radial artery that run along the underside of the BR. If needed, preserve and dissect (deepen the incision *lateral* to the biceps tendon to avoid compromising the radial artery). Ligate the recurrent radial artery just below the elbow joint under the proximal BR (provides increased mobility).
- *Deep Dissection:* To expose the distal third of the radius, supinate the forearm and incise the periosteum of the lateral aspect of the radius lateral to the pronator quadratus and flexor pollicis longus origins. Continue subperiosteal dissection, retracting the two muscles medially and lifting them off the radius. To expose the middle third, pronate the forearm and subperiosteally dissect away the PT insertion along the lateral aspect of the radius (this also detaches the insertion of the flexor digitorum superficialis [FDS] as well). The proximal third of the radius is covered by the supinator, through which the PIN passes on its way to the dorsal compartment of the forearm. **BEWARE the PIN!** To displace the nerve laterally and dorsally (away from the surgical area), fully supinate the forearm and expose the insertion of the supinator into the anterior aspect of the radius. Next, incise the supinator along its insertion along the radius and dissect subperiosteally, stripping the muscle off the bone. Gentle lateral retraction of the freed muscle will lift the PIN safely away from the surgical area. Finally, *do not* place retractors on the posterior surface of the radial neck (to displace the radius anteriorly) because they may compress the PIN against the bone (in 25% of patients).
- *Recap of Dangers:* PIN in the proximal third of the radius and the dorsal radial neck; superficial radial nerve under the BR when retracted; radial artery running down the middle of the forearm under the BR at two points: (1) when mobilizing the BR and (2) in the proximal third as it passes medially to the biceps tendon.
- You can extend the anterior approach distally to expose the wrist joint. It may also be extended into an anterolateral approach to the elbow/humerus (rarely required).
- A second internervous plane in the anterior forearm is between the median and ulnar nerves: a dissection between the flexor carpi ulnaris (FCU) and the FDS (used to expose the ulnar nerve).

Dorsal Approach of Thompson

- Provides excellent access to the entire dorsum of the radial shaft. The main goal is to isolate and retract the PIN before exposing the most proximal portions of the radius, thus protecting it at all stages of the operation from damage.
- *Patient Position:* Two are possible: Supine, arm with tourniquet and (1) in abduction and pronation or (2) across the chest and supinated (facilitates easier access to ulna through a second incision as described above).
- *Landmarks:* The lateral epicondyle of the humerus and Lister's tubercle (one third of the way across the dorsum of the wrist from the radial styloid).
- *Incision:* Gently curved incision along the dorsum of the forearm from a point anterior to the lateral epicondyle of the humerus to a point distal to the ulnar side of Lister's tubercle at the wrist.
- *Internervous Plane:* Proximally, ECRB and the EDC (their common aponeurosis is the cleavage plane); distally, the ECRB and EPL.

- *Superficial Dissection:* Incise the deep fascia in line with the skin incision and identify the proximal internervous plane. Dissect proximally to reveal the upper third of the radial shaft (covered by the supinator and containing the PIN). Distally, below the APL and EPB, identify the internervous plane between the ECRB and the EPL and separate the muscles to reveal the lateral radial shaft.
- *Deep Dissection:* Proximally, it is all about preserving the PIN. There are two methods to expose and preserve the nerve: (1) proximal to distal or (2) distal to proximal. In the former, detach and retract the origin of the ECRB and part of the ECRL to expose/identify the PIN before it enters the proximal supinator. Then, dissect the nerve out through the substance of the supinator in a proximal to distal fashion, preserving the multiple motor branches. In the latter, identify the nerve as it exits the supinator (~1 cm proximal to the distal end of the supinator muscle). Then, dissect the nerve out through the substance of the supinator in a distal to proximal fashion, again preserving all motor branches. Once the nerve is safe, fully supinate the arm and detach the insertion of the supinator muscle from the volar aspect of the radius subperiosteally to expose the upper third of the radial shaft (and shield the nerve from the procedure). Exposure of the middle third of the radius involves retracting/dissecting through the APL and EPB. Distally, separating the ECRB from the EPL (distal internervous plane) exposes the lateral border of the radius; subperiosteal dissection leads to the dorsal aspect of the bone.
- *Recap of Dangers:* The PIN, identify it! Remember that in 25% of cases, the PIN touches the dorsum of the bone opposite the bicipital tuberosity; thus, hardware placed high on the dorsal surface of the radius may trap the nerve underneath. *Identifying and preserving the nerve in the supinator is paramount* (if removing hardware via a dorsal approach, scarring makes visualization difficult, especially in the proximal third of the radius). The posterior interossius artery accompanying the PIN is small and of little consequence: if it is damaged, one need not be alarmed, because the anterior interossius artery will compensate via collateral circulation.
- To enlarge the exposure, detach the origin of the ECRB from the common extensor origin on the lateral epicondyle of the humerus. Furthermore, the approach itself can be extended distally into the dorsum of the wrist and proximally into the lateral aspect of the distal humerus (although these extensions are rarely required).

Approach to the Ulna

- Simplest of the three approaches. The ulna has a subcutaneous border that extends for its entire length; the bone can be reached simply and directly without endangering other structures.
- *Patient Position:* Supine, arm with tourniquet, and placed across the chest to expose the subcutaneous border of the ulna.
- *Landmarks:* The ulna is readily palpable along the entirety of its subcutaneous border.
- *Incision:* Linear, longitudinal incision, parallel and slightly volar to the subcutaneous crest of the ulna. More volarly placed incisions may cause incisional discomfort when the patient rests the forearm on a table (not the case with more dorsal incisions).
- *Internervous Plane:* Between the ECU and FCU (proximally may include the anconeus).
- *Superficial Dissection:* Beginning distally, incise the deep fascia as per the skin incision down to the subcutaneous border and divide any fibers of the ECU encountered.
- *Deep Dissection:* Incise the periosteum over the ulna longitudinally. Continue dissecting around the bone in the subperiosteal plane to expose flexor and extensor surfaces as necessary. Proximally, the insertion of the triceps will need to be detached to gain access to the bone.
- *Recap of Dangers:* The ulnar nerve travels under the FCU and atop the FDP; its safety relies on subperiosteal stripping of the FCU during deep dissection. It is most vulnerable during very proximal dissections and should be identified as it passes through the two heads of the FCU *before* the muscle is stripped from the bone; The ulnar artery runs radial to the ulnar nerve and is at risk along with the ulnar nerve.
- You can extend the approach proximally over the olecranon and into the distal humerus, but not distally.

Definition: A benign disorder characterized by metaplasia and proliferation of the synovial membrane.

Etiology: The etiology of this disorder is not known. Infection and trauma have been considered as possible etiologies.

Incidence: Synovial chondromatosis is not a common disorder and the true incidence is unknown.

Age: It usually affects patients in their second to fifth decades.

Gender: It is more common in the male population (male-to-female ratio 2 to 4:1).

Race: No racial predilection exists.

Signs and Symptoms: The patient usually complains of swelling, dull ache, locking, stiffness, limitation of joint motion, crepitus, or giving way. On physical examination, an effusion may be present. There may be tenderness of the joint or pain on range of motion. The range of motion may be limited. A palpable tender mass may also be present.

Diagnostic Studies: Plain x-ray studies show multiple (usually more than 5) calcified or osseous bodies within the joint or bursa. Pressure erosions (saucerization) and cyst formation can be seen in adjacent bone. A similar observation may be found in patients with pigmented villonodular synovitis. When radiographs are negative, Magnetic Resonance Imaging (MRI)

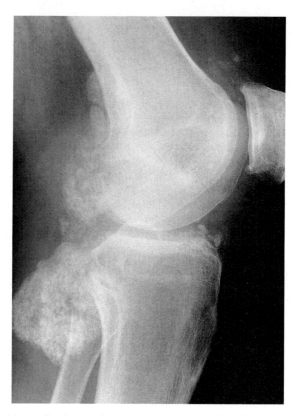

Fig. 217-1   Synovial osteochondromatosis. Lateral radiograph showing the fine cartilage calcifications of primary synovial osteochondromatosis. *(From Adam A, et al: Grainger & Allison's Diagnostic Radiology, 5th ed. Philadelphia, Saunders, 2008.)*

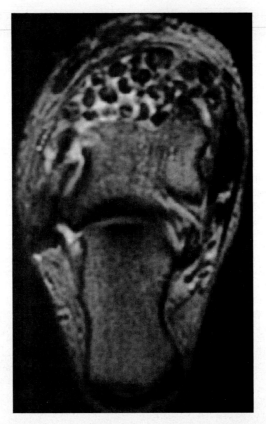

Fig. 217-2 Synovial osteochondroma tosus. Shown on MRI. The T2-weighted image shows the periphery of the nodules to remain dark, consistent with calcification or bone, and the centers of the nodules to remain intermediate in signal intensity. The joint fluid is very bright. *(From Harris ED, Jr: Kelley's Textbook of Rheunatology, 7th ed. Philadelphia, Saunders, 2005.)*

may show cartilaginous bodies. MRI shows high signal on T2-weighted images. Additionally, computed tomography scans are used in visualizing the location of such tumors.

Macropathology: More than one half of cases occur in the knee. The next most cases occur in the elbow. Other common sites include the hip, shoulder, wrist, and ankle. Microscopic evaluation of the joint shows synovial membrane metaplasia, hyperplasia, and hyaline or myxoid change. The synovial lining of a joint, bursa, or tendon sheath undergoes nodular proliferation, and fragments may break off from the synovial surface into the joint. Cartilaginous bodies are initially enveloped and then break free to form loose bodies. Many of the loose bodies are sequestered in the posterior aspect of the knee.

Micropathology: Composed often of a core of normal bone, surrounded by cartilage. Both the cartilage and bone are histologically benign.

Treatment: Total open synovectomy is the treatment of choice. Arthroscopy is another option to remove loose bodies. The recurrence rate after surgery is more than 25%.

Definition: Synovial sarcoma is a malignant soft tissue tumor. It is a high-grade tumor and is associated with poor prognosis. Oddly, it does not develop from the synovium. It typically occurs either in a monophasic or biphasic form. The most common site is surrounding the knee. Of all soft tissue sarcomas, this type is the most likely to metastasize to bone.

Incidence: Accounts for 7% of all patients presenting with a soft tissue sarcoma.

Age: Often seen in adolescents and children with a peak incidence in the third decade of life (median age, 36 years).

Gender: More common in females.

Race: No known differences.

Etiology and Pathophysiology: Ninety percent of cases of synovial sarcoma have a t(x;18)(p11;q11) translocation. This causes a fusion of the *SYT* gene with the *SSX* gene, resulting in a loss of repression and an increase in transcription.

Associations: Synovial sarcomas have a high tendency to metastasize to the lungs and bones.

Signs and Symptoms: Unlike other soft tissue sarcomas, synovial sarcoma is associated with pain.

Diagnostic Studies: Cytogenically analyzing the tumor cells for the t(x;18)(p11;q11) translocation has become a very accurate way to test for synovial sarcoma. Imaging studies can provide valuable information such as whether or not the tumor has invaded the surrounding bone.

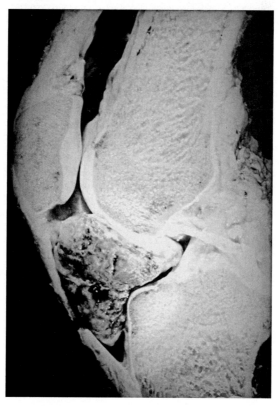

Fig. 218-1   The gross specimen shows that the tan, hemorrhagic tumor bulges into the joint but is covered by synovium. *(From Harris ED Jr: Kelley's Textbook of Rheumatology, 7th ed. Philadelphia, Saunders, 2005.)*

455

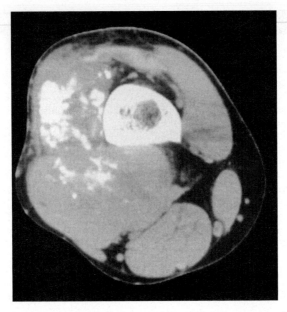

Fig. 218-2 Synovial sarcoma. Axial CT scan demonstrating a soft tissue mass lateral and posterior to the femur containing calcifications. *(From Adam A, et al: Grainger & Allison's Diagnostic Radiology, 5th ed. Philadelphia, Saunders, 2008.)*

Micropathology: The tumor is composed of ovoid and spindle cells. Three growth patterns have been identified: (1) monophasic, composed of spindle and ovoid cell sheets, (2) biphasic, in which sheets or cords of ovoid cells wind through a background of spindle cells, and (3) biphasic, in which the ovoid cells form glands. In all patterns the cells are usually positive for keratin and epithelial membrane antigens.

Macropathology: The tumor usually manifests as an isolated painful mass. Fifty-five percent of the time it is found in the lower extremity. Occasionally it is found in unusual sites such as the diaphragm. The tumor itself is grayish-white and often has a greasy feel.

Treatment: Complete surgical resection remains the treatment of choice. There is much controversy about whether or not chemotherapy provides any benefits. Because the tumor tends to extend along fascial planes, it is important to carefully plan the surgery. The tumor also tends to occur around proximal limb girdles, requiring dissection in and around neurovascular structures making it difficult to successfully salvage limbs.

Definition: As the name states, this is a fracture of the talus. In 50% of cases, the fracture is of the talar neck; in 5% of cases, the fracture is of the talar head. The rest of the time the fracture occurs in the talar body. The talus sits between the calcaneus, tibia, and fibula. These three bones along with the talus comprise the ankle joint. The talus' odd humped shape allows the body to transfer weight and pressure evenly when standing and walking. Motor vehicle accidents, falls, and snowboarding are the most frequently cited causes of the fracture.

Mechanism: Fractures in which the inferior fracture line propagates in front of the lateral process are considered talar neck fractures, whereas fractures in which the inferior fracture line propagates behind the lateral process, therefore involving the posterior facet of the subtalar joint, are considered talar body fractures. Fractures of the talar neck occur most frequently following the forced dorsiflexion of the foot. This forces the neck of the talus to strike the tibial crest, leading to a subluxation and/or dislocation of the body from the subtalar and tibiotalar articulations. Fractures of the talar head are due to compressive forces through the talar head.

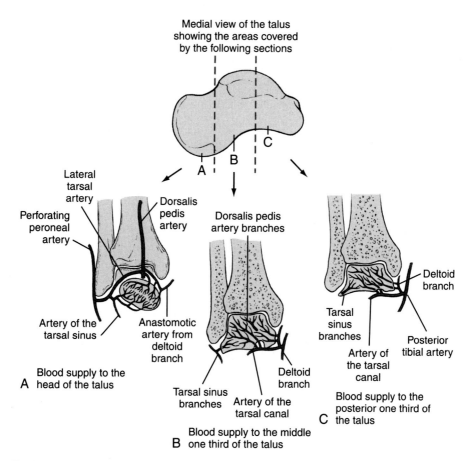

Fig. 219-1   Diagram showing the blood supply to the talus in coronal sections. *(From Mulfinger GL, Trueta J: The blood supply of the talus. J Bone Joint Surg Br 52:160, 1970.)*

Associations: Talar head fractures are associated with subtalar dislocations. Talar neck fractures are associated with medial/lateral malleoli, which suggests a possible rotational component. Often talus fractures are also associated with lower back injuries. In a majority of causes, osteonecrosis occurs due to the poor blood supply in the foot. This often causes problems for the patient later on, often resulting in the need for talonavicular joint arthrodesis.

Signs and Symptoms: Acute pain, inability to bear weight, considerable swelling, and tenderness. Because these symptoms are somewhat general, talus fractures are often mistaken for ankle sprains. Occasionally the fracture results in bone penetrating the skin.

Diagnostic Studies: Anteroposterior, lateral, and oblique radiographic studies of the foot and ankle are standard. Occasionally, radiographs will not show the fracture and therefore computed tomography scans and magnetic resonance imaging scans are often ordered in conjunction with radiographs. Postoperatively, checking for Hawkin's sign is the best way to determine whether avascular necrosis has occurred. This is done by checking for the appearance of decreased subchondral bone density in the dome of talus 6 to 8 weeks following injury. This indicates that there is sufficient vascular supply to bone thereby preventing osteopenia from occurring.

Treatment: The course of treatment varies depending on severity of the fracture. If the fracture did not result in displacement of the bone (type 1), cast immobilization and non–weight-bearing status for 6 to 8 weeks is indicated. If the bones are displaced as little as 1 mm (type 2), prompt reduction is required to avoid compromising the soft tissue surrounding the talus. This is accomplished by plantar-flexing the foot into either inversion or eversion, depending on the nature of the displacement. Open reduction and internal fixation may also become necessary due to displacement of the bones. Usually, K-wires, small fragment lag screws, and/or cannulated, bioabsorbable, headless/countersunk screws are used. Bone grafting also is often required to restore structural integrity. More severe cases of talus fracture (type 3) necessitate open reduction to mitigate compression caused by displacement and to decrease osteonecrosis. For very severe fractures (type 4), an external fixator becomes required to alleviate the pressure on the ankle joint. The surgeons then use a percutaneous pin to fix the bones in their anatomic positions. Sometimes a mortise, medial, or lateral malleolar osteotomy is necessary to gain exposure to fractures below the ankle joint.

Tendon injuries include tenosynovitis, tendonitis, partial tears, and rupture.

THE MUSCLES

Flexor: Flexor pollicis longus (FPL), flexor digitorum profundus (FDP), flexor digitorum superficialis (FDS), flexor carpi ulnaris (FCU), flexor carpi radialis (FCR), palmaris longus (PL)

Extensor: Abductor pollicis longus (APL), extensor pollicis brevis (EPB), extensor carpi radialis longus (ECRL), extensor carpi radialis brevis (ECRB), extensor pollicis longus (EPL), extensor digitorum (ED), extensor indicis proprius (EIP), extensor digiti minimi (EDM), extensor carpi ulnaris (ECU) (Fig. 220-1).

Intrinsic: Thenar, lumbricals, interosseous, hypothenar.

Tenosynovitis: Inflammatory response within the tendon sheath, most often due to repetitive stress or infection.

*Imaging: T2-weighted magnetic resonance imaging (MRI): fluid signal intensity is seen within the tendon sheath.

De Quervain's Tenosynovitis: APL + EPB.

Physical Examination: Positive Finkelstein's—pain in radial thumb with closed fist placed in passive ulnar deviation.

Treatment: Nonsteroidal anti-inflammatory drugs (NSAIDs), ice, immobilization, and cortisone injections. Surgery is indicated when conservative measures fail to work after 1 month (cutting of diseased tendon sheath).

Trigger Finger: Inflammation at MCP or PIP and nodule formation in the tendon sheath with periodic "locking" with movement.

Physical Examination: Palpable click at the site of the nodule; often finger cannot extend.

Treatment: Surgery to open the pulley that is being obstructed by the nodule.

Flexor Tenosynovitis: Disruption of normal flexor tendon movement most often due to infection, with inflammation and aggregation of inciting agent within the sheath.

Physical Examination: Inability to flex/extend IP joints, pain, fullness.

Treatment: Surgical drainage and débridement if not improved within 12 hours of beginning medical management and antibiotics.

Tendonitis: Inflammation, irritation, and swelling of the tendon, most commonly from repetitive mechanical motion.

*Imaging: T1- and T2-weighted MRI. Tendon is typically thickened and may have increased signal intensity.

Treatment: Splinting, NSAIDs, possible surgical release.

FCU Tendonitis: Palmar ulnar wrist pain.

Physical Examination: Pain with wrist flexion.

FCR Tendonitis: Palmar radial wrist pain.

Physical Examination: Pain on resisted wrist flexion.

ECU Tendonitis: Dorsal ulnar wrist pain.

Physical Examination: Pain on resisted dorsiflexion with the wrist in ulnar deviation and forearm supination.

Intersection Syndrome: Inflammation at the crossing point of the APL and EPB with the ECRL and ECRB 6-to 8-cm proximal to the radiocarpal joint in the dorsal forearm.

Physical Examination: Palpable crepitus with motion; tender and swollen at the site.

Partial Tear/Rupture: Tendons are still functional at 70% to 90% laceration. Most common etiologies are direct trauma, weakness due to natural aging, eccentric loading, or steroid injection for tendonitis.

*Imaging: T2-weighted MRI—malposition of the tendon and inflammation of the tendon sheath with discontinuity of the tendon fibers on complete rupture.

Rupture Treatment: Surgery using graft if greater than or equal to 30 mm between retracted ends.

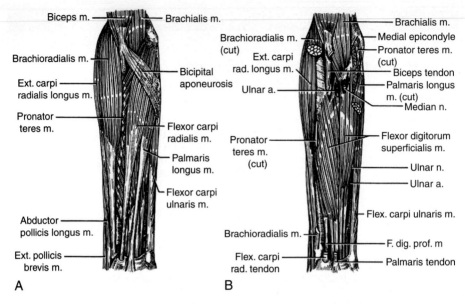

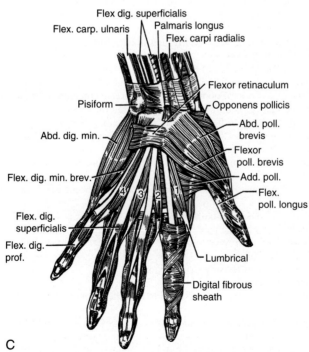

Fig. 220-1 Flexor tendons of the right forearm, wrist, and hand. **A,** Superficial forearm layer. **B,** Deep forearm layer. **C,** Left wrist and palm. Proper function of the flexor tendons requires defect-free tendons and smooth tendon sheaths for easy gliding, and an intact pulley system; hence, flexor tendon lacerations are seldom repaired in the emergency department. *(Modified from Pansky B: Upper extremity. In Pansky B [ed]: Review of Gross Anatomy, 4th ed. New York, Macmillan Publishing, 1979, pp 219, 243. Used with permission from Roberts J: Clinical Procedures in Emergency Medicine, 4th ed. Philadelphia, Saunders, 2004.)*

SITE OF INJURY

Flexors:
Treatment: Surgery preferred for all flexor tears/ruptures as soon as possible after the injury.
FDP (Jersey Finger): Seventy-five percent ring finger, due to forced extension of digit while DIP flexed.
Physical Examination: Pain, swelling, inability to flex DIP joint of digit while PIP held extended.
FPL: Cannot bend tip of thumb against resistance.
FDS: Holding all other digits in extension, patient cannot flex middle joint of digit.

Extensors:
Treatment: Conservative with NSAIDs, ice, and elevation for partial tears, but surgery required if conservative treatment fails or if tear is complete.
APL, EPB: Cannot move thumb away from other digits.
ECRL, ECRB: Cannot extended fisted hand at the wrist.
EPL: Cannot raise thumb off flat surface with hand prone.
MCP Joint Extensors (Mallet Finger): Rupture of distal extensor tendon/fracture distal phalanx.
Physical Examination: Cannot extend DIP.
Treatment: Surgical fixation if bone fragment greater than or equal to one third the articular surface of DIP; otherwise, splint dorsally 6 to 8 weeks.
Boutonnière Injury: Same as Mallet but cannot extend PIP.
Pseudoboutonnière: PIP hypertext with PIP flexion contracture.
Physical Examination: PIP in constant flexion.
EIP: Cannot extend index finger while rest of hand in fist.
EDM: Cannot extend little finger while rest of hand in fist.
ECU: Cannot deviate hand in ulnar direction.

Intrinsic:
Treatment: Conservative measures, then surgery if not improved within 1 month or if complete tear.
Thenar: Cannot touch thumb to other digits.
Interosseous/Lumbricals: Cannot abduct or adduct digits with palm on surface.
Hypothenar: Cannot deviate small fingers in ulnar direction.

Basics:
- Standard implants either employ cement or biologic interdigitation (press fit) for long-term fixation of both acetabular and femoral components.
- With cement fixation there is static mechanical interlock of the cement polymethyl-methacrylate (PMMA) to the interstices of bone.
- Biologic fixation is accomplished by either on-growth with a grit-blasted metallic surface or in-growth with a porous-coated surface.

Incidence: Fifteen percent of cemented THA has to be revised. Eleven percent of the revisions were for aseptic loosening. The rate of loosening for the femoral component was 3% and the rate for the acetabluar component was 10%.

Signs and Symptoms of Failure:
- Postoperative groin and thigh pain.
- Mechanical type of pain, increasing with weight bearing and relieved by rest.
- When a previously pain-free hip becomes painful, suspect loosening.
- Acetabular loosening tends to cause groin pain, femoral loosening tends to cause thigh pain.

Controversy: The trend toward the use of noncemented fixation in THA is justified by reports of higher rates of loosening in young active patients with cemented implants.

PMMA:
- Compared with cortical bone, it has a lower elastic modulus and significantly inferior mechanical strength properties.
- Tensile strength similar to that of cancellous bone.
- Poor fatigue strength attributed to porosity.
- Newer techniques employ pressurization and vacuum preparation techniques to avoid air pores in the cement that could crack.

Mode of Failure of Cemented Fixation:
- If increased cyclic loading leads to microfracture of the cement, the cement will not remodel because it is not alive and the implant will ultimately loosen.
- Successful bone in-growth requires an initial rigid fixation with micromotion of the prosthesis below 150 microns to prevent fibrous in-growth.
- As fibrous in-growth sets in, continued prosthetic micromotion and loosening cause decreased remodeling potential and ultimately pain will ensue.
- If a fibrous capsule forms around the prosthesis, it will settle and become biomechanically unstable.

Debonding:
- In femoral component failure, debonding—the deterioration of the stem-cement bond—occurs early.
- Debonding often leads to high peak stresses in the cement mantle, which can result in fractures, most of which occur proximally.
- Once this occurs, the thin mantles, as well as the defects and pores in the cement associated with most mantle fractures, make the implant more susceptible to biologic factors.

Treatment:
- Prevention, press fitting
- Revision arthroplasty

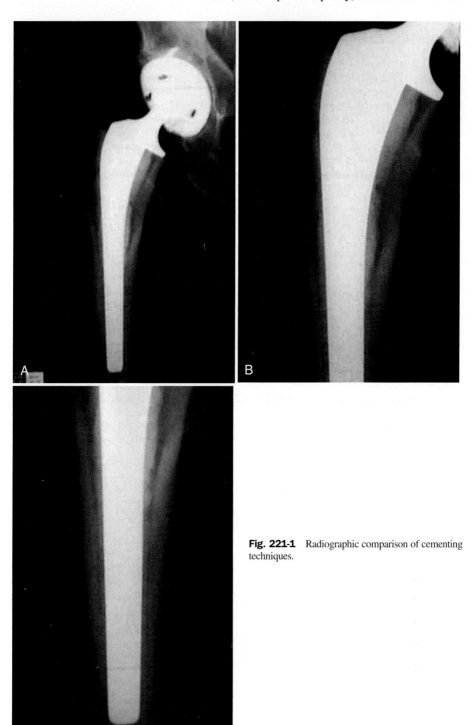

Fig. 221-1 Radiographic comparison of cementing techniques.

Definition: Localized cold injury related to tissue freezing and destruction (90% hands and feet).
Epidemiology and History: Average age 38 to 41 years. More common in males and those unaccustomed to cold (African Americans, Middle Eastern individuals). First described by Napoleon's surgeon, Dominique Larrey.
Pathophysiology: Cold causes extracellular ice crystal formation, cellular dehydration, protein denaturation, inhibition of DNA synthesis, abnormal cell wall permeability with resultant osmotic changes, damage to capillaries, and pH changes.

Rewarming causes cell swelling, erythrocyte and platelet aggregation, endothelial cell damage, thrombosis, tissue edema, increased compartment space pressure, bleb formation, localized ischemia, and tissue death.
"Hunting Reaction:" Alternating cycles of vasoconstriction and vasodilatation, causing partial thawing and refreezing; with increasing blood viscosity comes progressive thrombosis.
Jackson's Zone of Stasis: Endothelial injury from decreased dermal blood flow.
Classification (after Rewarming): Superficial (first and second degree) or deep (third and fourth degree).
• First Degree—anesthetic central white plaque with peripheral erythema
• Second Degree—clear/milky blisters with surrounding erythema/edema (first 24 hours)
• Third Degree—hemorrhagic blisters, form hard black eschar at approximately 2 weeks
• Fourth Degree—complete necrosis and tissue loss
Physical: Sensitivity to light touch and pain, change in color, tissue deformability
Imaging: Magnetic resonance imaging (MRI) and MR angiography (MRA) show occluded vessels and delineate ischemic soft tissue, allowing for earlier surgical intervention. Two-phase Tc-99 bone scan is used for prognosis. Initial scan on day 3 evaluates severity; second scan on day 7 has increased sensitivity. Correlation has been shown between demarcation zone of uptake in phalanges and level of amputation.
Treatment (Three Phases):
Prethaw/Field Care/Prehospital: Protect from mechanical injury with padding, **avoid thawing** until definite rewarming assured.

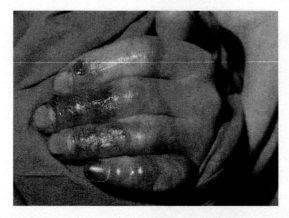

Fig. 222-1 Frostbite of the hand in a mountaineer. On rewarming, the hand became painful, red, and edematous, with signs of probable gangrene in the fifth finger. *(From Forbes CD, Jackson WF: Color Atlas and Text of Clinical Medicine, 3rd ed. London, Mosby, 2003.)*

464

Table 222-1. MULTISYSTEMIC FEATURES OF HYPOTHERMIA AND REWARMING TECHNIQUES

System*	Mild Hypothermia (Core > 32°C)	Moderate Hypothermia (Core 28°C–32°C)	Severe Hypothermia (Core < 28°C)
Thermoregulatory	Shivering intact	Shivering lost, rapid cooling	Shivering lost, rapid cooling
Respiratory	Tachypnea	Hypoventilation, respiratory acidosis, hypoxemia, aspiration pneumonia, atelectasis	Apnea, adult respiratory distress syndrome
Cardiovascular	Tachycardia, hypertension	Hypotension, bradycardia, prolonged QT interval, J waves (leads II and V_6)	Pulseless electrical activity, atrial fibrillation, heart block, ventricular fibrillation, asystole
Gastrointestinal	Ileus	Pancreatitis, gastric erosions	Pancreatitis, gastric erosions
Genitourinary and fluids/electrolytes	Bladder atony, cold diuresis	Hyperkalemia, hyperglycemia, lactic acidosis	Hyperkalemia, hyperglycemia, lactic acidosis
Muscular	Hypertonia	Rigidity	Rhabdomyolysis
Hematologic	—	Hemoconcentration, hypercoagulability	Disseminated intravascular coagulation, bleeding
Neurologic	Hyperreflexia, disorientation, ataxia, dysarthria	Hyporeflexia, agitation, hallucination, dilated pupils	Areflexia, coma, absent pupil responses, brain-dead—like state
Rewarming technique†	Passive rewarming (active external rewarming may be required if the patient is unable to generate heat through shivering because of exhaustion or advanced age)	Active external and noninvasive internal rewarming (invasive internal rewarming may be required if there is cardiovascular compromise)	Active external, noninvasive internal, invasive internal or extracorporeal blood rewarming (venovenous or arteriovenous hemodialysis, cardiopulmonary bypass)

* The systemic effects are a continuum and depend not only on core temperature but also on patient features. Rewarming methods need to be decided on an individual basis.
† Passive, blanket (covering body and head). Active external, forced air or heating blanket; warm baths are not recommended because they make monitoring difficult. Noninvasive internal, warmed oxygen and warmed intravenous fluids. Active internal, peritoneal lavage, pleural lavage, esophageal warming tubes.
From Koehncke N, Dosman J: Out of the cold: management of hypothermia and frostbite. CMAJ 168:305-311, 2003.

Immediate Hospital/Rewarming: **Rapid**, 40° to 42° C water until thawing complete (red/purple indicates the end of vasoconstriction), narrow temperature range (too cold reduces tissue survival, too warm causes thermal damage).

Post-thaw Care: **Débride white** blisters (blister fluid has high levels of prostaglandin $F_2\alpha$ and thromboxane A_2) but **leave hemorrhagic blisters intact** (avoid desiccation); coat both with **aloe vera** q6 (inhibits thromboxane and tissue necrosis) or Silvadene (opens wounds).

- ASA/nonsteroidal anti-inflammatory drugs prevent thrombosis and retard inflammation
- Antitetanus prophylaxis, analgesia, ibuprofen, benzyl PCN 48 to 72 hours
- Daily hydrotherapy 30 to 40 minutes at 40° C
- Elevate parts and splint, prevent smoking

Surgical Care:
- Early limited débridement of blisters and necrotic tissue
- Fasciotomy for compartment syndrome
- Delay amputation/aggressive débridement until progressive ischemia is complete and see final demarcation (1 to 3 months) unless infected

Late Sequelae: Cold insensitivity, sensory loss, vasospastic syndromes with **increased sympathetic tone** (pain, hyperhidrosis, coldness or edema, trophic changes, Raynaud's; may require regional sympathetectomy), osteoarthritis of interphalangeal joints, intrinsic muscle atrophy, epiphyseal destruction, heterotopic calcification.

Table 222-2. LOCAL COLD-INDUCED INJURIES

Injury	Symptoms and Signs
Axonal degeneration	Numbness, dysesthesia, cutaneous vasomotor instability; sensitivity to cold may persist for years
Chilblains (pernio)	Pruritic patches of erythema and cyanosis, especially on hands and feet, that may blister, ulcerate, scar or atrophy
Cold-contact adhesion[†]	Erosion or ulcer on forcible separation
Frostbite	
Superficial	Pallor, edema, blistering, desquamation
Deep	Hemorrhagic blisters and anesthesia, followed later by hyperesthesia, ulceration and gangrene
Frostnip	Transient numbness and tingling without residual tissue damage
Immersion syndrome (trench foot)[*]	Alternating vasoconstriction (cold, pallor, cyanosis, and pulselessness) and vasodilatation (warmth, erythema, and edema), ecchymosis, blistering, lymphangitis, cellulitis, thrombophlebitis, gangrene

[*] Limb, often inactive, is immersed for prolonged period in non-freezing cold water or mud.
[†] Contact between metal and moist skin or mucosa.
From Koehncke N, Dosman J: Out of the cold: management of hypothermia and frostbite. CMAJ 168:305-311, 2003.

These fractures are often *high-energy* with *severe soft tissue injury* and *articular comminution,* leading to *increased complications* and *worse outcomes.*
- Relatively uncommon fracture—7% to 10% of all tibia fractures
- More common in males and patients ages 35 to 40 years
- Most commonly result from motor vehicle accidents or falls from a height
- Unlike rotational ankle fractures, the principal load is *axial*

Imaging:
- Standard ankle radiographs (anteroposterior, lateral, mortise) and full-length tibia films if fracture extends proximally
- As with most intraarticular fractures, *CT is generally required* for assessment of the articular surface and surgical planning

Classification:
Ruedi-Allgower: Based on degree of comminution

Type I—nondisplaced

Type II—displaced, minimal comminution

Type III—displaced, extensive comminution

AO/OTA: 27 subtypes

Type A—nonarticular

Type B—partial articular

Type C—total articular

Fracture classification does not always correlate with the amount of soft-tissue injury, which must be repeatedly assessed and used as a guide for timing of surgery

Treatment: Emphasis has changed in recent years from anatomic reduction and rigid fixation to the limitation of complications due to many devastating problems with early open reduction and internal fixation.

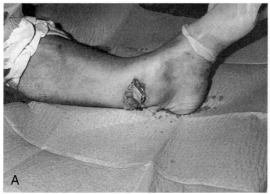 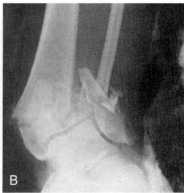

Fig. 223-1 **A** and **B,** A type IIIB open pilon (tibial plafond) fracture. *(From Browner BD, et al: Skeletal Trauma: Basic Science, Management and Reconstruction, 3rd ed. Philadelphia, Saunders, 2002.)*

467

Technique	Advantages	Disadvantages
Ankle spanning external fixation	Easiest to apply Avoids zone of injury	Immobilizes ankle Articular reduction difficult
External fixation on same side of joint	Allows ankle motion Stabilizes metaphysis	Technically difficult Disrupts zone of injury Cannot be used in all fractures
Open reduction and internal fixation	Better articular reduction Allows ankle motion	Highest incidence of wound complications and amputation

Current trend is temporary spanning external fixation with or without limited fixation of the articular surface and fibular plating followed by delayed (7 to 14 days) open reduction and internal fixation if needed after soft tissue injury has improved (return of skin wrinkles is one method of assessment)

Complications:

Malunion—more common with external fixation/limited reduction (30%) than with delayed plating (14%)

Nonunion/Delayed Union—about 5%, increased with higher energy/severe soft tissue injury

Wound Complication/Infection—very high with immediate plating (37% to 67%), generally less than 10% with newer techniques

Ankle Arthrosis—Common (up to 50%); does not correlate well with clinical results

Definition: Transient osteoporosis of the hip (TOH) is an uncommon clinical syndrome characterized by pain in the involved joint with temporary osteopenia without joint space destruction in the absence of recognizable causes of synovitis or osteoporosis.

Etiology: Unknown. Some have postulated that it is a form of nontraumatic reflex sympathetic dystrophy or due to an ischemic insult. Others hypothesize that there exists a viral stimulus of osteoclasts to increase resorption of bone.

Association: There are no predisposing factors except pregnancy.

Incidence: TOH is uncommon, with close to 200 cases having been reported in the literature since its first description.

Demographics: Two thirds of the patients are middle-aged men, whereas the remaining are women exclusively in their third trimester of pregnancy. TOH is rare in children. The age of the patients at presentation ranges from 24 to 75 years, with most patients between 40 and 60 years of age.

Signs and Symptoms: Classically, it is characterized by acute, disabling, progressive hip pain located mostly in the groin or anterior aspect of the thigh, accompanied by an antalgic gait and functional disability in the affected extremity. This pain is exacerbated by weight bearing and relieved by rest, and it is rarely present at night.

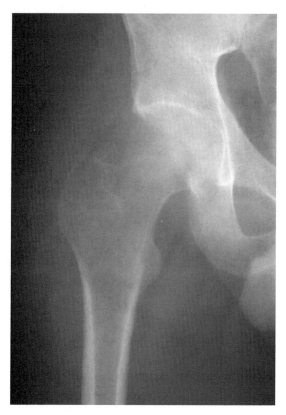

Fig. 224-1   Idiopathic transient osteoporosis of hip. (*Courtesy of James L. Guyton, MD. From Canale ST, Beaty JH [eds]: Campbell's Operative Orthopaedics, 11th ed. Philadelphia, Mosby, 2007.*)

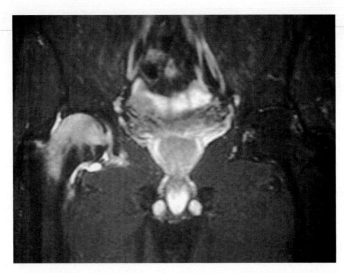

Fig. 224-2 Transient osteoporosis of the hip in 30-year-old man. Coronal inversion recovery sequence shows hyperintense bone marrow edema in more diffuse pattern than seen in osteonecrosis. *(From Canale ST, Beaty JH [eds]: Campbell's Operative Orthopaedics, 11th ed. Philadelphia, Mosby, 2007.)*

Diagnostic Studies: The characteristic radiographic appearance reveals diffuse osteopenia of the entire femoral head and neck and is present within 4 to 8 weeks after onset of symptoms. Rarely are the trochanters, the acetabula, and even iliac wings affected. The joint space is preserved without osseous erosion or subchondral collapse. Radionuclide bone scans reveal a diffuse, increased uptake involving the entire femoral head and neck extending to the intertrochanteric line. T1-weighted images reveal low signal intensity, whereas matching T2-weighted images show high signal extending from the femoral head to the intertrochanteric region.

Micropathology: There is substantial cell death of hematopoietic and fatty elements, but limited death of osteocytes. Inflammation, osteoporosis, and edema with spaced trabeculae and marrow elements, fat necrosis, and reactive bone formation are also present.

Treatment: TOH is usually self-limited and resolves spontaneously within 6 to 8 months, although many physicians recommend protected weight-bearing with nonsteroidal anti-inflammatory drugs as a treatment. Oral and intra-articular administrations of corticosteroids, sympathetic blocks, and calcitonin have all been attempted, but none has altered the course of the disease.

Definition: Triplanar fracture is a physeal fracture of the distal tibia that results from injury during the final phase of maturation and cessation of growth. It is a severe injury and a complex combination of Salter-Harris III and IV fractures. Fracture planes are in the sagittal, coronal, and transverse planes.

Etiology: External rotation mechanism.

Incidence: Accounts for 7% of ankle fractures in girls and 15% of ankle fractures in boys younger than 18 years of age.

Age and Gender: Triplanar fracture occurs in males more often than in females between the ages of 10 and 17 years of age.

Clinical findings: Inability to weight bear and ankle hematoma and hemarthrosis—-may have an associated fibular fracture. It is often difficult to distinguish from a simple ankle sprain.

Classification: Usually classified intra-articularly. Two-part fracture occurs when the medial malleolus region has closed and the lateral physis detaches in a SH IV pattern (lateral epiphysis may be comminuted). Three-part fracture occurs when the middle of the physis has closed and appears as SH type III injury on AP view and type II on lateral radiographs. This type may be associated with a fibular fracture

Treatment: Plain radiography tends to underestimate fracture pattern complexity and displacement. Computed tomographic (CT) imaging is therefore indicated to evaluate properly. If it is truly undisplaced or less than 2 mm displaced with a congruous articular surface, conservative management with a long leg splint should be considered. Surveillance is required, because the fracture may displace further when swelling subsides.

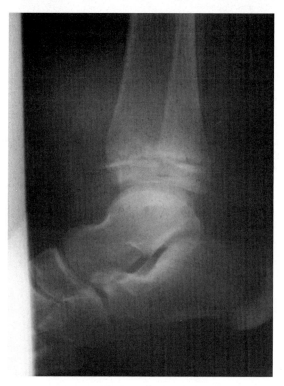

Fig. 225-1 Triplanar fracture.

471

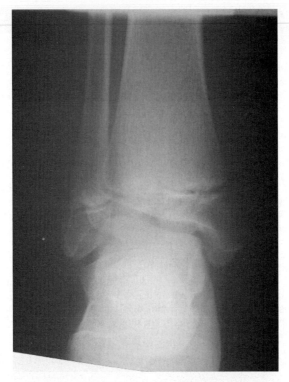

Fig. 225-2 Triplanar fracture. The fracture has two vertical extensions and a horizontal extension.

Surgical Care: Anatomic reduction is manadatory if displacement is greater than 2 mm. For intra-articular fractures—generally 3.5 to 4.5 mm—cannulated screws are employed to reconstruct the joint surface using the CT to plan the procedure.

Complications: Growth arrest is relatively common and depends on severity; any residual growth may require corrective osteotomy. The incidence of arrest and future symptoms may be reduced by anatomic surgical reduction. Overall, anatomic reduction results in satisfactory outcomes for two thirds of patients.

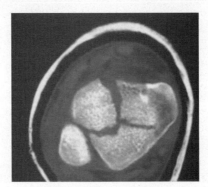

Fig. 225-3 CT scan showing extent of triplanar fracture.

Definition: Tuberculosis (TB) is an inhaled infectious disease that primarily affects the lungs; however, it may also affect the central nervous system, lymphatic and circulatory systems, bones, and tissues. TB was the cause of the "white plague" in the seventeenth and eighteenth centuries in Europe.

Incidence: Eight million people globally develop TB and 3 million die from the disease. In 1998, there were about 18,000 new cases in the United States.

Age and Gender: TB is not age or gender specific.

Etiology and Pathophysiology: Tuberculosis is caused by an acid-fast, aerobic bacilli bacterium—*Mycobacterium tuberculosis*. The disease is initiated when the bacilli reach the pulmonary alveoli after inhalation. TB is a granulomatous inflammatory condition causing periods of tissue destruction and necrosis followed by healing and fibrosis.

Associations and Predispositions: Infection with human immunodeficiency virus, acquired immunodeficiency syndrome, poor nutrition and environmental conditions, intravenous drug use, and alcoholism.

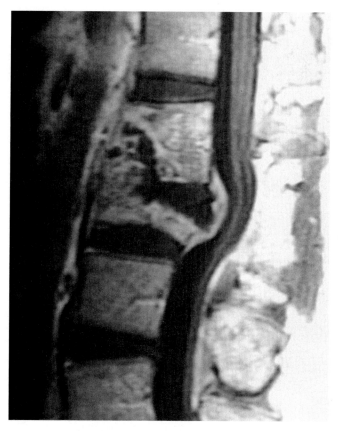

Fig. 226-1 Magnetic resonance imaging study showing extensive destruction of L1 and L2 vertebral bodies and the intervening disk with posterior extension in a Pakistani man with Pott's disease. *(From Mandell GL, Bennett JE, Dolin R [eds.]: Principles and Practice of Infectious Diseases, 6th ed. Philadelphia, Saunders, 2005.)*

473

Signs and Symptoms: Signs and symptoms include a persistent dry cough, significant weight loss, a decrease in energy, fever, and night sweats. For advanced stage tuberculosis, symptoms include chest pain and difficulty breathing.

Diagnostic Studies: Diagnostic tests include chest x-ray examination, computed tomography scan, sputum cultures, tuberculin skin test, bronchoscopy, interferon (IFN)-gamma blood test, and QuantiFERON-TB Gold, which has more recently been used instead of the tuberculin skin test.

Macropathology: An individual with stage IV TB disease presents with either exudative lesions resulting from polymorphonuclear leukocytes around *M.tuberculosis* or granulomatous lesions due to hypersensitivity of the host to tuberculoproteins. These lesions appear in the well-aerated upper lobes of the lungs because *M. tuberculosis* is an obligate aerobe.

Micropathology: Once *M. tuberculosis* is inhaled, activated macrophages surround tubercles; this complex often serves as a breeding ground, hence promoting growth of *M. tuberculosis*.

Treatment: If active TB is diagnosed or strongly suspected, treatment is initiated with isoniazid, rifampin, pyrazinamide, and ethambutol. Dosage and drug of choice are altered per case, gender, and age. Second-line drugs include cycloserine, ethionamide, streptomycin, and levofloxacin.

Definition: Also known as athletic foot injury, it is defined as a plantar-capsular-ligamentous sprain due to forced hyperdorsiflexion.

Etiology: Rapid warmup, intense workout, overuse, playing on artificial surfaces, and wearing soft-soled shoes are predisposing factors.

Incidence: It has been more common since artificial surfaces have become popular in sports. It is mostly seen in football players.

Signs and Symptoms: A grade 1 sprain involves stretching and minor tearing of the capsuloligamentous structures. Typical symptoms include pain, stiffness, and swelling. Physical findings are mild swelling, ecchymosis, and mild pain with weight bearing and motion. A grade 2 sprain is a moderate injury to the joint. The signs and symptoms are more severe pain, swelling, or stiffness greater than a grade 1 sprain. A grade 3 sprain is more severe and can have associated fracture, such as a compression fracture of the metatarsal head or an avulsion fracture with a complete tear of the capsuloligamentous structures.

Diagnostic Studies: Plain radiographs, including anteroposterior, lateral, and sesamoid views should be ordered to assess any injuries to bony structure. In professional athletes, magnetic resonance imaging can help the orthopaedist better evaluate the hard and soft tissue.

Pathology: Occurs when an axial load is put on a foot, fixed in equinus position, which is mostly seen in football linemen. Capsular strain/tears occur at the ventral surface of the metatarsal neck and injury occurs at the dorsal articular surface of the metatarsal head. Sometimes, valgus and varus injuries happen at the same time, with injuries to the lateral and medial capsule.

Treatment: Treatment begins with nonoperative measures, such as instructing the patient to wear shoes with a wide toe box, perhaps extra depth, and stiff soles. Activity modification and the use of nonsteroidal anti-inflammatory drugs are usually helpful in decreasing symptoms. Surgery can be an option for persistent symptoms, sesamoid fracture, instability, hallux rigidus, and loose body in the metatarsophalangeal joint.

Prognosis: In most cases, patients can return to their previous level of function with surgical or nonsurgical treatment. However, some disability can be seen.

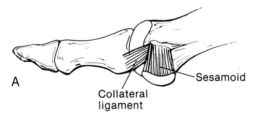

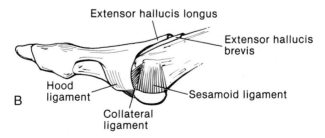

Fig. 227-1   A, The sesamoid and collateral ligaments stabilize the medial and lateral aspects of the first metatarsophalangeal joint. **B,** The hood ligament of the extensor expansion reinforces the dorsal aspect of the first metatarsophalangeal joint. *(From DeLee D, Drez D [eds]: DeLee and Drez's Orthopaedic Sports Medicine, 2nd ed. Philadelphia, Saunders, 2003.)*

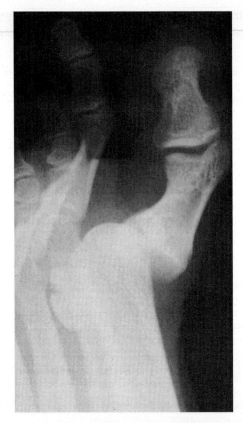

Fig 227-2 Fracture-dislocation of the metatarsophalangeal-sesamoid joint (grade III injury). *(From Clanton TO, Butler JE, Eggert A: Injuries to the metatarsophalangeal joints in athletes. Foot Ankle 7:162-176, 1986. © American Orthopaedic Foot and Ankle Society, 1986.)*

ANATOMY

Path:
- Arises off medial cord with C7, C8, T1 distribution
- Courses down arm → cubital tunnel → medial forearm (beneath FCU) → gives off palmar branch → Guyon's canal → deep branch (courses around hook of the Hamate)/superficial branch

Motor:
- Flexor carpi ulnaris, one-half flexor digitorum profundus
- Deep branch supplies adductor pollicis, deep head of flexor pollicis brevis, interosseous muscles, third and fourth lumbricals, hypothenar (opponens digiti minimi, flexor digiti minimi brevis, abductor digiti minimi, palmaris brevis (superficial)

Sensory:
- Palmar—proximal medial palm
- Superficial—palmar/dorsal digital branch—fifth and one-half fourth

Pathology:
Ulnar Tunnel Syndrome:
- Guyon's Canal—compression
- Paresthesia and numbness involving the ring and little fingers
- Tinel's Sign—percussion of the ulnar nerve at the wrist will elicit a "pins and needles" sensation

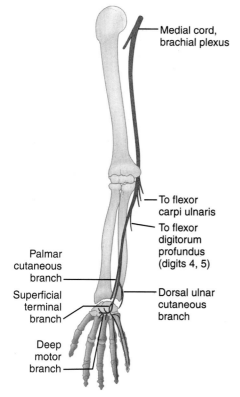

Medial cord, brachial plexus

To flexor carpi ulnaris

To flexor digitorum profundus (digits 4, 5)

Palmar cutaneous branch

Superficial terminal branch

Deep motor branch

Dorsal ulnar cutaneous branch

Fig. 228-1   Major branches of the ulnar nerve, right arm, anterior view. *(From Stewart JD: Focal Peripheral Neuropathies, 3rd ed. Philadelphia, Lippincott Williams & Wilkins, 2000.)*

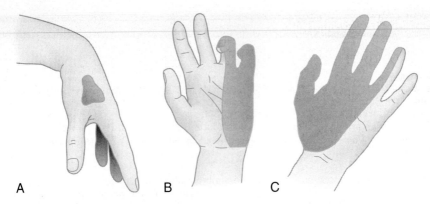

Fig. 228-2 Deformities of the hand. **A,** Radial palsy—wrist drop. **B,** Ulnar nerve palsy—main en griffe (clawhand). **C,** Median nerve palsy—main en singe (monkey hand). The shaded areas represent the usual distribution of anesthesia. *(From Ellis H: Clinical Anatomy: A Revision and Applied Anatomy for Clinical Students, 7th ed. Oxford, Blackwell Scientific, 1983.)*

- Electrodiagnostic studies can be preformed
- Treatment—splinting and decreased use; release
- If in concert with carpal tunnel, it is important that surgical resection includes transverse carpal ligament, because it covers both

Cubital Tunnel Syndrome:
- More common—second to carpal tunnel syndrome for nerve compressions
- Between the humeral and ulnar origins of the flexor carpi ulnaris
- Compression and straining occur with elbow flexion
- Present similar ulnar tunnel syndrome
- Tinel's sign over the elbow
- Electrodiagnostic may not be as accurate
- Treatment—simple padding or 45-degree splint
  - Decompression
  - Transposition out of the cubital tunnel
  - Cubital tunnel reconstruction; medial epicondyle may be detached

Signs of Ulnar Nerve Palsy:
- Claw hand—fourth and fifth digits hyperextended
- Ulnar guttering—interosseous wasting

Definition: Unicameral, or solitary, bone cyst, is a benign, fluid-filled lesion that occurs in long bones of children. The proximal humerus (50% to 60% of cases) and the proximal femur (25% to 30% of cases) are the most frequently involved bones. It was recognized as an entity apart from other cystic lesions of the bone by Bloodgood in 1910. Jaffe and Lichtenstein gave a detailed discussion of the lesions in 1942.

Etiology: The etiology of this disorder is unknown. Some studies have proposed possible vascular or genetic etiologies.

Incidence: They are found in 3% of biopsies.

Age and Gender: Unicameral bone cysts are mostly seen in children 5 to 15 years old. They are more common in boys than girls (2:1).

Signs and Symptoms: Patients are often asymptomatic unless there is a fracture. If the adjacent growth plate is affected, there may be an abnormal growth.

Diagnostic Studies: Plain x-ray films show a central, well-defined, symmetrical radiolucent defect in the intramedullary metaphyseal region immediately adjacent to the physis with no bony loculations.

Pathology: On gross examination, the cyst expands the cortex of the bone. An intact periosteum covers the cortical shell. The cyst usually contains clear serous fluid and, infrequently, blood products. Computed tomography and magnetic resonance imaging studies are usually done to evaluate the extent of the cyst and distinguish it from other types of bone cysts. Malignant transformation in the simple bone cysts is reportedly rare.

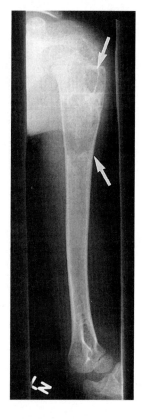

Fig. 229-1 Unicameral bone cyst. The proximal portion of the humerus is a common location for this lesion (*arrows*). The lesion is lucent, is quite well defined, and can be slightly expansile. A fracture can occur through this area owing to the weakened bone. (*From Mettler FA, Jr: Essentials of Radiology, 2nd ed. Philadelphia, Saunders, 2003.*)

479

Treatment: Treatment is aimed at preventing fracture. Curettage and bone grafting, injection of methylprednisolone, and bone marrow or a combination of the above methods, have been used as treatment methods. Lesion with cortical thinning may require surgical intervention. Additionally, multiple factors such as upper extremity (lower stress) versus lower extremity (higher stress) and younger children (more amenable to cast immobilization) versus older adolescents (less amenable to cast immobilization) should be considered before surgical decisions are made.

Complications: Injury to the growth plate (physis) may occur as a result of cyst expansion, pathologic fracture, or unintended disturbance during surgical intervention.

Definition: The upper C-spine includes the occiput, the atlas (C1), and the axis (C2). Injuries to this portion of the spine most commonly include atlas, odontoid, Jefferson, Hangman, occipital condyle, and lateral mass fractures as well as atlantoaxial subluxation and atlanto-occipital dislocation.

Etiology: The exact mechanism of upper C-spine injuries is often difficult to identify with certainty. Many of these injuries are the result of complex mechanisms. Most commonly, upper C-spine injuries are caused by motor vehicle accidents (MVAs), sporting activities, and ground level falls (GLFs). However, any traumatic event causing significant flexion, extension, rotation, or compression of the C-spine can result in injury.

Incidence: Twenty percent of all spinal injuries involve the cervical spine. One third of all cervical spine injuries involve the axis (C2). Five percent to 18% percent of patients brought to the emergency department after suffering severe trauma have an upper C-spine injury.

Age: Adults ages 15 to 24 years are most frequently involved in MVAs. The next most common group is adults over the age of 55 who suffer from osteoporosis and sustain a GLF.

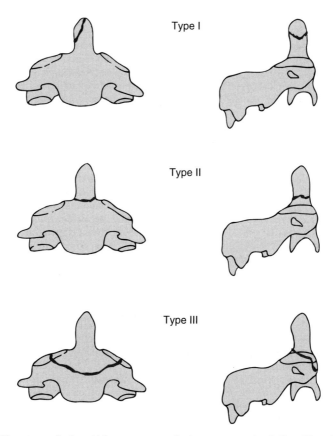

Fig. 230-1   Three types of odontoid fractures as seen in the anteroposterior *(left)* and lateral *(right)* planes. Type I is an oblique fracture through the upper part of the odontoid process itself. Type II is a fracture at the junction of the odontoid process and the vertebral body of the second cervical vertebra. Type III is really a fracture through the body of the atlas. *(Redrawn from Anderson LD, D'Alonzo RT: J Bone Joint Surg Am 56:1663–1674, 1974. In Browner BD: Skeletal Trauma: Basic Science, Management, and Reconstruction, 3rd ed. Philadelphia, Saunders.)*

Gender: In the age-group 15 to 24 years, males predominate. In the older group, females comprise the majority of cases.

Signs, Symptoms, and Clinical Findings: Presentation includes posterior neck pain, pain associated with rotation and weakness, and numbness and paresthesias in the extremities. However, symptoms are frequently nonexistent or nonspecific, including headache, apprehension, dysphagia, and speech changes. Physical examination findings include increased pain on palpation, neck stiffness, and facial/head trauma.

Staging: There is no clear staging for upper C-spine injuries. Both the Canadian C-Spine Rules (CCR) and the National Emergency X-Radiography Utilization Group (NEXUS) criteria enable clinicians to clear low-risk patients of C-spine injury.

Micropathology: Osteoporosis causes a change in the microarchitecture of bone. Porous bone leads to increased risk for fractures. With constant stress on the spine, compression fractures are some of the most common fractures associated with osteoporosis.

Medical Treatment: If a C-spine injury is suspected, the patient must be immobilized with a rigid collar and placed on a spine board. Steroids can be administered if neurologic symptoms exist and the injury is less than 8 hours old. A bolus of methylprednisolone (30 mg/kg IV) is given at 30 minutes followed by a continuous intravenous drip (5.4 mg/kg q1h) for 24 to 48 hours.

Surgical Treatment: If misalignment of the spine is confirmed through radiography, placement in skeletal traction with tongs positioned one finger-width above the earlobes in alignment with the external auditory canal maximizes patient safety. After closed or open reduction of the C-spine has been performed, the need for further surgical intervention can be determined based on the type and severity of the fractures and instability. If more severe instability results, halo immobilization for various lengths of time is the standard of care. Finally, if a collar or halo is deemed inadequate, surgical decompression and fixation from an anterior, posterior, or combined approach can be used. The halo can be left in place as needed postoperatively.

Diagnostic Studies: A lateral radiograph is most useful because 85% to 90% of cervical spine injuries are evident on this view. Acceptable lateral radiographs should exhibit all seven vertebral bodies and the cervicothoracic junction. The odontoid view complements the lateral view and provides evaluation of the lateral masses of C1 with respect to the odontoid process and axis-body.

Complications: A variety of complications are associated with C-spine injuries. These include spinal shock, neurogenic shock, complete and incomplete cord syndromes, anterior spinal cord syndrome, central spinal cord syndrome, Brown-Séquard syndrome, high cervical spinal cord syndrome, Horner's syndrome, posteroinferior cerebellar artery syndrome, and craniofacial injuries. Halo rings can become dislodged if placed above the maximum circumference of the skull, and eyelid closure can be compromised due to superior skin traction if the eyes are not closed when anterior halo pins are placed.

Halo Application: The application process for a halo consists of placing anterior pins in the anterolateral aspect of the skull 1 cm above the orbital rim, slightly lateral to the center of the orbit to avoid injury to the superior orbital nerve. Posterior pins are positioned on the posterolateral aspect of the skull maintaining the halo ring 1 cm above the top of the ear. Skin incisions are not necessary and all pins should be placed perpendicular to the skull. Eight inches per pound of torque should be used in placing the pins in the adult skull. The halo vest size is determined by chest circumference at the xiphoid process. The posterior aspect of the vest should be securely attached before attaching the anterior shell. Twenty-eight feet per pound of torque should be used on common vest bolts. Finally, all pin sites must be cleaned with saline or soap and water, radiographs should be taken to confirm spinal alignment and all pins and bolts must be checked for loosening at 24 to 48 hours. It is recommended to tighten loose pins on only one occasion. If loosening continues, replacing the pins through an adjacent hole in the halo-ring is preferred to maintain stability.

Legg-Calvé-Perthes Disease (Coxa Plana)

Osteonecrosis of the proximal femoral epiphysis.
Incidence: Increased in boys 4 to 8 years old with positive family history and low birth weight. Bilateral in 12% to 15% but generally not symmetrical or simultaneous.
Signs and Symptoms: Pain (often in knee), effusion, limp, decreased range-of-motion (ROM), Trendelenburg gait.
Radiographic Findings: Growth cessation of ossific nuclei, subchondral fracture (crescent sign), and medial joint space widening. Poor prognosis (Caterall's "head at risk" signs)—lateral calcification, Gage's sign—V-shaped defect at lateral physis, lateral subluxation, metaphyseal cyst formation, horizontal growth plate.
Prognosis: Worse with bone age greater than 6 years, deceased ROM, female gender, B or C lateral pillar classification.
Classification Systems: Wallenstraam's classification explains four phases: initial, fragmentation, reossification, healed or reossified. Herring classification—most prognostic: based on involvement of the lateral pillar and the capital femoral epiphysis.
Treatment: Nonsteroidal anti-inflammatory drugs (NSAIDs), traction, bracing, Petrie cast, partial weight bearing, osteotomy.

Hip Avascular Necrosis

Likely secondary to intravascular coagulation. Coagulation leads to generalized venous thrombosis resulting in arterial occlusion.
Steinberg Classification: Six stages based on femoral head involvement: (1) normal x-ray, abnormal magnetic resonance imaging (MRI) and/or bone scan, (2) abnormal x-ray showing cystic or sclerotic changes in femoral head, (3) subchondral collapse producing crescent sign, (4) flattening of femoral head, (5) joint narrowing with or without acetabular involvement, (6) advanced degenerative disease.
Treatment: Observation, core decompression (early stages), vascularized fibular strut grafting (contraindicated with whole head involvement), femoral head rotational osteotomy (less than 50% involvement of head), hip arthroplasty, fusion.

Scaphoid Avascular Necrosis

Common in contact sports causing scaphoid fracture. Vascular supply enters scaphoid distally, leading to a high rate of nonunion and avascular necrosis in proximal fractures.
Diagnosis: Bone scan has 100% sensitivity and 98% specificity for diagnosis of fracture.
Treatment:
• Nondisplaced/stable fractures—long arm/thumb spica cast
• Displaced/unstable fractures (displacement > 1 mm, capitolunate angle > 15 degrees, scapholunate angle > 60 degrees, proximal pole fracture)—open reduction and internal fixation. Local vascularized bone graft from the distal radius for failed surgery.
• Nonunion—inlay (Russe) graft when carpal collapse is not associated or interposition (Fisk) graft for carpal stabilization.

Kienböck's Disease

Avascular necrosis of the lunate. Secondary to overuse and negative ulnar wrist variation.
Treatment: Immobilization, NSAIDs, ulnar lengthening or radial shortening, fusion

Talar Avascular Necrosis

Nondisplaced/displaced talar body fractures (25%/40% to 50%) and types II, III, and IV talar neck fractures.
• Fractures secondary to dorsiflexion and inversion. Necrosis directly related to injury to vascular supply—artery of the tarsal canal (body), dorsalis pedis, and peroneal arteries (head and neck).
• Hawkins sign—subchondral radiolucency in talar dome on anteroposterior radiograph 6 to 8 weeks after talar neck fracture indicates adequate blood supply.
Treatment:
• Nondisplaced—non–weight bearing for 6 to 8 weeks
• Displaced > 2 mm—open reduction and internal fixation with possible medial malleolar osteotomy

Compartment Syndrome

Increased pressure in a closed fascial space that can lead to muscle ischemia and death
Symptoms and Signs: 5 Ps—pain, pallor, pulselessness, paresthesia, and paralysis.
Diagnosis: Pain worse with passive stretch is the most sensitive.
Evaluation: By 4 Cs—color, consistency, contracture, and capacity to bleed.
Treatment: Pressure > 30 mm Hg requires fasciotomy.

Volkmann's Contracture

Contracture of hand, wrist, and forearm musculature secondary to trauma. Flexor digitorum profundus and flexor digitorum longus most commonly involved.
Variations and Treatment:
• Mild—wrist flexors; dynamic splinting and tendon lengthening
• Moderate—wrist and digital flexors; excision of necrotic muscle, neurolysis, tendon transfers
• Severe—flexors and extensors; excision of necrotic muscle, neurolysis, tendon transfers, free muscle transfer

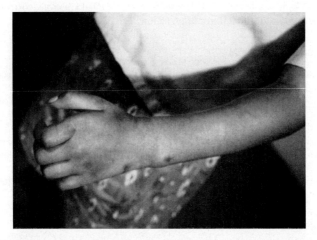

Fig. 231-1 Volkmann's ischemic contracture of the forearm after treatment of a both-bones fracture and unrecognized compartment syndrome. Note the contracture of the fingers, which are partially insensitive. *(From Green NE, Swiontkowski MF: Skeletal Trauma in Children, 3rd ed. Philadelphia, Saunders, 2003.)*

Definition: Vertical talus, also referred to as *congenital convex pes valgus,* is a congenital condition characterized by an irreducible and rigid dorsal dislocation of the navicular on the talus. This results in a rigid rocker bottom flatfoot. The calcaneus is in fixed equinus, and the Achilles tendon is very tight. The hindfoot also is in valgus, while the head of the talus is found medially in the sole, creating the rocker bottom appearance. The forefoot is abducted and dorsiflexed.

Incidence: This is a very rare disorder with an estimated rate of 1 in 10,000.

Gender: Equal between genders.

Etiology and Pathophysiology: The exact etiology is unknown. It is believed that this disorder may be the result of trisomy of chromosomes 13, 15 or 18. It has been proposed that vertical talus is due to a contracture of the Achilles tendon, which causes an equinus of the calcaneus. Vertical talus may also be the result of contracture of the extensor digitorum longus, extensor hallucis longus, or tibialis anterior. This contracture pulls the navicular onto the dorsum of the navicular, creating the dislocation.

Associations: Often vertical talus is associated with neuromuscular disorders and neural tube defects. It has also been associated with myelomeningocele, arthrogryposis, spina bifida, neurofibromatosis, cerebral palsy, poliomyelitis, spinal muscular atrophy, and tethered cord syndrome.

Diagnostic Studies: Radiography reveals the talus parallel to the tibia, the calcaneus in an equinus position, and the navicular dislocated on the neck of the talus. The diagnosis is confirmed by a lateral view of the foot during maximum plantarflexion and maximum dorsiflexion. The plantarflexion view reveals an irreducible talonavicular joint and the dorsiflexion view reveals fixed equinus.

Classification: Type 1 vertical talus is stiffer and is associated with a calcaneocuboid dislocation. Type 2 is not associated with such a dislocation. Treatment of type 1 deformities must focus on releasing the calcaneocuboid joint.

Treatment: The first step in treating vertical talus is serial casting and manipulation. This stretches the skin, tendons, ligaments, and muscles. On very rare occasions this will resolve the problem; however, in almost all cases, reconstructive surgery is required. The surgery consists of lengthening the extensor hallucis longus and peroneus tertius. The talonavicular joint is then reduced and held with K-wire. Occasionally capsulotomies of the talonavicular and calcaneocuboid joints are required. The final phase of the surgery is to percutaneously lengthen the Achilles tendon.

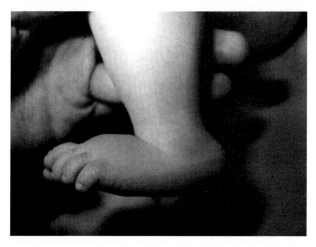

Fig. 232-1　Rocker-bottom foot in congenital vertical talus. *(From Kliegman RM, et al: Nelson Textbook of Pediatrics, 18th ed. Philadelphia, Saunders, 2007.)*

The complex anatomy of the wrist joint in addition to its multiplanar capabilities has provided diagnosticians with numerous challenges in assessing the structure and function of the wrist in an acute and chronic pathologic setting. There are many noninvasive modalities available to evaluate wrist pain; however, when the diagnosis remains unclear or conservative measures fail in the presence of significant wrist pain, more invasive procedures need to be considered. Diagnostic tools such as magnetic resonance imaging, although useful for soft tissue injuries, have been shown to have weaknesses in the accurate evaluation of certain wrist injuries. Alternatively, wrist arthroscopy allows greater three-dimensional visualization of wrist structures, decreasing the rate of false-negative results encountered in obscure causes of wrist pain. The greatest degree of sensitivity and specificity for evaluating wrist pain is achieved when the various analytic assessments are used in conjunction with one another. The decision to perform arthroscopy is comprised of intertwined factors involving cost and the activity level of the patient. These various elements should be evaluated on a case-by-case circumstance, and a clinical decision made after the full picture is taken into account. For example, the decision to perform such a procedure on an athlete would encompass whether or not the patient's sport was in season and their competitive level within the sport.

Indications:
1. Evaluation and treatment of ligamentous injury
2. Triangular fibrocartilage complex lesions
3. Examination of joint articular surfaces
4. Removal of loose bodies
5. Biopsy of synovium
6. Irrigation and debridement of carpal joints
7. Confirmation and supplementation of wrist arthrography
8. Intra-articular fractures of the distal radius, ulna, and carpal bones

Complications: Wrist traction performed during arthroscopic evaluation of the wrist is the source of many complications that may include joint edema, stiffness, ligamental strain, and stretching of peripheral nerves. In addition, the portal placement may cause damage to peripheral arteries, veins, or nerves, and increase the risk of articular cartilage, ligament, and tendon laceration. The majority of these problems result in an inability to restore proper functioning of the joint or inadequate relief of symptoms. A less commonly encountered complication is joint effusion resulting in forearm compartment syndrome, which can be avoided by compression of the forearm during the procedure.

Positioning and Setup: Wrist arthroscopy can be performed under general or regional block anesthesia, and a tourniquet around the mid arm provides a blood-free surgical field during the operation. The wrist to be scoped is placed in sterile finger-traps and suspended from a vertical

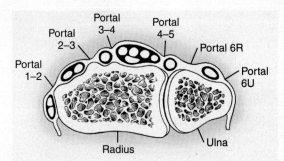

Fig. 233-1   Cross-section of wrist at level of distal radius showing compartments and portals used for examination of radiocarpal and ulnocarpal joints. *(Redrawn from Botte MJ, Cooney WP, Linscheid RL: Arthroscopy of the wrist: anatomy and technique. J Hand Surg 14A:313, 1989.)*

Table 233-1.

Name	Location	Visualization/Use	Danger
1st Portal	• Between 1st (abductor pollicis longus and extensor pollicis brevis) and 2nd (extensor carpi radialis longus and brevis) extensor compartments	• Evaluation of articular surface of distal radius	
2nd Portal	• Between 2nd (extensor carpi radialis longus and brevis) and 3rd (extensor pollicis longus) extensor compartments	• Evaluation of the radial palmar ligaments	
3-4 Radiocarpal portals	• 1 cm distal to Lister's tubercle • Palpated between the 3rd (extensor pollicis longus tendon) and 4th (extensor digitorum communis tendon) extensor compartments	• Main radiocarpal arthroscopic viewing portals • Intercarpal and volar radiocarpal ligaments • Scaphoid and lunate facets	
4-5 Radiocarpal portals	• Located between the 4th (extensor digitorum communis tendon) and 5th (extensor digiti minimi tendon) extensor compartments	• Midportion of the triangular fibrocartilage complex • Lunate bone • Lunotriquetral joint • Volar ulnocarpal ligaments	
6-R Portal	• Located on the dorsoradial aspect of the extensor carpi ulnaris tendon • The proximal border of the triquetrum should be used as a landmark rather than the distal ulna to avoid injuring the triangular fibrocartilage complex	• Ulnar-sided wrist disease • Extensor carpi ulnaris tendon • Frequently used for irrigation	• Triangular fibrocartilage complex • Dorsal sensory branch of the ulnar nerve

Portal	Location	Uses
6-U Portal	• Ulnar to the extensor carpi radialis tendon • Enters the joint through the prestyloid recess next to the ulnar styloid	• Triangular fibrocartilage complex • Ulnocarpal ligaments • Can be used as outflow • Dorsal sensory branch of the ulnar nerve
Radial midcarpal portal	• Lies to radial side of the 3rd metacarpal axis proximal to the capitate in a soft depression between the capitate and scaphoid (1 cm distal from 3-4 portal). • In line with Lister's tubercle	• Evaluation of the scaphocapitate and capitohamate joint and associated ligaments • Distal scaphoid, the lunate, and proximal pole of the capitate • Midcarpal disease
Ulnar midcarpal portal	• Another location is in the center of the axis of the 4th metacarpal and proximal to the capitohamate joint (1 cm distal from 4-5 portal).	• Evaluation of the scaphocapitate and capitohamate joint and associated ligaments • Distal ends of the lunate and triquetrum and the proximal portions of the capitate and hamate • Midcarpal disease

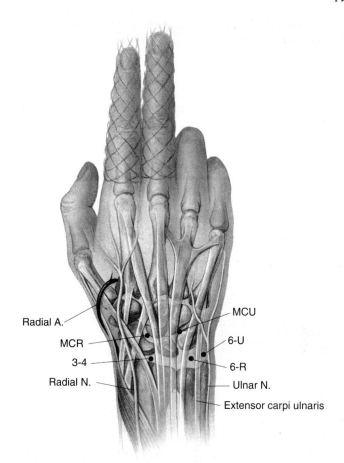

Radial A.

MCR

3-4

Radial N.

MCU

6-U

6-R

Ulnar N.

Extensor carpi ulnaris

Fig. 233-2 The 3-4, 6-U, and 6-R portals provide the access and visibility needed for basic diagnostic wrist arthroscopy. The midcarpal (MC) portals provide a view of the midcarpal joint. R, radial; U, ulnar. *(From Wrist Arthroscopy: Portals to Progress, as described by Gary Poehling. Andover, Mass, Dyonics Inc., 1989.)*

traction apparatus above the operating table. Seven to 10 pounds of traction may be used to provide adequate distraction force needed for the procedure. A forearm clamp stabilizes the forearm and maintains the elbow in 80 to 90 degrees of flexion. Alternatively, traction may be placed longitudinally with the elbow in extension on the operating table.

Anatomic Landmarks:

Osseous Structures: Lister's tubercle, radial styloid, dorsal lip of radius, ulnar styloid, and the distal radioulnar joint.

Soft Tissue Structures: Extensor tendons.

Soft Tissue Structures at Risk of Injury during the Procedure: Radial artery, sensory branch of the radial nerve, and the dorsal sensory branch of ulnar nerve.

Portal Placement: Portal placement is determined by the goals of the operation and the suspicion of the attending physician. They are numbered according to the extensor tendon compartments immediately lateral to them and the surrounding osseous structures (Table 233-1).

Aftertreatment: The exact procedure and extent of injury will ultimately determine the treatment outcome; however, in general the splint is normally removed and mobilization reassumed 7 to 10 days after arthroscopy. The more extensive the injury, the more prolonged the immobilization and rehabilitation required.

Definition: A beam of electromagnetic waves generated by accelerating electrons toward a high-voltage anode in an x-ray tube. Some of the beam is absorbed or scattered by various tissues or materials in the body in different amounts while the rest passes through the body and strikes a fluorescent screen, producing light that exposes a film.

Characteristics:

Four basic visible shades on plain films.

- Air: Black; very dark
- Fat: Gray; darker than blood/soft tissue
- Water (blood and soft tissue): Light gray/light white; lighter than bone
- Bone: Almost white; bright

Metal/contrast is white and very bright.

Standard Views: Anteroposterior (AP), lateral, and oblique

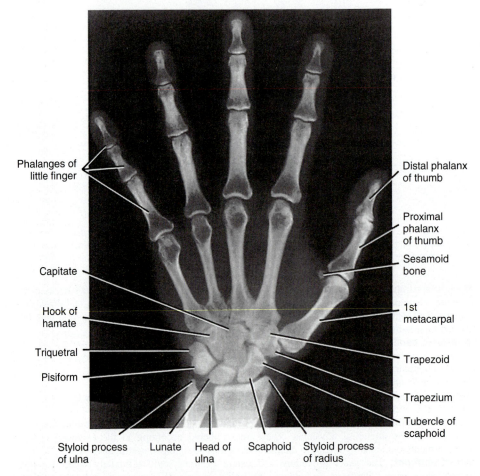

Fig. 234-1   Posteroanterior radiograph of the wrist and hand with the forearm pronated. *(From Marx J: Rosen's Emergency Medicine: Concepts and Clinical Practice, 6th ed. Philadelphia, Mosby, 2006.)*

Special Views:
- Cervical spine—odontoid view
- Collateral ligament avulsions of the hand—Brewerton view
- Scaphoid fracture—scaphoid view
- Lunate fracture—coned view
- Hamate hook fracture—carpal tunnel view
- Proximal humerus fracture/dislocation—axillary and scapular views
- Pelvic fracture—inlet, outlet, Judet views
- Hip fracture/dislocation—internal and external rotation views
- Proximal tibial fracture—tibial plateau and tunnel views
- Patellar fracture—axial view
- Ankle fracture—mortis view
- Calcaneal fracture—axial view

Sequelae: Potentially damaging to tissues and DNA, resulting in possible carcinogenesis and genetic mutation (caused by gonadal irradiation).
- Most radiosensitive organ—thyroid gland
- Most common cancers following exposure to ionizing radiation:
  - Leukemia
  - Thyroid tumors
  - Breast tumors
  - Lung tumors
  - Skin tumors

Index

Page numbers followed by *f, t,* and *b* indicate figures, tables, and boxes, respectively.